Balance Disorders:
A Case-Study Approach

Joseph M. Furman, MD, PhD
Associate Professor
Departments of Otolaryngology,
Neurology, and Electrical Engineering
University of Pittsburgh
Pittsburgh, Pennsylvania

Stephen P. Cass, MD, MPH
Assistant Professor
Department of Otolaryngology
University of Pittsburgh
Pittsburgh, Pennsylvania

 F. A. DAVIS COMPANY • Philadelphia

F. A. Davis Company
1915 Arch Street
Philadelphia, PA 19103

Printed in the United States of America

Last digit indicates print number: 10 9 8 7 6 5 4 3 2 1

Medical Editor: Robert W. Reinhardt
Medical Developmental Editor: Bernice M. Wissler
Medical Production Editor: Jessica Howie Martin
Cover Designer: Louis J. Forgione

As new scientific information becomes available through basic and clinical research, recommended treatments and drug therapies undergo changes. The authors and publisher have done everything possible to make this book accurate, up to date, and in accord with accepted standards at the time of publication. The authors, editors, and publisher are not responsible for errors or omissions or for consequences from application of the book, and make no warranty, expressed or implied, in regard to the contents of the book. Any practice described in this book should be applied by the reader in accordance with professional standards of care used in regard to the unique circumstances that may apply in each situation. The reader is advised always to check product information (package inserts) for changes and new information regarding dose and contra-indications before administering any drug. Caution is especially urged when using new or infrequently ordered drugs.

Library of Congress Cataloging in Publication Data
Furman, Joseph M., 1952–
Balance disorders : a case-study approach / Joseph M. Furman, Stephen P. Cass.
p. cm.
Includes bibliographical references and index.
ISBN 0-8036-0166-2 (hardcover)
1. Vestibular apparatus—Diseases—Case studies.   2. Dizziness—Case studies.   3. Equilibrium (Physiology)—Case studies.
I. Cass, Stephen P., 1957– . II. Title.
[DNLM: 1 Vestibular Diseases—case studies.   2. Equilibrium. 3. Dizziness. WV 255 F986b 1996]
RF260.F87 1996
617.8′82—dc20
DNLM/DLC
for Library of Congress
95-52576
CIP

Preface

Dizziness is one of the most common complaints that patients bring to their doctors. As many as 40 percent of adults experience clinically significant dizziness at some time in their lives,[2] and nearly 1 in 4 emergency room visits includes a complaint of dizziness.[3] Even though dizziness is common, it remains a perplexing problem for most physicians. It can be a symptom of disease in almost any organ system, and the constellation of symptoms presented by patients with dizziness often seems complex. Moreover, the same disorder may present differently, depending on the patient's personality and his or her response to disease, lifestyle, and age.

Many patients with dizziness have an abnormality related to vestibular function or to central nervous system processing of sensory information that is important for spatial orientation. The pathophysiology underlying a balance disorder can be baffling because much of vestibular physiology is grounded in physics and applied engineering, topics that are remote to most physicians. This mix of basic science and complex patient presentations makes the field of balance disorders challenging. Nevertheless, deducing the origin of dizziness and implementing appropriate treatment is a skill that will benefit any physician who encounters patients complaining of dizziness, especially primary care physicians, otolaryngologists, neurologists, and physiatrists.

We have chosen to use a case-study approach to outline the principles and practice of the care of patients with balance disorders. The use of a case-study approach is consistent with the recent evolution of problem-based learning in the medical sciences. In particular, the University of Pittsburgh School of Medicine recently instituted problem-based learning as a major focus of its preclinical curriculum. We play an active role in the education of medical students and residents in otolaryngology and neurology and have tailored the case-study approach used in the book so that it can be used as part of training programs.

Our approach to balance disorders reflects the merging of ideas from the combined experience of a neurologist (Dr. Furman) and a neurotologic surgeon (Dr. Cass). We hope that this dual perspective makes this book enlightening to its readers. Each case study contains relevant material regarding history, physical examination, laboratory testing, diagnosis, and treatment. This material provides a springboard for discussion of either a concept in the field of balance disorders or the diagnosis or treatment of a particular disease state. Practical, specific treatment options are discussed throughout the book.

Because of the importance of understanding the underlying physiology and pathophysiology of the conditions being discussed, Part I provides essential background information concerning vestibular physiology, vestibular laboratory testing, audiology, and vestibular rehabilitation. Parts II, III, and IV consist of case studies. In Part II, each of nine *tutorial* cases elucidates an essential principle or major issue in the field of balance disorders. In Part III, 26 *common disease* cases review disorders that are frequently encountered. Particularly common disorders are discussed in multiple cases, with different specific issues addressed in each case. Part IV contains 17 case studies pertaining to *unusual* disorders. These cases provide the reader with an appreciation for the breadth of the field and an awareness of the rarer causes of dizziness.

This book is not meant as a substitute for other texts that deal specifically with the

iii

anatomy and physiology of the vestibular system, the details of the ocular motion system, or vestibular rehabilitation. Excellent texts are available on each of these topics. Rather, this book spans the gap between these in-depth texts and the problems that arise whenever a patient presents with dizziness.

Joseph M. Furman, MD, PhD
Stephen P. Cass, MD, MPH

References

1. NIH Publication No. 86-76: Dizziness: Hope through Research. Prepared by the Office of Scientific and Health Reports, NICDS, September 1986, pp 5–6.
2. National Institute on Deafness and Other Communication Disorders, NIH: A Report of the Task Force on the National Strategic Research Plan. April 1989, p 74.
3. Koziol-McLain J et al: Orthostatic vital signs in emergency department patients. Ann Emerg Med 20:806–810, 1991.

Acknowledgments

We wish to acknowledge our families for their patience and support during the writing of this book. We also thank Dr. Eugene N. Myers, Professor and Chairman, Department of Otolaryngology, University of Pittsburgh School of Medicine, for his foresight and wisdom in creating an environment that fosters multidisciplinary collaboration. Special thanks go to Mr. Del Bloem, President of ICS Medical Corporation, who accepted and encouraged the idea of a case-study approach for the continuing education course that he sponsors. Many of the illustrations in the book were generated as part of a slide series entitled "Evaluation of the Dizzy Patient," developed by us for the American Academy of Otolaryngology—Head and Neck Surgery, which graciously allowed us to reprint many illustrations. We are grateful to the F. A. Davis Company for publishing the book, especially to Mr. Sandy Reinhardt for his encouragement and helpful suggestions. Dr. David Shoemaker provided helpful suggestions regarding the manuscript. We also thank Ms. Karen Anderson for her secretarial support.

Contents

Introduction: Guide for the Reader

The text is divided into four parts. Part I includes background information common to many of the case studies. Chapters 1 through 4 discuss anatomy and physiology of the vestibular system, vestibular laboratory testing, audiometric testing, and vestibular rehabilitation. Parts II, III, and IV include 52 case studies. In Part II, 9 cases illustrate major themes in the field of balance disorders; in Part III, 26 cases illustrate commonly encountered disease states; and in Part IV, 17 cases illustrate unusual disorders.

The material in this book can be used in several ways. For individuals with minimal background in the area of balance disorders, Part I should be read thoroughly before beginning the case studies, which should be read in order. An alternative approach, better suited to a more knowledgeable reader, is to read Part II, the tutorial cases, first and refer to the material in Part I as needed. The reader can then study the common disease cases in Part III and the unusual disease cases in Part IV. More experienced clinicians can approach the material by referring to the cases as they arise in their practice or in their own order of interest. The Appendix of Diagnoses and Index should allow the reader to find sought-after material directly. The cases are also cross-referenced extensively so that relevant material that appears elsewhere in the text can be easily accessed.

Background
for Case Studies

CHAPTER

1

Vestibular Anatomy and Physiology

The vestibular labyrinth contains two types of sensors, the semicircular canals and the otolith organs (Fig. 1–1). The semicircular canals sense rotational movement; the otolith organs sense linear motion and orientation with respect to gravity. There are three semicircular canals, each sensitive to rotation in a particular plane. These three planes are more or less perpendicular to one another, allowing the labyrinth to sense rotations about any spatial axis because one or more semicircular canals are stimulated by any particular rotation. For example, turning the head to the left and right stimulates predominantly the horizontal semicircular canals, whereas moving the head up and down stimulates the vertical semicircular canals. Figure 1–2 depicts the orientation of the semicircular canals.

The otolith organs include the utricle and saccule. The utricle senses motion in the horizontal plane, that is, naso-occipital (forward-backward) movement, left-right movement, and combinations thereof. The saccule senses motion in the sagittal plane, such as naso-occipital movement, up-down movement, and combinations of these movements. The utricle and saccule also sense changes in orientation to gravity resulting from pitch and roll of the head, for example, in movements like putting the chin on the chest or touching the ear to the shoulder. As can be seen in Figure 1–1, the cochlea is immediately adjacent to the vestibular labyrinth. In fact, the endolymph of the vestibular labyrinth and the cochlea are in communication with one another. The perilymphatic spaces of the vestibular labyrinth and the cochlea also communicate. The vestibular and auditory portions of the inner ear share a common blood supply as well. Because of their propinquity, common fluid spaces, and shared blood supply, it is not surprising that disorders affecting the vestibular labyrinth often also affect the cochlea, so that dizziness and disequilibrium are often accompanied by hearing loss and/or tinnitus.

Each of the three semicircular canals contains an enlarged area known as the ampulla, which is important for the transduction of rotational motion into neural activity (Fig. 1–3). Within each ampulla is a cupula, a gelatinous membrane that completely seals the semicircular canal. During head movement, the cupula bows like a drum head. This cupular movement, the first step in the transduction process, activates the under-

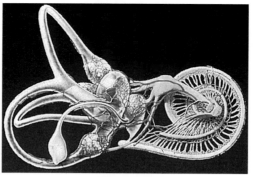

Figure 1–1.
The vestibular labyrinth contains two types of sensors, the semicircular canals and the otolith organs. There are three semicircular canals, the horizontal, the superior (anterior), and posterior (inferior). Each semicircular canal is sensitive to rotation in the plane of the canals. The otolith organs include the utricle and saccule. The utricle senses motion both to and fro and left and right, and also senses static pitch and roll of the head, i.e., movements such as putting the chin on the chest and touching the ear to the shoulder. The saccule senses up-and-down motion, to-and-fro motion, and static pitch of the head. Note the proximity of the cochlea to the vestibular labyrinth. The vestibular and auditory portions of the inner ear share a common blood supply and inner-ear fluid metabolism. (Adapted with permission from Platzer, W (ed): PERNKOPF, Atlas der topographischen und angewandten Anatomie des Menschen (3rd ed). Baltimore: Urban & Schwarzenberg, Inc., 1989, p. 148.[4])

lying hair cells, which in turn are innervated by a semicircular canal nerve, which itself is a branch of the vestibular portion of the eighth cranial nerve.

The maculae of the vestibular labyrinth are the sensory transduction regions of the otolith organs, the utricle and saccule. The maculae are organized so that individual hair cells sense motion in a particular direction known as its polarization vector. The arrows shown in Figure 1–4 represent the most sensitive directions for individual hair cells on the surface of the utricular and saccular maculae. Note that for each macula there is a complete representation of directions of motion in the horizontal and sagittal planes for the utricle and saccule, respectively. For example, a hair cell in the utricular macula whose polarization vector points toward the left ear is stimulated by left-ear down-tilt or by linear acceleration to the right.

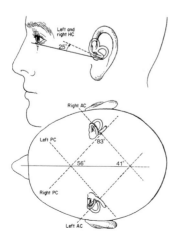

Figure 1–2.
The vestibular labyrinth is oriented in the temporal bone in such a way that the lateralmost semicircular canal, which is the horizontal semicircular canal, is more or less in the head-horizontal plane. The other two semicircular canals are oriented more or less vertically and optimally sense oblique pitch-and-roll rotations of the head. The utricle lies more or less in the same plane as the horizontal semicircular canals, which allows it to transduce translational motion forward and backward and left and right. The saccule is oriented vertically.

Figure 1–3.
Ampulla of a semicircular canal. The ampulla of each semicircular canal is an enlarged area that is important to the transduction of rotational movement into neural activity. Within each ampulla is a cupula, a gelatinous membrane that completely seals the semicircular canal. During head movement, the cupula bows like a drum head; it does not flap like a swinging door. This cupular movement, the first step in the transduction process, activates the underlying hair cells. (With permission from Harada, Y (ed): The Vestibular Organs. Amsterdam: Kugler & Guedini Publications, 1988.[5])

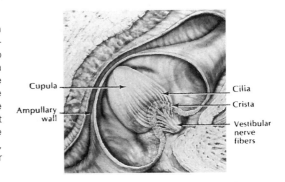

A component of each macula is the otolithic membrane, which contains otoconia (literally, "ear stones"), pebblelike structures composed of crystallized calcium carbonate (Figs. 1–5 and 1–6). Otoconia are constantly being formed and reabsorbed in a process involving the macular supporting cells and surrounding dark cells. This process of formation and absorption is probably important in the pathophysiology of benign positional vertigo (see Cases T1 and C9).

Hair-cell stimulation results from the bending of an array of surface "hairs," or stereocilia. Bending the array *toward* the tallest hair (kinocilium) causes hair-cell depolarization, whereas bending the array of stereocilia *away from* the kinocilium causes hyperpolarization. Depolarization of the hair cells results in an increase in the firing rate of the eighth nerve afferents that innervate the hair cells, whereas hyperpolarization causes decreased activity.

Each neuron in the vestibular portion of the eighth cranial nerve has a so-called resting discharge. That is, numerous action potentials (about 90 per second) occur even

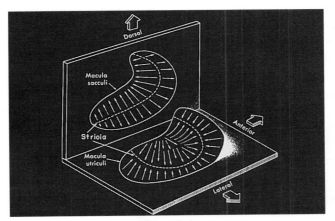

Figure 1–4.
Maculae of the utricle and saccule. The maculae are the sensory transduction regions of the utricle and saccule. They are organized so that individual hair cells lie in various orientations, allowing them to optimally sense motion in a particular direction. The arrows indicate the most sensitive direction for individual hair cells on the surface of the maculae. At the center of each macula is a region called the striola, where the orientation of the hair cells changes abruptly. (With permission from Baloh, RW (ed): Dizziness, Hearing Loss, and Tinnitus: The Essentials of Neurotology. Philadelphia: FA Davis Company, 1984, p. 22.[6])

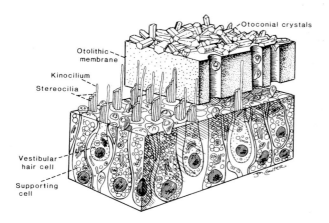

Figure 1–5.
Otolithic macula. A component of each macula is an otolithic membrane containing otoconia (otoconial crystals). The otoconia add mass to the otolithic membrane. The heavy otolithic membrane deforms in response to linear motion and changes of orientation with respect to gravity. This deformation bends the hairs of the underlying hair cells. The directional sensitivity of each hair cell is determined by the location of the kinocilium with respect to the stereocilia.

with the head at rest. This is unique for sensory organs of the body. Although requiring an expenditure of energy even while the head is still, the constant high-level firing rate of these neurons is quite useful because such cells can sense motion in both the excitatory and the inhibitory direction. Vestibular neurons (Fig. 1–7) increase or decrease their firing rate as a result of depolarization or hyperpolarization, respectively, of the hair cells that they innervate.

The information regarding head movement transduced by the peripheral vestibular organs is relayed by the eighth cranial nerve, which traverses the internal auditory canal and cerebellopontine angle before entering the brainstem at the pontomedullary junction. The vestibular nerve synapses on cells in the vestibular nuclei and other central nervous system structures such as the cerebellum. Information from the vestibular nuclei both ascends and descends in the central nervous system. Ascending pathways are important for vestibulo-ocular reflexes and for perception of vestibular sensations. Descending pathways are important for vestibulospinal reflexes.

Also included in the vestibular nerve are the vestibular *efferents*, which are neurons that project *from* the central nervous system *to* the labyrinth. Their function is uncertain; they may modulate the sensitivity of the labyrinth.

The vestibular nucleus on each side of the brain is comprised of at least four anatomic subdivisions named the superior, medial, lateral, and inferior vestibular nuclei.

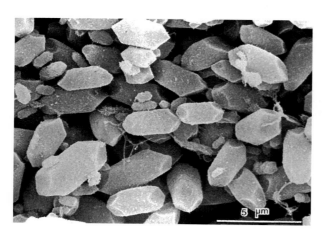

Figure 1–6.
Scanning electron micrograph of otoconia, pebble-like structures composed of crystallized calcium carbonate ($CaCO_3$) that are constantly being formed and reabsorbed in a process involving the macular supporting cells and surrounding dark cells. (With permission from Harada, Y (ed): The Vestibular Organs. Amsterdam: Kugler & Guedini Publications, 1988.[5])

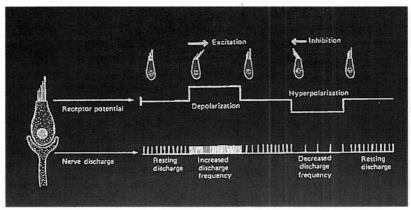

Figure 1–7.
Each neuron in the vestibular portion of the eighth cranial nerve has a so-called "resting discharge." That is, numerous action potentials (about 90 per second) occur even with the head at rest. Although requiring expenditure of energy even while the head is still, the constant high-level firing rate of these neurons is useful because such cells can sense motion in both the excitatory and the inhibitory directions via depolarization or hyperpolarization that increases and decreases eighth-nerve firing rate respectively. (Adapted with permission from Kelly, JP: Vestibular system. In Kandel, ER, Schwartz, JH, and Jessell, TM (eds): Principles of Neural Science (3rd ed). Norwalk, CT: Appleton & Lange, 1991, p. 506.[7])

The vestibular nuclei receive inputs not only from the vestibular labyrinth but also from other sensory modalities including vision, somatic sensation, and audition. As a result of these varied sensory inputs, the name *vestibular* nuclei is somewhat misleading. These structures are, in fact, *sensory integration* nuclei whose output influences eye movements, truncal stability, and spatial orientation.

VESTIBULO-OCULAR REFLEX

The vestibulo-ocular reflex is a mechanism whereby head movement automatically results in an eye movement equal and opposite to the head movement so that the eyes stay on target. For example, a leftward head movement is associated with a rightward eye movement and vice versa. The vestibulo-ocular reflex works for all types of head movements, including rotation and translation. The vestibulo-ocular reflex is mediated by a three-neuron arc that includes the eighth cranial nerve (neuron 1), an interneuron from the vestibular nucleus to the abducens nucleus (neuron 2), and the motoneuron to the eye muscles (neuron 3) (Fig. 1–8). One remarkable feature of the vestibulo-ocular reflex is that it is produced by the coordinated action of the *two* vestibular nuclear complexes, one on each side of the brainstem, which cooperate with one another such that when one is excited, the other is inhibited. This "push-pull" behavior is a direct result of the tonic vestibular activity in the eighth cranial nerve that allows both an increase and a decrease in neural activity during head movement. For example, when the head is turned to the left, the activity in the left eighth cranial nerve and left vestibular nuclei is increased, whereas the right eighth nerve and right vestibular nuclei activity is decreased (Fig. 1–9). This reciprocal effect increases the sensitivity of the vestibulo-ocular reflex greatly.

Operationally, the central nervous system responds to *differences* in activity between the two vestibular nuclear complexes. For example, when there is no head move-

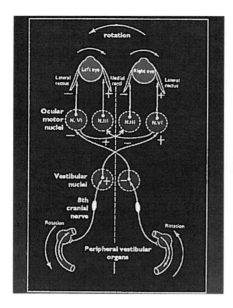

Figure 1–8.
Horizontal vestibulo-ocular reflex pathways. The vestibulo-ocular reflex is mediated by a three-neuron arc that includes the eighth cranial nerve, an interneuron from the vestibular nucleus to the abducens nucleus (N.VI), and the motoneuron to the lateral rectus muscles. To coordinate the movement of the two eyes, an interneuron connects the abducens nucleus to the oculomotor nucleus (N.III), which contains the cell bodies of the motoneurons to the medial rectus muscle. (With permission from Kelly, JP: Vestibular system. In Kandel, ER, Schwartz, JH, and Jessell, TM (eds): Principles of Neural Science (3rd ed). Norwalk, CT: Appleton & Lange, 1991.[7])

ment, resting neural activity within the vestibular nuclei is symmetric. However, during movement, there is asymmetric activity in the vestibular nuclei. A left-right asymmetry in the vestibular nuclei is interpreted by the central nervous system as a head movement, even when such asymmetries are a result of pathology.

VESTIBULOSPINAL AND NECK-RELATED REFLEXES

Information from the vestibular labyrinth descends in the nervous system to control head position, truncal stability, and limb position. The medial and lateral vestibulo-spinal tracts (MVST and LVST) and reticulospinal tract (RST) carry information from the vestibular nuclei into the brainstem and spinal cord. The neck also sends neural signals to the central nervous system regarding head position. These signals, coupled with vestibular signals, provide information regarding head and trunk position.[1] Signals from the neck can cause eye movements via the cervico-ocular reflex, which is normally almost completely inactive. Possibly, in patients with vestibular deficits, the cervico-ocular reflex becomes more active.[2] Another important reflex is the vestibulo-colic reflex, whereby vestibular signals are relayed to neck muscles to stabilize the head. This reflex may account for the neck stiffness experienced by many patients with vestibular asymmetries.

VESTIBULOAUTONOMIC PROJECTIONS

An additional projection of the vestibular system is to the autonomic nervous system, predominantly to the sympathetic nervous system and to structures that control respiration. Through these projections, patients with vestibular imbalance may experience

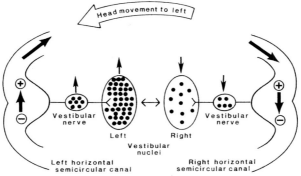

Figure 1–9.
Push-pull action of the horizontal vestibulo-ocular reflex. With head movement to the left, endolymph flow produces an excitatory stimulus in the left horizontal semicircular canal and an inhibitory stimulus in the right horizontal semicircular canal. The excitatory stimulus increases neural activity in the vestibular nerve and vestibular nuclei, and the inhibitory stimulus decreases such activity. The brain interprets the difference in neural activity between the vestibular nuclei as a head movement to the left and generates appropriate vestibulo-ocular and postural responses.

nausea and vomiting. The physiologic necessity for the vestibuloautonomic system, especially the need for vestibular imbalance to induce nausea and vomiting, is unknown.

EFFECT OF UNILATERAL PERIPHERAL VESTIBULAR INJURY

Unilateral labyrinthine injury disrupts the reciprocal, push-pull interaction of the two labyrinths. Following the acute loss of unilateral peripheral vestibular function, there is a loss of resting neural activity in the vestibular nuclei ipsilateral to the lesion. Because the brain normally detects *differences* in activity between the two vestibular nuclear complexes, an acute loss of unilateral peripheral vestibular function is interpreted as a continuous rapid head movement (Fig. 1–10). The brain responds with "corrective" eye movements manifested as vestibular nystagmus.

With complete loss of unilateral vestibular function, the three semicircular canals and the two otolith organs on one side become inactive and the resulting eye movement and body postures reflect the unopposed action of the contralateral labyrinth. In the case of eye movement, there is nystagmus. The direction of the nystagmus, which is

Figure 1–10.
The reciprocal "push-pull" interaction of the two labyrinths is disrupted after labyrinthine injury. Following the acute loss of unilateral peripheral vestibular function, there is a loss of resting neural activity in the vestibular nerve and unilateral vestibular nuclei. Because the brain normally detects differences in activity between the two vestibular nuclear complexes, this situation is interpreted as a rapid head movement, in this case to the left.

Right Acute Peripheral Vestibular Injury

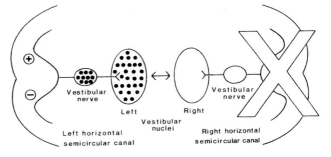

predominantly horizontal-torsional, can be explained as follows: the remaining horizontal semicircular canal is unopposed, thus accounting for the horizontal component; the orientation of the two remaining vertical canals is such that their torsional (roll) influences add to each other, but their vertical (pitch) components cancel one another. The vestibulospinal manifestation of acute unilateral peripheral vestibular loss may include head tilt. Most patients, however, do not have a static head tilt but do experience disequilibrium and postural instability that includes leaning and veering of gait to the side of the lesion.

The nystagmus, postural instability, and severe vegetative symptoms (e.g., nausea, vomiting, and diaphoresis) that are associated with acute vestibular injury gradually abate through compensatory mechanisms. This process, known as *vestibular compensation,* involves restoring the lost resting activity within the ipsilateral vestibular nucleus and thereby reducing the asymmetry in neural activity between the left and right vestibular nuclei (Fig. 1–11). Such changes restore the function of the vestibulo-ocular and vestibulospinal reflexes. Also, the vegetative symptoms and signs resulting from vestibuloautonomic projections are less severe.

Once the process of vestibular compensation has occurred, the neural activity in a *single* vestibular nerve influences the neural activity within *both* vestibular nuclei. Although compensation acts to rebalance brainstem vestibular activity, patients with chronic unilateral peripheral vestibular loss have a reduced vestibulo-ocular reflex magnitude, abnormal timing of the vestibulo-ocular reflex (see Chap. 2 regarding rotational testing), and an asymmetry of vestibulo-ocular responses during quick head movements. Occasionally, patients may overcompensate for a peripheral vestibular lesion and manifest a "recovery nystagmus," which beats in the opposite direction from that which occurred initially. Also, such patients are susceptible to decompensation, leading to a remanifestation of all or part of their acute vestibular syndrome.

The central vestibular system is profoundly influenced by the cerebellum.[3] Particular regions of the cerebellum, including the vestibulocerebellum (the flocculo-nodular lobe and the cerebellar vermis), are particularly important for control of eye movements and body position. Important and powerful connections between the vestibular nuclei and the cerebellum enable the cerebellum to influence vestibular-induced eye and trunk movements. As a result, lesions of the cerebellum are frequently associated with symptoms and signs such as gait instability and nystagmus that are indistinguishable from those seen with peripheral vestibular lesions.

The vestibular nuclear projection to the thalamus and to the cerebral cortex allows vestibular sensations to reach consciousness. However, these projections are not solely vestibular because they are mixed with somatic sensation. As a result, the distinctions

Chronic Right Peripheral Vestibular Injury

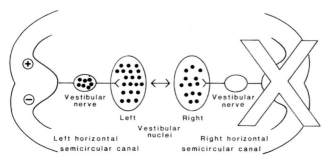

Figure 1–11.
When injury is chronic, the central nervous system is able, through vestibular compensation, to partially restore the lost resting activity within the deafferented vestibular nucleus and thus reduce the asymmetry of neural activity between the vestibular nuclei and partially restore the function of the vestibulo-ocular reflex.

that patients can make regarding other sensory systems, such as brightness, color, loudness, and pitch, are not possible for vestibular sensation. The diffuse character of the vestibulocortical projection may underlie the difficulty that patients experience when trying to describe vestibular ailments.

REFERENCES

1. Melvill Jones, G, and Berthoz, A (eds): Adaptive Mechanisms in Gaze Control: Reviews in Oculomotor Research. Amsterdam: Elsevier, 1985.
2. Kasai, T, and Zee, DS: Eye-head coordination in labyrinthine-defective human beings. Brain Res 144:123–141, 1978.
3. Ito, M (ed): The Cerebellum and Neural Control. New York: Raven Press, 1984.
4. Platzer, W (ed): PERNKOPF, Atlas der topographischen und angewandten Anatomie des Menschen (3rd ed). München–Wien–Baltimore: Urban & Schwarzenberg, 1989.
5. Harada, Y (ed): The Vestibular Organs. Amsterdam: Kugler & Guedini Publications, 1988.
6. Baloh, RW (ed): Dizziness, Hearing Loss, and Tinnitus: The Essentials of Neurotology. Philadelphia: FA Davis Company, 1984.
7. Kelly, JP: Vestibular system. In Kandel, ER, Schwartz, JH, and Jessell, TM (eds): Principles of Neural Science (3rd ed). Norwalk, CT: Appleton & Lange, 1991.

CHAPTER

2

Vestibular Laboratory Testing

Vestibular laboratory testing of the dizzy patient should be reserved for those in whom such testing may be useful in establishing a diagnosis. Laboratory testing is most useful when a thorough history has been obtained and a physical examination has been performed to guide both the selection of appropriate tests and the interpretation of those tests. Vestibular laboratory testing may be helpful in distinguishing between a peripheral vestibular abnormality and a central vestibular abnormality. Also, for disorders thought to be peripheral, vestibular laboratory testing may enable lateralization of the abnormality, which is often helpful when designing and monitoring therapy. Vestibular laboratory testing is also useful in allowing documentation of an abnormality suspected as the result of a bedside evaluation. This is particularly helpful when patients are being evaluated by several physicians and may also be useful for medical/legal situations.

In patients who are undergoing treatment either specifically for a balance disorder or for another condition that requires potentially ototoxic medication, vestibular laboratory testing may be useful because it allows patients to be evaluated during their course of treatment. Certain tests, such as rotational testing and posturography, lend themselves more to serial evaluation than does caloric testing.

Vestibular laboratory tests can be divided into vestibulo-ocular tests and vestibulospinal tests. Each type of testing relies on a measure of motor response or output resulting from vestibular sensory input. Because of this reliance on measuring a motor output, either eye movements or postural sway, currently available vestibular laboratory tests provide only an *indirect* measure of vestibular end-organ function.

Vestibulo-ocular testing is well established and relies on the vestibulo-ocular reflex. To properly evaluate the vestibulo-ocular reflex, it is necessary first to assess the neural motor output, that is, the ocular motor system, independent of the vestibular system. Because eye movement abnormalities, if undetected, could lead to an erroneous conclusion that an abnormality was a result of a vestibular system lesion, an ocular motor screening battery is performed to identify difficulties with the neural control of eye movements. Vestibulo-ocular reflex tests, which include caloric, positional, and rotational testing, are described in the remainder of this chapter.

The vestibulospinal reflexes are not as well understood as the vestibulo-ocular reflex, and, to date, vestibulospinal testing consists mostly of using a moving posture platform to record sway. As with testing the vestibulo-ocular reflex, vestibulospinal testing requires an assessment of the neural motor output (i.e., postural sway, independent of the vestibular system) before assessment of the vestibular effects on posture. The neural motor output (i.e., the postural motor control system) is evaluated by exposing patients to both translation and rotation of the platform while postural responses are recorded. The vestibulospinal system is then studied by altering vision and somatic sensation so that patients must rely on vestibular sensation to maintain balance.

OCULAR MOTOR TESTING

Ocular motor testing is designed to uncover abnormalities in ocular motor control in both the rapid and slow eye-movement systems. Ocular motor testing consists of (1) a search for nystagmus with fixation, (2) a search for gaze nystagmus with both horizontal and vertical gaze deviation, (3) a search for spontaneous vestibular nystagmus with loss of fixation using both eyes open in the dark and eyes closed, (4) an assessment of saccadic eye movements, (5) a recording of ocular pursuit, and (6) a recording of optokinetic nystagmus.

Electro-oculography is the most commonly used method for recording eye movements. The physiologic basis for electro-oculography is the corneal-retinal dipole potential, which is created by the metabolic activity of the retina, which causes the eye to act as a dipole oriented more or less along the visual axis (Fig. 2–1). Other eye-movement measuring techniques are occasionally used, especially for research purposes.[1,2] Video-based eye-movement recording using computerized digital image processing is a promising new technique.

The electro-oculographic signal is recorded by placing surface electrodes either (1) bitemporally to record the combined motion of the two eyes or (2) medially to the medial canthus and laterally to the lateral canthus of each eye to record the movements of each eye separately. The signals recorded from the electrodes are typically amplified using a DC-coupled optically isolated amplifier, the output of which is connected to a chart recorder and often to a digital computer. By convention, for horizontal recordings,

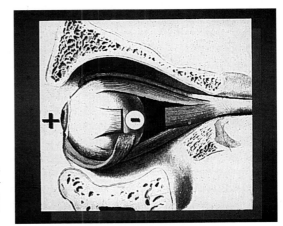

Figure 2–1.
The physiologic basis for electro-oculography is the corneal-retinal dipole potential, which is created by the metabolic activity of the retina causing the eye to act as a dipole oriented more or less along the visual axis.

Components of Nystagmus

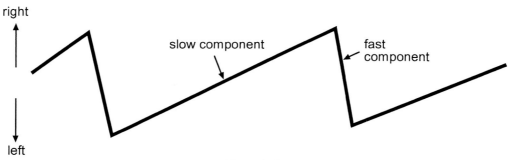

Figure 2–2.

Shown diagrammatically are the two components of nystagmus, the slow component and the fast component. By convention, for horizontal eye movements, upward deflections on the eye movement record correspond to rightward eye movements, and downward deflections on the record correspond to leftward eye movement. Note that the velocity of the slow component is lower than the velocity of the fast component, as evidenced by the slope of the lines representing these components of nystagmus.

upward deflections of the chart recorder pen denote rightward eye movement and downward deflections denote leftward eye movement. For vertical recordings, upward deflections denote upward eye movement and downward deflections denote downward eye movements. An example of nystagmus recorded with electro-oculography is shown in Figure 2–2.

POSITIONAL TESTING

Positional testing is performed by placing the patient in the following positions: supine, head left while supine, left lateral, head right while supine, and right lateral, while recording eye movements in the dark. Positional testing is designed to search for "static" positional nystagmus. Static positional nystagmus is not paroxysmal in that it is present as soon as the patient assumes the provocative position and persists for as long as the patient stays in that position. When nystagmus of this type is seen, it is critical that the effect of visual fixation be determined to help localize the disorder because failure to suppress static positional nystagmus with visual fixation strongly suggests a central nervous system lesion. Otherwise, static positional nystagmus is a nonspecific, nonlocalizing sign.

Paroxysmal positional nystagmus, that is, nystagmus induced by the Dix-Hallpike maneuver, may have the typical characteristics of benign paroxysmal positional nystagmus; that is, it (1) appears predominantly torsional and upbeating (that is, beating toward the forehead), (2) has a brief latency of 5 to 10 seconds prior to its appearance, (3) lasts for 15 to 45 seconds, (4) is typically associated with vertigo, and (5) does not occur on repeated provocation. Because electro-oculography is insensitive to torsional eye movements and vertical electro-oculography is plagued by artifacts and poor signal-to-noise ratio, typical benign paroxysmal positional nystagmus is difficult to record in the vestibular laboratory. Newer video-based techniques will help to alleviate this deficiency of the vestibular laboratory. If a nystagmus is recorded during the Dix-Hallpike maneuver that does not conform in every respect to the typical pattern seen with benign paroxysmal positional nystagmus, it should be considered the result of a central nervous system abnormality until proven otherwise.

CALORIC TESTING

Caloric irrigation of the labyrinth is the mainstay of vestibular laboratory testing and forms the basis for so-called electronystagmography. The basis for caloric testing is the establishment of a thermal gradient across the horizontal semicircular canal. By positioning the patient in such a way that the horizontal semicircular canal lies in the vertical plane, a convection current is developed that is thought to induce a change in activity in the vestibular nerve. Although research from microgravity (outer space) experiments has indicated that the thermal stimulus, *independent of the convection current,* actually generates a portion of the caloric response,[3] the convection current theory still accounts for the majority of the caloric response (Fig. 2–3).

The caloric stimulus to the labyrinth can be delivered into the external auditory canal using either water or air. Water irrigation can use either direct irrigation of the external auditory canal or a small distensible balloon that fills with cold or warm water from a reservoir (Fig. 2–4). This so-called closed-loop irrigation has many advantages: the stimulus can be reproduced; caloric testing can be performed despite perforations in the tympanic membrane; and testing is well tolerated, even by children.

Nystagmus responses induced by caloric irrigation are analyzed by measuring the velocity of the slow component of the nystagmus, whose magnitude reflects the intensity of the vestibular response. Many studies have shown that the *peak* slow component velocity attained following caloric irrigation is the best determinant of the intensity of a particular response.[3]

To compare the responsiveness of one ear to that of the other ear, established practice is to use Jongkees' formula to compute a percent "reduced vestibular response." Quite simply, the peak slow component velocities are summed for each ear and then subtracted from the sum of responses to irrigation of the opposite ear. The difference is normalized by dividing by the sum of the four responses and then multiplying by 100 to develop a measure of reduced vestibular response in percent. Each vestibular laboratory should establish its own normative values. For many laboratories, a reduced vestibular response of less than 25 is considered within normal limits.

A unilateral caloric reduction almost always signifies a "peripheral" vestibular lesion, which by definition includes a lesion localized to the vestibular end organ, the

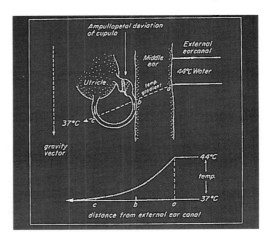

Figure 2–3.
Caloric testing. The physiologic basis for caloric testing is the establishment of a thermal gradient across the horizontal semicircular canal and placement of the horizontal canal in the vertical plane such that a convection current is developed. (Adapted with permission from Baloh, RW, and Honrubia, V (eds): Clinical Neurophysiology of the Vestibular System (2nd ed). Philadelphia: FA Davis Company, 1990, p. 138.[8])

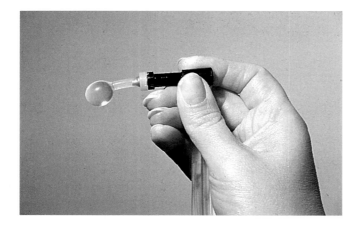

Figure 2–4.
The thermal stimulus to the laby-rinth can be delivered into the exter-nal auditory canal using a small dis-tensible balloon that fills with cold or warm water from a reservoir. Closed-loop irrigation has many advantages: the stimulus is repro-ducible; caloric testing can be per-formed despite perforations in the tympanic membrane; and the test-ing is well tolerated, even by children.

vestibular nerve, or the vestibular nerve root entry zone. Typically, the side of the reduced vestibular response is the lesion side. Rarely, however, the lesion side may have a *hyperactive* rather than a *hypoactive* response as the result of an excitatory rather than a ablative lesion. In such cases, the lesion side may actually be *contralateral* to the side of the caloric reduction.

When responses in an ear to warm and cool irrigation are absent, it is the standard practice in most laboratories to use ice-water irrigation to provoke a response. As with any alerting stimulus, ice-water irrigation may unmask a latent spontaneous nystag-mus. Thus, caloric responses induced by ice-water irrigation should be recorded with the patient both supine (head up 30 degrees) and prone (head down 30 degrees) in order to invert the orientation of the horizontal semicircular canal. Only if the direction of the caloric nystagmus reverses is it certain that the ear truly has a caloric response.

In patients with bilateral vestibular loss, caloric responses are reduced or absent in both ears. Some patients require ice-water irrigation of both ears (sequentially) to as-certain the overall level of unresponsiveness. However, some patients may have re-duced or even absent caloric responses and preserved rotational responses. This ap-parent contradiction can be explained by understanding that caloric stimulation is a nonphysiologic but useful laboratory curiosity and rotation is the natural stimulus to the labyrinth. Also, because it increases slowly, caloric stimulation is a very low fre-quency stimulus with an equivalent frequency of about 0.003 Hz.[4] Some patients may respond poorly at this very low frequency and still have robust responses during ro-tational testing, which uses much higher frequencies.[5]

Rarely, patients may exhibit increased caloric responses. As in the case of increased *gain* on rotational testing (see below), increased responses usually signify cerebellar disease.

Also available from the caloric response is a measure of so-called directional pre-ponderance, which expresses numerically whether the amount of right-beating nystag-mus exceeds the amount of left-beating nystagmus or vice versa. Unlike the measure of reduced vestibular response, the directional preponderance of caloric testing is a nonspecific and nonlocalizing sign of vestibular dysfunction. Moreover, the measure is more variable than reduced vestibular response. Most laboratories use a value of 30 percent directional preponderance as a threshold of normality.

The great advantage of caloric testing is that it provides lateralizing information that is not available from any other vestibular laboratory test. Disadvantages of the caloric test include its variability, its propensity for inducing nausea and occasional vomiting, and the unwillingness of most patients to undergo repeated caloric testing even when such testing would be helpful for management.

ROTATIONAL TESTING

Rotational testing relies on natural stimulation of the labyrinth, namely angular acceleration. Rotational testing typically uses so-called earth-vertical axis rotation, in which a subject sits on a computer-controlled turntable and is turned left and right in a prescribed fashion (Fig. 2–5). Assessment of the vestibulo-ocular reflex independent of vision is accomplished by rotating a patient with eyes open in the dark. Rotational testing can also be used to assess visual-vestibular interaction by rotating patients in various visual conditions.

Unlike caloric testing, rotational testing stimulates *both* semicircular canals simultaneously; one is inhibited while the other is excited. Many different trajectories of rotation can be used for rotational testing. The most common trajectories are sinusoidal profiles, also called sinusoidal harmonic acceleration. With this type of stimulus, subjects are rotated first to the right and then to the left, then right, then left, and so on in a smoothly, sinusoidally varying pattern of velocity and acceleration. Also, patients may be rotated at a constant velocity followed by an abrupt deceleration to a stop.

To analyze the nystagmus induced by rotational testing, it is necessary to identify the slow components, because these reflect the influence of vestibular stimulation. The slow components induced by rotational stimulation are pieced together to generate a so-called cumulative slow-component eye *position*. This response measure is typically differentiated mathematically to yield slow-component eye *velocity*, which can be compared with the turntable velocity to establish the response parameters of *gain, phase,* and *symmetry* (directional preponderance).

The *gain* of the response to sinusoidal earth-vertical axis rotation is, by definition,

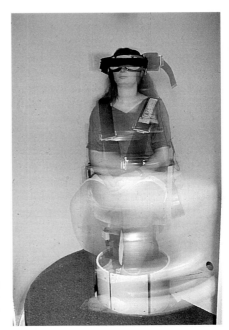

Figure 2–5.
Earth-vertical axis rotational testing is usually performed using a test chair located inside an enclosure with a computer-controlled turntable. Testing of the vestibulo-ocular reflex is performed with eyes open behind opaque goggles.

the ratio of the magnitude of the response to the *magnitude* of the stimulus. The estimate of gain is obtained by using a computer to fit the best sinusoid through the slow-component eye velocity and then by dividing the magnitude of that best fit by the peak velocity of the sinusoidal rotational stimulus.

Reduced gain indicates decreased vestibular sensitivity. Unilateral vestibular loss may not reduce gain below normal. Thus, reduced gain usually indicates bilateral vestibular loss. Rarely, gain can be abnormally large, usually as a result of a cerebellar lesion.

The *phase* of the response to sinusoidal earth-vertical axis rotation is also determined following generation of the best-fit sinusoid through the slow-component eye velocity response. Phase represents the *timing* relationship between the eye velocity response and turntable velocity. Phase is a highly sensitive but nonspecific measure of vestibular system abnormality. Phase commonly changes with peripheral vestibular injury, and the changes are often permanent. Another measure, comparable to phase, can be obtained from constant velocity rather than sinusoidal rotations. That measure, the so-called time constant of the vestibulo-ocular reflex, is a measure of how rapidly the vestibular nystagmus decays following an abrupt stop of the rotational chair. Like phase, the vestibulo-ocular reflex *time constant* is a sensitive but nonspecific measure of vestibular system abnormality.

Many patients, especially those who are symptomatic at the time of testing, display an *asymmetric* response, that is, a *directional preponderance*. Despite a symmetric stimulus with equal rotations to the right and to the left, patients with a directional preponderance display an excessive amount of either right-beating or left-beating nystagmus. Such an asymmetry of response can manifest simply as a shift in the average velocity of the response, or the slow-component velocity may have a nonsinusoidal shape with a higher velocity in one direction or the other. A rotational response asymmetry indicates an ongoing vestibulo-ocular imbalance but does not provide localizing information.

Another type of rotational testing, visual-vestibular interaction, which is usually reserved for detailed testing of patients suspected of having a central vestibular lesion, is performed by asking patients to look at a small target that rotates with them or by having them view earth-fixed full-field stripes or dots while undergoing earth-vertical axis rotation. In this way, vision is used to either reduce or augment the vestibular response, respectively. Visual-vestibular interaction testing is particularly useful when assessing central vestibular abnormalities because appropriately combining visual and vestibular information depends upon the normal functioning of brainstem and cerebellar structures. Typically, patients are rotated at a single sinusoidal frequency: (1) in the dark, (2) with a fixation target, and (3) with earth-fixed stripes. A sinusoidal optokinetic stimulus while the patient is stationary may be a pure visual stimulus. The response to these visual, vestibular, and combined visual-vestibular stimuli is recorded and analyzed in a manner similar to the response to sinusoidal rotational acceleration in the dark, that is, to yield *gain* and *phase*.

Yet another test of central vestibular function is an assessment of so-called tilt suppression of postrotatory nystagmus. For this assessment, immediately on cessation of rotation, a patient is tilted forward by about 45 degrees. Normally, such a reorientation of a patient immediately on cessation of rotation results in a shortening of the *time constant* (see previous text) of the vestibulo-ocular reflex. If this expected decrease in the time constant of the vestibulo-ocular reflex does not occur, that is, if tilt suppression is abnormal, a vestibulo-cerebellar lesion, specifically a lesion of the caudal midline cerebellum, should be considered.[6]

Rotational testing has several advantages: (1) the stimulus can be controlled precisely; (2) rotation consists of the natural stimulation to the labyrinth, that is, angular acceleration; (3) rotation is rarely bothersome; (4) rotation can be used for serial evaluations; and (5) in special circumstances, visual-vestibular interaction and tilt suppression can be assessed. Testing can be performed at several rotational frequencies and amplitudes, allowing flexibility in the design of the stimulus so that patients with particular types of abnormalities, such as bilateral vestibular loss, can be evaluated more thoroughly. In particular, higher frequencies and amplitudes of rotation can be used to determine the degree, if any, of remaining vestibular function in patients who have suffered bilateral vestibular loss either from ototoxic medication or an underlying disease state.[7]

The great disadvantage of rotational testing is that it does not provide lateralizing information; *both* labyrinths are stimulated simultaneously. Thus, rotational testing is best used as an adjunct to conventional electronystagmography.

POSTUROGRAPHY

Posturography is now performed in many vestibular laboratories using the commercially available EquiTest device.[3] Testing is divided into two broad types, which have been named motor control (formerly "movement coordination") testing and "sensory organization" testing. Motor control testing employs repeated translations and rotations of the support surface that are designed to assess a patient's ability to maintain balance.

The sensory organization test is designed to manipulate vision and somatic sensation, which constitute two of the three sensory modalities important in maintaining upright balance. Using a technique called "sway referencing," the platform and the

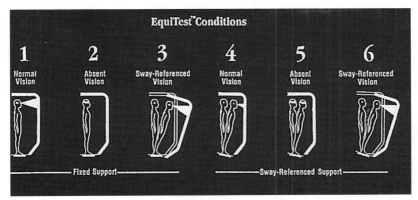

Figure 2–6.
The sensory organization portion of computerized dynamic posturography includes six paradigms: (1) eyes open, platform stable; (2) eyes closed, platform stable; (3) eyes open with visual surroundings moving and platform stable; (4) eyes open, platform moving; (5) eyes closed, platform moving; and (6) both visual surroundings and platform moving. The movements of the visual surroundings, the platform, or both are designed to parallel movements of the patient's center of mass, so-called "sway-referencing," thereby providing a distorted visual or proprioceptive input. The fifth and sixth conditions, wherein the patient's eyes are closed or the patient is viewing moving visual surroundings while the floor moves, force the patient to rely on the vestibulospinal system to maintain balance. (With permission from NeuroCom International Inc., Clackamas, Oregon.)

20

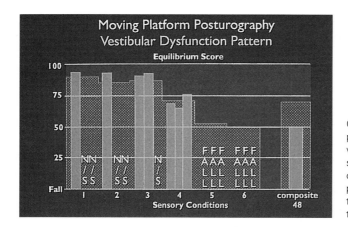

Figure 2–7.
Computer analysis of postural sway provided by EquiTest for a patient who was able to stand during the first four sensory conditions but unable to stand on the fifth and sixth conditions. This patient has a vestibular pattern on posturography, suggesting an ongoing vestibulospinal abnormality.

visual surroundings are rotated in the same way that the patient is swaying, thereby distorting these sensory inputs. Sway referencing the platform and visual surroundings in various combinations can force patients to rely primarily on their vestibular system to maintain upright balance. Thus, the sensory organization portion of the posturography evaluation includes six paradigms, illustrated in Figure 2–6.

Figure 2–7 shows an example of the computer analysis of postural sway provided by the EquiTest device. This patient was able to stand during the first four sensory conditions but was unable to stand during the fifth and sixth conditions; the patient lost balance and put tension on the safety harness. This patient therefore has a vestibular pattern on posturography suggesting an ongoing vestibulospinal abnormality. Another pattern of abnormality, shown in Figure 2–8, is called a "surface-dependent pattern" and suggests a combined visual and vestibular abnormality regarding postural control. Only when provided with reliable proprioceptive input can such an individual stand.

An advantage of dynamic posturography is that it evaluates upright "balance" and thus provides a functional evaluation that depends on vestibulospinal function. In this regard, dynamic posturography provides information distinctly different from that provided by caloric and rotational testing, which assess vestibulo-ocular responses. Dynamic posturography is noninvasive and has been shown to be repeatable. Although a lack of patient cooperation and effort will lead to abnormal responses, only with great sophistication can particular patterns of abnormalities be spuriously produced.

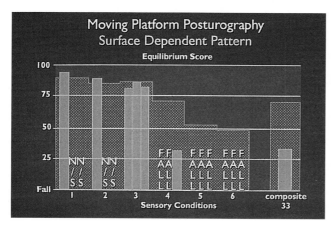

Figure 2–8.
Computer analysis of postural sway by EquiTest for a patient who was able to stand during the first three sensory conditions but unable to stand on the fourth, fifth, and sixth conditions. This patient has a surface-dependent pattern on posturography, suggesting a combined visual/vestibular abnormality regarding postural control. Such an individual can stand only with reliable proprioceptive input.

A disadvantage of dynamic posturography is that results are somewhat nonspecific and may indicate vestibular disease even when not present. Some neurologic abnormalities are undetected by dynamic posturography; patients with cerebellar and basal ganglia disease may have normal responses. Also, dynamic posturography does not provide localizing information with regard to central nervous system abnormalities.

REFERENCES

1. Young, L, and Shenna, D: Eye movement measurement techniques. Am Psychol 30(3):315–330, 1975.
2. Robinson, D: A method of measuring eye movement using a scleral search coil in a magnetic field. IEEE Trans Biomed Electr 10:137–145, 1963.
3. Jacobson, GP, and Newman, CW: Handbook of Balance Function Testing. St. Louis: Mosby Year Book, 1993.
4. Hamid, M, Hughes, G, and Kinney, S: Criteria for diagnosing bilateral vestibular dysfunction. In Graham, MD, and Kemink, JL (eds): The Vestibular System: Neurophysiologic and Clinical Research. New York: Raven Press, 1987, pp 115–118.
5. Furman, JM, and Kamerer, DB: Rotational responses in patients with bilateral caloric reduction. Acta Otolaryngol (Stockh) 108:355–361, 1989.
6. Hain, TC, Zee, DS, and Maria, BL: Tilt suppression of vestibulo-ocular reflex in patients with cerebellar lesions. Acta Otolaryngol (Stockh) 105:13–20, 1988.
7. Baloh, RW, et al: Changes in the human vestibulo-ocular reflex after loss of peripheral sensitivity. Ann Neurol 16:222–228, 1984.
8. Baloh, RW, and Honrubia, V (eds): Clinical Neurophysiology of the Vestibular System (2nd ed). Philadelphia: FA Davis Company, 1990.

3

Auditory System and Testing

The cochlea, the human organ of hearing, consists of a membranous structure called the cochlear duct, which is approximately 33 mm in length and twisted into a spiral with 2¾ turns (Fig. 3–1). The cochlear duct is supported by a bony skeleton consisting of a central modiolus and surrounding otic capsule. The afferent auditory neuronal cell bodies form the spiral ganglion, which is located inside the modiolus of the cochlea. The spiral arrangement of the cochlear duct results in a spiral arrangement of neurons within the spiral ganglion. The auditory nerve, which is a component of the eighth cranial nerve, carries approximately 30,000 primary afferent neurons and about 1000 efferent nerve fibers, whose function is unknown. Because the vestibular and auditory apparatus share common inner ear fluids, nerves, blood supply, and location within the temporal bone, disorders that affect the peripheral vestibular apparatus often affect hearing. Vertigo associated with a unilateral hearing loss suggests a peripheral vestibular abnormality on the side with the hearing loss. Thus, it is important to assess hearing in the evaluation of the dizzy patient because hearing loss may help to localize a vestibular system disorder to the labyrinth and also may help to lateralize the problem to a particular ear.

Many vertigo syndromes have characteristic associated audiologic findings that can help with establishing a specific diagnosis. For example, a fluctuating low-frequency sensorineural hearing loss is characteristic of endolymphatic hydrops, that is, Meniere's disease. Acute vestibular neuritis is characterized by the absence of auditory symptoms and normal hearing. Compression of the vestibular-cochlear nerve within the internal auditory canal or cerebellopontine angle by a neoplasm can produce symptoms of unsteadiness and dysequilibrium as well as a sensorineural hearing loss, which typically presents at high frequencies and is slowly progressive. Such lesions also cause diminished word recognition. Otosclerosis, which may cause dizziness, produces a characteristic *conductive* hearing loss.

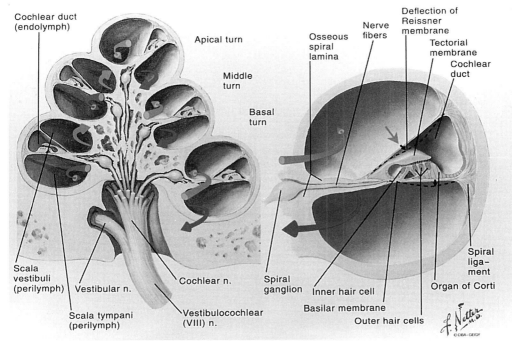

Figure 3–1.
Two views of the anatomy of the cochlea. The left panel shows the three turns of the cochlear duct. The cochlear nerve enters the center of the cochlea from the internal auditory canal. The right panel shows one turn of the cochlea in greater detail. The organ of Corti contains the hair cells involved in transduction of sound to neural activity. (With permission from Silverstein, H, Wolfson, RJ, and Rosenberg, S: Diagnosis and management of hearing loss. Clinical Symposia 44(3):5, 1992.[10])

LABORATORY ASSESSMENT OF HEARING

AUDIOGRAM AND WORD RECOGNITION TEST

The mainstay of hearing assessment consists of two psychophysical tests: the *audiogram* and the *word recognition test*.[1,2] The audiogram summarizes hearing thresholds compared to those of normal persons at standardized pure tone frequencies that range from 250 to 8000 Hz. These hearing thresholds are plotted in a graphic format, wherein the abscissa (horizontal axis) is frequency and the ordinate (vertical axis) is hearing threshold in units of decibels (dB) referenced to the sound pressure level of normal hearing at each test frequency (Fig. 3–2). The word recognition test measures the ability of a patient to correctly repeat words represented at 30 to 40 dB louder than the patient's hearing threshold. The percentage of words correctly recognized is reported for each ear separately.

Normally, hearing thresholds are symmetric in the two ears. When one ear is found to have significantly worse hearing than the other ear, further evaluation of the auditory system is warranted, especially to rule out eighth nerve or cerebellopontine angle lesions. Although there are no strict guidelines as to when to pursue further evaluation of asymmetric hearing loss, a significant hearing difference is considered to be 10 dB or more at two adjacent test frequencies or a 15 percent or greater difference in word

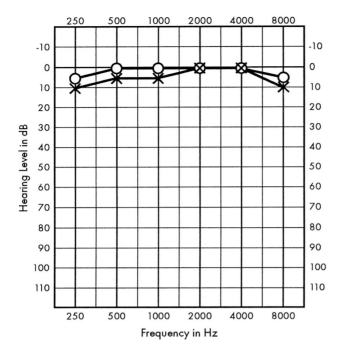

Figure 3–2. Audiogram.

		Right	Left
Air	unmasked	o—o	x—x
	masked	△—△	□—□
Bone	unmasked	←---<	>---→
	masked	⊢---⊏	⊣---⊐

Word Recognition Score

Right : 100%
Left : 100%

recognition scores. It is recommended that, whenever a significant hearing asymmetry is present that cannot be explained by other clinical circumstances, such as unilateral noise-induced hearing loss, either brainstem auditory-evoked potential testing (see later text) or brain imaging be performed to rule out a structural lesion of the auditory system.[3]

TYMPANOMETRY AND ACOUSTIC REFLEX TESTING

Tympanometry and acoustic reflex testing are commonly used audiologic screening tests.[4] Tympanometry assesses the compliance (acoustic resistance) of the tympanic membrane and middle ear ossicles and is largely used to help diagnose middle ear infection. Tympanometry is also used as part of the electronystagmographic perilymphatic fistula test. This test consists of changing external auditory canal pressure while recording eye movements. Patients with a perilymphatic fistula may develop nystagmus or eye deviation in response to pressure changes. Acoustic reflex testing assesses the integrity of the *stapedius reflex* by exposing the ear to loud sound and then assessing changes in acoustic resistance and, thus, provides information about the afferent sensory (auditory) and efferent motor (facial nerve) limbs of this reflex. Historically, acoustic reflex testing has been used as part of a "site-of-lesion" test battery. However, more advanced audiologic tests (see below), such as brainstem auditory-evoked potential testing and electrocochleography, have superseded acoustic reflex testing and other previously used site-of-lesion tests for localizing disorders of the auditory system.

BRAINSTEM AUDITORY-EVOKED POTENTIAL TESTING

Brainstem auditory-evoked potential testing is an electrophysiologic test used to evaluate the integrity of the auditory pathway from the cochlea through several brainstem auditory relay centers.[5] In the brainstem auditory-evoked potential testing procedure, auditory clicks or brief tone bursts are delivered through headphones to evoke a highly synchronous and repeatable neural response. This response is measured using surface electrodes and standard signal averaging techniques. The evoked neural potentials that occur early, that is, within 1 to 12 milliseconds, reflect cochlear nerve and brainstem activity and are collectively called *brainstem* auditory-evoked potentials or the auditory brainstem response. The brainstem auditory-evoked potential is characterized by a series of five vertex-positive waves (I to V) that are thought to correspond to relay centers

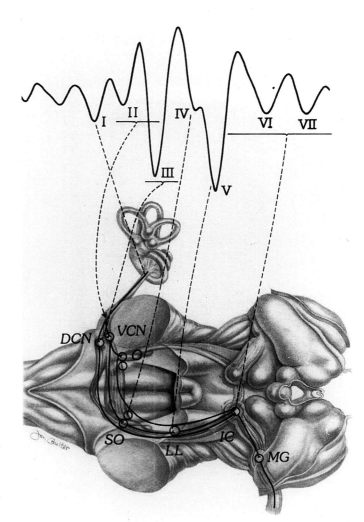

Figure 3–3.
Neural generators of brainstem auditory evoked potentials. VCN = ventral cochlear nucleus; DCN = dorsal cochlear nucleus; SO = superior olive; LL = lateral lemniscus; IC = inferior colliculus; MG = medial geniculate. (With permission from Moller, AR, and Jannetta, PJ: Neural generators of the brainstem auditory evoked potentials. In Nodar, RH, and Barber, C (eds): Evoked Potentials II: The Second International Evoked Potentials Symposium. Butterworth Publishers, Boston, 1984, p. 144.[11])

within the auditory pathway: wave I–cochlear nerve at the level of the spiral ganglion; wave II–cochlear nerve/brainstem junction; wave III–cochlear nucleus; wave IV–superior olive complex; and wave V–lateral lemniscus (Fig. 3–3). The interpretation of the brainstem auditory-evoked potential is based on the qualitative morphology of the waveforms and quantitative latency and amplitude of each wave.

Brainstem auditory-evoked potential testing can be used for site-of-lesion testing since the latencies of waves I to V can be compared between the two ears and to normative data[6,7] (Fig. 3–4). These measurements can be used to determine whether abnormal wave latencies exist and the likely anatomic site of such delays. Disruption of auditory neural transduction may be caused by neoplasia, by compression or invasion of the eighth cranial nerve or brainstem, or by demyelination anywhere along the central auditory pathway. Auditory system abnormalities may be associated with concomitant vestibular abnormalities caused by the close anatomic relationship between the vestibular nerve and the auditory nerve and between the vestibular nuclei and the cochlear nuclei. Thus, brainstem auditory-evoked potential testing, which provides information regarding the integrity of central auditory pathways, also provides information regarding central vestibular pathways. Brainstem auditory-evoked potential testing can also be used for determining auditory thresholds in patients who cannot otherwise cooperate, such as adults with altered mental status and infants.

ELECTROCOCHLEOGRAPHY

Electrocochleography is a modification of the brainstem auditory-evoked potential test in which wave I is amplified to reveal both the "action potential" of the cochlear nerve, also called N1, as well as another wave preceding the action potential referred to as the "summating potential." Normally the ratio of the summating potential to the action potential is less than one third. However, when endolymphatic hydrops is present, the summating potential increases relative to the action potential (Fig. 3–5). When the ratio of the summating potential to action potential amplitude exceeds 0.5, it is considered

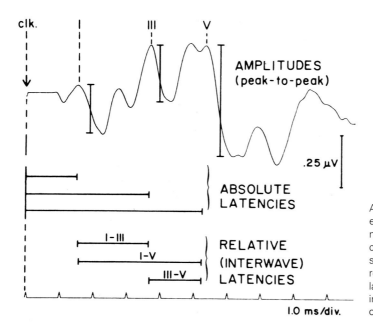

Figure 3–4.
Analysis of brainstem auditory evoked potentials (BAEP). Latency measurements are used more commonly than amplitude measurements. Absolute latencies, relative latencies, and interaural latencies (not shown) can be used in the analysis and interpretation of BAEP.

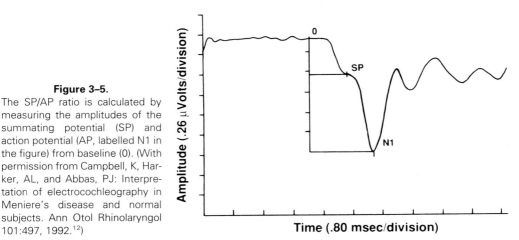

Figure 3–5.
The SP/AP ratio is calculated by measuring the amplitudes of the summating potential (SP) and action potential (AP, labelled N1 in the figure) from baseline (0). (With permission from Campbell, K, Harker, AL, and Abbas, PJ: Interpretation of electrocochleography in Meniere's disease and normal subjects. Ann Otol Rhinolaryngol 101:497, 1992.[12])

abnormal and indicative of endolymphatic hydrops. The association of an elevated summating potential/action potential ratio with endolymphatic hydrops has been substantiated both experimentally and clinically.[8,9] Thus, electrocochleography can be helpful in diagnosing endolymphatic hydrops as the underlying cause of a balance disorder. Electrocochleography is particularly useful in patients whose symptoms are not characteristic of a particular disorder. Also, in cases in which both ears appear to be affected, electrocochleography may be helpful in localizing underlying endolymphatic hydrops to an actively pathological ear.

REFERENCES

1. Katz, J (ed): Handbook of Clinical Audiology. Baltimore: Williams & Wilkins, 1994.
2. Rintelmann, WF (ed): Hearing Assessment. Perspectives in Audiology Series, Austin: Pro-ed, 1991.
3. Selesnick, SH, and Jackler, RK: Atypical hearing loss in acoustic neuroma patients. Laryngoscope 103:437–446, 1993.
4. Sheehy, JL, and Hughes, RL: The ABC's of impedance audiometry. Laryngoscope 134(11):1935–1949, 1974.
5. Moller, AR: Auditory neurophysiology. J Clin Neurophysiol 11(3):284–308, 1994.
6. Selters, WA, and Brackmann, DE: Acoustic tumor detection with brain stem electric response audiometry. Arch Otolaryngol 103:181–187, 1977.
7. Wilson, DF, et al: The sensitivity of auditory brainstem response testing in small acoustic neuromas. Laryngoscope 102:961–964, 1992.
8. Ferraro, JA, Arenberg, K, and Hassanein, S: Electrocochleography and symptoms of inner ear dysfunction. Arch Otolaryngol 111:71–74, 1985.
9. Arenberg, IK, et al: ECoG results in perilymphatic fistula: Clinical and experimental studies. Otolaryngol Head Neck Surg 99(5):435–443, 1988.
10. Silverstein, H, Wolfson, RJ, and Rosenberg, S: Diagnosis and management of hearing loss. Clinical Symposia 44(3):5, 1992.
11. Moller, AR, and Jannetta, PJ: Neural generators of the brainstem auditory evoked potentials. In Nodar, RH, and Barber, C (eds): Evoked Potentials II: The Second International Evoked Potentials Symposium. Boston: Butterworth Publishers, 1984.
12. Campbell, K, Harker, AL, and Abbas, PJ: Interpretation of electrocochleography in Meniere's disease and normal subjects. Ann Otol Rhinolaryngol 101:497, 1992.

CHAPTER

4

Vestibular Rehabilitation

Physical therapy evaluation and treatment have become an important resource to the practicing otolaryngologist. In the early 1940s, Cawthorne,[1] Cooksey,[2] and Dix and Hood[3] recognized that patients who actively moved their heads recovered more quickly and completely from acute peripheral lesions than those who did not. These early clinical observations have engendered a large body of experimental and clinical data that support the concept that vestibular exercises promote functional balance recovery and compensation following vestibular system injury. More recently, the writings of Shumway-Cook and Horak[4] and Herdman[5] have focused the expertise of therapists on the problem of functional recovery following vestibular system injury. Attention to the specific problems of each patient has improved the quality of such intervention. The formerly common practice of dispensing a generic list of head movement exercises has evolved into a referral for a comprehensive sensory and motor evaluation by a skilled therapist with specialized training in balance disorders who then develops a treatment plan for a program of vestibular rehabilitation. The goal of vestibular rehabilitation is to develop a specific program of movements directed at improving a patient's specific functional balance deficits, decreasing dizziness, increasing activity level, and improving functional abilities in general.

Who is a candidate for vestibular rehabilitation? Very few patients do not obtain some benefit from it. Ideal patients for vestibular rehabilitation include those with chronic uncompensated peripheral vestibulopathy. Other disease states that respond to vestibular rehabilitation include multisensory disequilibrium, drug-induced vestibulopathy, head trauma, panic/anxiety disorders, and the vestibular imbalance that follows a destructive surgical procedure. Patients with episodic vertigo who have otherwise normal balance (e.g., many patients with Meniere's disease) are not candidates for therapy because exercises do not influence the frequency or severity of episodes. Also, patients with benign positional vertigo do not require vestibular rehabilitation unless their evaluation uncovers evidence for an ongoing vestibulo-ocular or vestibulospinal imbalance.

Despite the fact that some disorders are easier to treat than others and that some disorders have poorer prognoses than others, vestibular rehabilitation has few contra-indications. The therapist should be informed of the patient's medical problems, results of vestibular testing, medications, and contraindicated exercises such as vigorous neck exercises in patients with vertebral vascular disease. Patients should be reassured that they must often be willing to "feel worse before they begin to feel better." Although elderly individuals are generally less stable, there is no age limit for a trial of vestibular rehabilitation.

THEORETIC BASIS FOR PHYSICAL THERAPY

Although considered primarily reflexive, vestibular responses are actually quite malleable. For example, the capability to alter the vestibulo-ocular reflex forms one of the theoretic bases for vestibular rehabilitation. Physiologic alterations of the vestibulo-ocular reflex (VOR) can be brought about by (1) changing the *magnitude* of the VOR using an altered visual environment such as that produced by magnifying or miniaturizing lenses[6]; (2) changing the *timing* of the VOR using repeated rotations[7,8]; and (3) altering vestibulo-ocular responses by imagining an earth-fixed visual target or imagining a head-fixed visual target.[9] This capacity for vestibulo-ocular responses to change, depending on the demands of the situation, provides the therapist with a modifiable substrate.

As discussed in Chapter 1, in response to peripheral vestibular injury, the vestibular system is known to alter its responses to produce a more functional response. Unilateral vestibular injury is known to be followed immediately by an acute vestibular syndrome. However, in a matter of hours or days, depending on age and central nervous system status, the patient improves so much that vestibular reflex responses are almost symmetric. This process of central nervous system compensation for unilateral peripheral injury occurs by mechanisms as yet unknown. However, certain types of movement and exposure to visual surroundings potentiate this compensation process.[10] Also, certain pharmaceutic agents (e.g., meclizine) may slow this process.[11] Neurophysiologically, the response to unilateral peripheral vestibular injury undoubtedly includes changes in the neural activity in the vestibular nuclei. The crossed pathways of the vestibular commissures may be important for the compensatory process.[12] After compensation, if a subsequent injury occurs to the contralateral vestibular system, some individuals appear to have only an acute vestibular injury on the newly affected side. This is known as Becterew's phenomenon.

Bilateral peripheral vestibular injury is a more challenging problem than unilateral vestibular injury. Proprioceptive and visual influences may assume a more important role in stabilization of the eyes and the body following severe bilateral vestibular deficits. This process can be exploited by the therapist during vestibular rehabilitation.

TECHNIQUE OF VESTIBULAR REHABILITATION

A thorough discussion of the technique of vestibular rehabilitation is beyond the scope of this book. However, a brief overview follows. For an in-depth discussion of this topic, the reader is referred to the excellent text entitled *Vestibular Rehabilitation Therapy*.[5]

VESTIBULAR REHABILITATION ASSESSMENT

A thorough evaluation of each patient by the therapist on an individualized basis precedes the development of a treatment plan for vestibular rehabilitation. This evaluation begins by reviewing material supplied by the referring physician, which typically includes the diagnosis/differential diagnosis and past medical history including medications, recently prescribed medications, and laboratory test results. Even though a diagnostic evaluation by the referring physician has already been undertaken, the therapist personally evaluates the patient's vestibular, proprioceptive, and visual systems from his or her own perspective to uncover any deficits that may be affecting the patient's balance. Then, using the environmental context as a basis, the therapist evaluates changes in the patient's ability to maintain adequate postural control. This is done because some patients are able to balance without difficulty if they are in an environment with little extraneous movement and yet have marked problems in a more dynamic environment that contains extraneous movement. Evaluation of body morphology is also essential. The patient's height, weight, strength, posture, coordination, and range of motion can all affect balance.

During the vestibular rehabilitation assessment, patients are given a monthly calendar and asked to report the frequency and intensity of symptoms on a daily basis because it is very important for the patient's self-confidence to document progress. Also, patients are asked to fill out a Dizziness Handicap Inventory[13] to assess their perception of handicap. The Dizziness Handicap Inventory attempts to quantify the effects of dizziness on a patient's function, physical status, and emotional well-being.

The therapist then elicits a detailed social history to determine whether or not the patient is living in a safe environment. The therapist may then make recommendations that attempt to improve the level of safety in the patient's home environment. For example, it may be suggested that a patient use a night light in the bedroom, remove throw rugs, or install handrails. It is also helpful to know whether any family members can assist the patient in a home exercise program.

After these factors are assessed, the therapist assesses the patient's ability to perform functional movements with the eyes open, eyes closed, and at various speeds. Transitional movements that are tested include rolling, sitting, reaching, standing, and Dix-Hallpike maneuvers (see Case T2). Then the therapist assesses head and eye movements. This assessment parallels that of the physical examination performed by the physician. However, the patient's symptoms, such as dizziness and blurred vision, are especially important during these movements. Finally, the therapist performs a balance assessment, that is, an assessment of the patient's ability to sit, stand, and walk in different situations. "Static" balance measures include Romberg testing, single leg stance, and tandem Romberg testing. Sensory inputs for static balance are modified using compliant foam and a visual conflict dome,[14] which qualitatively simulate computerized platform posturography (see Chap. 2). Dynamic balance measures in common use include the standing reach task[15] and the Fukuda stepping test,[16] which is also used by many physicians. Gait is usually assessed qualitatively by observing base and speed, looking for veering, and noting any unsteadiness, especially during turns. Also, patients are asked to walk while making head movements, which is a particularly difficult task.

VESTIBULAR REHABILITATION TREATMENT

Herdman and associates[5] recommend that therapists identify the specific problems and functional limitations of each patient so that a list of vestibular rehabilitation goals can

TABLE 4–1
Comparison of Different Vestibular Rehabilitation Approaches for the Patient with a Peripheral Vestibular Disorder

Movement	Cawthorne and Cooksey	Norre	Herdman	UPMC*
Incorporates head and neck exercises into the treatment approach	X	X	X	X
Uses eye exercises	X		X	X
Uses a functional evaluation to assess the symptoms of the patient	X	X	X	X
Incorporates principles of motor control and learning into designing a treatment program			X	X
Practices mental exercises to increase concentration	X		X	X
Has the patient work in a variety of environments and task contexts	X		X	X

*University of Pittsburgh Medical Center.
Source: Adapted from Herdman, SJ (ed): Vestibular Rehabilitation. FA Davis, Philadelphia, 1994.[5]

be constructed. Once these goals are established, the therapist has numerous movements from which to choose to develop a program for each patient. Many of these movements can be performed by the patient at home. They are designed to potentiate compensation for peripheral vestibular lesions and to help patients learn how to substitute other sensory inputs, such as vision and somatosensory inputs, for vestibular sensation. Substitution of other sensory modalities is especially important in patients with bilateral vestibular deficits.

TABLE 4–2
Balance and Gait Exercises

1. Perform the following exercises while standing. Stand near a kitchen counter, but hold on only if needed.
   a. Walk sideways 15 ft. Repeat in both left and right directions _____ times, twice a day.
   b. Walk backward 15 ft. Repeat _____ times, twice a day.
2. Perform the following exercises while standing. Stand with a wall behind you. Have a family member stand nearby if needed. Stand on a pillow or couch cushion for _____ seconds.
   a. Do this with your eyes open. Repeat _____ times, twice a day.
   b. Do this with your eyes closed. Repeat _____ times, twice a day.
   c. Stand on one leg with your eyes open. Repeat _____ times, twice a day.
3. Walk down a corridor and practice moving your head left and right. Keep your head turned in each direction for about 3 steps. Walk _____ ft. Repeat _____ times, twice a day. Also repeat by moving your head up and down.
4. Set up an obstacle course. Use chairs, pillows, and furniture as obstacles. Place smaller objects on the floor that you must step over. Change the course each time so that you do not get used to the same routine.

   You can incorporate stair climbing, sitting to standing, or picking up and carrying objects during the obstacle course. Set a timer or clock yourself to see how quickly you can finish.

   To add difficulty, have a family member give commands (i.e., ''Turn left now'') or throw a ball toward you unexpectedly.
5. Walk around a darkened room (preferably carpeted) in your house for _____ minutes.
6. Go grocery shopping, as tolerated.
7. Do your walking program at a shopping mall 1 to 2 times a week.

Source: Adapted from Herdman, SJ (ed): Vestibular Rehabilitation. FA Davis, Philadelphia, 1994.[5]

TABLE 4–3
Factors that Affect the Outcome of
Vestibular Rehabilitation

Duration and chronicity of illness
Pre-existing orthopedic conditions
Age
Ongoing litigation
Pre-existing or associated psychiatric disorders
Combined central and peripheral vestibular disorders

Herdman and associates[5] state that "The goals of physical therapy intervention are to improve the patient's mobility, overall general physical condition and activity level, functional balance, safety for gait and gait-related activities, and the magnitude of the patient's symptoms" (p. 290). Because many patients feel worse symptomatically when they begin vestibular rehabilitation, vestibular suppressants may be prescribed when therapy begins. Subsequently, these medications, which may actually impair vestibular rehabilitation (see Case C1), should be discontinued.

Various approaches use vestibular rehabilitation to treat patients with a vestibular deficit. Table 4–1 provides an overview of the most commonly used approaches. Table 4–2 lists balance and gait exercises used at the University of Pittsburgh Medical Center.

Patients with bilateral vestibular reduction have a more serious balance problem and a worse prognosis than those with a unilateral vestibular loss. Many of the principles that underlie the vestibular rehabilitation of patients with unilateral vestibular loss also apply to patients with bilateral vestibular loss, but there are several special considerations: recovery is slower; sensory substitution is the primary means of rehabilitation; exercises may be needed chronically; visual input (proper lighting) is critical; and a cane or walker may provide a great deal of help, especially early in the rehabilitation process.[5] After assessment and development of a treatment plan, patients are typically seen in follow-up every 2 to 3 weeks for a total of 6 visits so that progress can be monitored and the treatment program modified as needed.

Factors that affect the outcome of vestibular rehabilitation are listed in Table 4–3. Although studies that address the efficacy of vestibular rehabilitation are still under way, a study by Kamerer and coworkers[17] at the University of Pittsburgh Medical Center indicated that about 75 percent of patients who were enrolled in a vestibular rehabilitation program experienced subjective improvement; slightly less than 50 percent of the patients manifested objective improvement. Patients with peripheral vestibular ailments fared best. The patients least likely to benefit included those with fluctuating conditions, those with pure central disorders, those with mixed central and peripheral disorders, and those involved in litigation.

REFERENCES

1. Cawthorne, TE: Vestibular injuries. Proc R Soc Med 39:270–273, 1945.
2. Cooksey, FS: Rehabilitation in vestibular injuries. Proc R Soc Med 39:275, 1945.
3. Dix, MR, and Hood, JD: Vestibular habituation: Its clinical significance and relationship to vestibular neuronitis. Laryngoscope 80:226–232, 1970.
4. Shumway-Cook, A, and Horak, FB: Rehabilitation strategies for patients with vestibular deficits. In Arenberg, IK (ed): Dizziness and Balance Disorders. New York: Kugler Publications, 1993, pp 667–691.
5. Herdman, SJ (ed): Vestibular Rehabilitation. Philadelphia: FA Davis, 1994.

6. Melvill Jones, G: Adaptive modulation of VOR parameters by vision. In Berthoz, A, and Melvill Jones, G (eds): Adaptive Mechanisms in Gaze Control: Reviews in Oculomotor Research. Amsterdam: Elsevier, 1985, pp 21–50.

7. Schmid, R, and Jeannerod, M: Vestibular habituation: An adaptive process? In Berthoz, A, and Melvill Jones, G (eds): Adaptive Mechanisms in Gaze Control. Amsterdam: Elsevier, 1985.

8. Baloh, RW, Henn, V, and Jager, J: Habituation of the human vestibulo-ocular reflex by low frequency harmonic acceleration. Am J Otolaryngol 3:235, 1982.

9. Melvill Jones, G, and Berthoz, A: Mental control of the adaptive process. In Berthoz, A, and Melvill Jones, G (eds): Adaptive Mechanisms in Gaze Control. Amsterdam: Elsevier, 1985.

10. Igarashi, M: Physical exercise and acceleration of vestibular compensation. In Lacour, M, et al (eds): Vestibular Compensation. Amsterdam: Elsevier, 1989.

11. Peppard, SB: Effect of drug therapy on compensation from vestibular injury. Laryngoscope 96:878–898, 1986.

12. Bienhold, H, and Flohr, H: Role of commissural connexions between vestibular nuclei in compensation following unilateral labyrinthectomy. J Physiol 284:178, 1978.

13. Jacobson, GP, and Newman, CW: The development of the Dizziness Handicap Inventory. Arch Otolaryngol Head Neck Surg 116:424–427, 1990.

14. Shumway-Cook, A, and Horak, FB: Assessing the influence of sensory interaction on balance. J Am Phys Ther Assoc 66(10):1548–1550, 1986.

15. Duncan, P, et al: Functional reach: A new clinical measure of balance. J Gerontol 45:192–197, 1990.

16. Uemura, T, et al: Neuro-Otological Examination. Baltimore: University Park Press, 1977.

17. Kamerer, DB, Furman, JM, and Whitney, SL: Vestibular System Evaluation and Rehabilitation. St. Louis: Mosby Year Book, 1991.

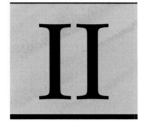

Tutorial Case Studies

C A S E
T1

History of the Dizzy Patient

HISTORY

A 65-year-old woman complained of positional dizziness that had begun 6 months before her evaluation. The patient's symptoms were a sense of spinning that was induced only when changing head position. Provocative changes included tipping her head obliquely back and to the right and rolling over in bed from left to right. Symptoms occurred daily and seemed to be exacerbated by fatigue.

There were no complaints of hearing loss, tinnitus, abnormal vision, or changes in strength or sensation. The patient had no clumsiness but noticed some mild disequilibrium when walking.

Question 1: What is meant by *dizziness?* What is meant by *vertigo?*

Answer 1: *Dizziness* means different things to different people. Thus, sensations described by a patient as dizziness should be further defined. Many patients use dizziness to mean that they feel lightheaded, have a swimming sensation in the head, or have a sense of giddiness. They may also mean that they have imbalance or, in fact, *vertigo*. *Vertigo* is an illusory sensation of motion of either self or surroundings. This illusory motion can be rotational (a sense of spinning), translational (a sense of rising), or static reorientation of the visual world (tilting of self or surroundings).

Question 2: Why is interviewing a patient who suffers from dizziness often difficult, and what steps can be taken to yield a more satisfactory history?

Answer 2: Patients are often unable to describe their dizziness. This difficulty is probably related to the comparatively meager and impure neural projection from the peripheral vestibular system to the cerebral cortex. As a result, patients do not have a vocabulary for vestibular sensations, as they do for auditory and visual stimuli. Moreover, the vestibular information at cerebral levels is mixed with somatic sensation, which further degrades the specificity of vestibular complaints. Nevertheless, an attempt should be made to understand what a patient means by dizziness. Ask the patient to describe the symptoms in his or her own words, but be ready to assist the patient in learning a new vocabulary to describe the symptoms by providing descriptors such as spinning, lightheadedness, giddiness, swimming, and gait instability. A little extra time spent in educating the patient about different subjective manifestations of dizziness can help develop a mutual understanding of what is meant by dizziness, which will improve physician-patient communication, help the physician focus on the patient's functional complaint, and save time and potential frustration later.

Question 3: What types of information should be elicited in the history of a dizzy patient?

Answer 3: The history should include an inquiry into (1) the *characteristics* of the patient's dizziness, (2) the *time course* and *aggravating factors* regarding the dizziness, (3) associated *otologic* symptoms, and (4) associated *neurologic* symptoms.

The first episode of dizziness is often vivid and the most typical for a particular disorder. Over time, either normal or maladaptive compensatory mechanisms can change the character of dizziness and obscure the diagnosis. Thus, it is often useful to begin the history focused on the first episode of dizziness. Once the character of the first episode is established, review the time course of the dizziness from its inception to the present. Is the dizziness episodic or constant? If the dizziness is episodic, note the duration, severity, and frequency of the episodes. If it is constant, determine whether the symptoms are getting progressively worse, slowly improving, or remaining static.

The discovery of factors that provoke or aggravate the patient's symptoms can provide important clues to the diagnosis. Vertigo may be provoked in some people by lying down, rolling over in bed (as in this patient), or pitching the head back to look up. In others, dizziness is associated with rising quickly from supine or seated positions. Particular environmental or social situations provoke vertigo in some individuals.

Because the hearing and vestibular apparatuses are closely linked anatomically and functionally, an inquiry into otologic symptoms is critical. Hearing loss, tinnitus, and aural fullness or pressure suggest involvement of the inner ear and may provide clues regarding laterality.

An inquiry into the presence of neurologic symptoms is important because of the common association of dizziness with central nervous system disorders such as cerebellopontine angle neoplasms, multiple sclerosis, migraine, and vertebrobasilar artery insufficiency. Visual symptoms can be caused by both peripheral and central vestibular abnormalities and by nonvestibular central nervous system abnormalities. Blurred vision is particularly nonspecific and can be caused by an abnormality anywhere in the vestibular, visual, or ocular motor pathways. However, blurred vision that occurs only during or immediately after head movement strongly suggests a vestibular abnormality with an impaired vestibulo-ocular reflex. Double vision strongly suggests an ocular motor abnormality but can also be seen with vestibular system abnormalities, especially during or just after a head movement. Loss of vision definitely points to a visual pathway abnormality or to an alteration in level of consciousness.

Figure T1–1 is a "dizziness questionnaire" that may be used to aid in eliciting the history. This questionnaire does *not* replace eliciting a history personally; rather, it focuses the patient's thinking and ensures that none of the essential elements of the history are omitted.

DIZZINESS QUESTIONNAIRE - CHARACTERISTICS OF DIZZINESS

IS YOUR DIZZINESS ASSOCIATED WITH ANY OF THE FOLLOWING SENSATIONS? PLEASE READ THE
ENTIRE LIST FIRST. THEN CIRCLE <u>YES</u> OR <u>NO</u> TO DESCRIBE YOUR FEELINGS MOST ACCURATELY.

Yes	No	1.	Lightheadedness or swimming sensation in the head.
Yes	No	2.	Blacking out or loss of consciousness.
Yes	No	3.	Tendency to fall.
Yes	No	4.	Objects spinning or turning around you.
Yes	No	5.	Sensation that you are turning or spinning inside, with outside objects remaining stationary.
Yes	No	6.	Loss of balance when walking in the light: Veering to the: Right? Left?
Yes	No	7.	Loss of balance when walking in the dark: Veering to the: Right? Left?
Yes	No	8.	Headache.
Yes	No	9.	Nausea.
Yes	No	10.	Vomiting.
Yes	No	11.	Pressure in the head.
Yes	No	12.	Tingling in the fingers or toes?
Yes	No	13.	Tingling around the mouth?

DIZZINESS QUESTIONNAIRE - TIME COURSE & AGGRAVATING FACTORS

		1.	When did your dizziness first occur? _____
		2.	How often do you become dizzy? _____
		3.	If in attacks, how long does an attack last? _____
Yes	No	4.	Do you have any warning that the attack is about to start?
Yes	No	5.	Do they occur at any particular time of day or night?
Yes	No	6.	Are you completely free of dizziness between attacks?
Yes	No	7.	Does change of position make you dizzy? Which movements?
Yes	No	8.	Do you become dizzy when rolling over in bed? _____
			To the right? To the left?
Yes	No	9.	Do you know of any possible cause for your dizziness? What? _____
	10.		Do you know of anything that will:
Yes	No		a. Stop your dizziness or make it better? _____
Yes	No		b. Make your dizziness worse? _____
Yes	No	11.	Do you become dizzy when you bend your head forward? _____ backward? _____
Yes	No	12.	Do you become dizzy when you cough? _____
			When you sneeze? _____
			When you have a bowel movement? _____
		13.	Can any of the following make your dizziness worse or precipitate an attack?
Yes	No		Fatigue?
Yes	No		Exertion?
Yes	No		Hunger?
Yes	No		Menstrual Period?
Yes	No		Stress?
Yes	No		Emotional Upset?
Yes	No		Alcohol?
Yes	No	14.	Do you have any allergies? What? _____

DIZZINESS QUESTIONNAIRE - ASSOCIATED OTOLOGIC SYMPTOMS

Do you have any of the following symptoms? Please circle <u>Yes</u> or <u>No</u> and circle the ear involved, if appropriate.

Yes	No	1.	Dizziness. Describe dizziness _____			
Yes	No	2.	Difficulty in hearing?	Both Ears	Right	Left
Yes	No	3.	Does your hearing change with dizziness?	Yes	No	
			If so, how? _____			
Yes	No	4.	Do you have noise in your ears? Both Ears		Right	Left
			Describe the noise:			
Yes	No	5.	Does noise change with dizziness?	Yes	No	
			If so, how? _____			
Yes	No	6.	Do you have fullness or stuffiness			
			in your ears?	Both Ears	Right	Left
Yes	No	7.	Do you have pain in your ears?	Both Ears	Right	Left
Yes	No	8.	Do you have discharge from your ears?	Both Ears	Right	Left

Figure T1–1
Dizziness
questionnaire.

Question 4: Which elements of the general medical history (past medical history, current and previous medication use, family history, and review of systems) are important in evaluating the patient with dizziness?

Answer 4: Each of the areas of the history, including the general medical history, is extremely important because all provide clues as to diagnosis and can be helpful in

DIZZINESS QUESTIONNAIRE - ASSOCIATED NEUROLOGIC SYMPTOMS

HAVE YOU EXPERIENCED ANY OF THE FOLLOWING SYMPTOMS? PLEASE CIRCLE <u>YES</u> OR <u>NO</u> AND CIRCLE IF <u>CONSTANT</u> OR <u>IN EPISODES</u>.

Yes	No	1.	Double vision.	Constant	In Episodes
Yes	No	2.	Blurred vision.	Constant	In Episodes
Yes	No	3.	Blindness.	Constant	In Episodes
Yes	No	4.	Numbness of the face or extremities.	Constant	In Episodes
Yes	No	5.	Weakness in the arms or legs.	Constant	In Episodes
Yes	No	6.	Clumsiness of the arms or legs.	Constant	In Episodes
Yes	No	7.	Confusion or loss of consciousness.	Constant	In Episodes
Yes	No	8.	Difficulty with speech.	Constant	In Episodes
Yes	No	9.	Difficulty with swallowing.	Constant	In Episodes
Yes	No	10.	Pain in the neck or shoulders.	Constant	In Episodes

DIZZINESS QUESTIONNAIRE - PAST MEDICAL HISTORY

Yes	No	15.	Do you have a history of earaches or ear infections as a child?
Yes	No	16.	Did you ever injure your head? When?
Yes	No	17.	Were you ever unconscious? When
Yes	No	18.	Did you suffer from motion sickness before age 12?
Yes	No	19.	Have you suffered from motion sickness in the last 10 years?
Yes	No	20.	Do you now take any medications regularly? What?
Yes	No	21.	Have you taken medications in the past for dizziness?
Yes	No	22.	Do you use tobacco in any form? What kind? How much?
Yes	No	23.	Does caffeine affect your dizziness? How?
Yes	No	24.	Does alcohol affect your dizziness? How?
Yes	No	25.	Do you have a past medical history of: Diabetes? Heart disease? High blood pressure? Kidney disease? Thyroid disease? Migraine headache?
Yes	No	26.	Do you have a family history of: Ear disease? Neurologic disease? Migraine headaches?

Figure T1–1
(Continued)

planning further management of the patient. For example, the review of systems may provide clues suggesting autoimmune inner ear disease, hormonal dysfunction (reactive hypoglycemia, diabetes mellitus, thyroid dysfunction), renal disease, neurologic disease (especially multiple sclerosis and migraine), or chronic infection (HIV, syphilis, Epstein-Barr). Patients should be asked specifically about exposure to potentially ototoxic medications (e.g., aminoglycoside antibiotics, certain chemotherapeutic agents, and loop diuretics).

PHYSICAL EXAMINATION

Because this patient had a history of positional dizziness and indicated that a spinning sensation accompanied tipping the head back and to the right, a Dix-Hallpike maneuver (see Case T2) was performed in addition to the general examination, a neurologic examination, and an otologic examination. The physical examination of the dizzy patient is discussed fully in Case T2.

General examination was normal. Neurologic examination included Romberg's test and an evaluation of eye movements, cranial nerves, motor system, coordination, sensation, and gait, all of which were entirely normal. Otoscopic examination was also normal. The Dix-Hallpike maneuver using Frenzel glasses (see Case T2) was positive with head-hanging right: paroxysmal positional nystagmus and vertigo were elicited with the right ear down. The nystagmus was upbeating (toward the forehead) and torsional with the upper poles (superior aspect) of the eyes beating toward the right ear. The nystagmus began approximately 5 seconds after positioning, was accompanied by a sense of spinning, and lasted for 15 to 20 seconds. The cessation of nystagmus was accompanied by an abatement of the spinning sensed by the patient. No signs or symptoms were elicited with the Dix-Hallpike maneuver with the left ear down.

Question 5: How does the physical examination help explain this patient's history?

Answer 5: The patient's symptoms were reproduced by the Dix-Hallpike maneuver. It is likely that the patient's presenting complaints of dizziness were associated with maneuvers that placed the posterior semicircular canal in a dependent position, much like the action of the Dix-Hallpike maneuver.

Laboratory Testing

Vestibular Laboratory Testing

ELECTRONYSTAGMOGRAPHY:	Not performed
ROTATIONAL TESTING:	Not performed
POSTUROGRAPHY:	Not performed

Audiometric Testing: Not performed

Imaging: Not performed

Other: None

DIAGNOSIS/DIFFERENTIAL DIAGNOSIS

Question 6: Based on the patient's history, where is the abnormality? Is the abnormality in the vestibular system or in some nonvestibular structure; if the problem is vestibular, is it otologic ("peripheral") or neurologic ("central")?

Answer 6: This patient's problem is almost certainly localized to the vestibular system. The patient's description of spinning is quite common for vestibular system abnormalities. Nonvestibular dizziness is more frequently described as a sensation of floating, swimming, dissociation, or lightheadedness. The episodic nature of the symptoms is also suggestive of a vestibular system abnormality; the dizziness associated with nonvestibular ailments is more often constant. Position change was a precipitating factor for this patient's dizziness. This, too, is highly suggestive of a vestibular system disorder. Despite the lack of associated otologic symptoms, because the patient had no associated neurologic symptoms, the localization of the patient's abnormality is more likely to be peripheral than central.

Question 7: Based on the history and physical examination, what is the differential diagnosis? What is the most likely diagnosis?

Answer 7: The most likely diagnosis is benign paroxysmal positional nystagmus and vertigo (BPPN or BPPV). Some physicians use the term benign *positional* vertigo (BPV) to describe this condition. This disorder is thought to be the result of either free-floating debris in the posterior semicircular canal (canalithiasis) or debris adhering to the cupula of the posterior semicircular canal (cupulolithiasis). Regardless of the exact mechanism, benign positional vertigo is characterized by a labyrinthine malfunction that causes the peripheral vestibular system to signal motion even when the patient's head is still.

Few other conditions reproduce the signs and symptoms of benign paroxysmal positional nystagmus and vertigo. Extremely rare cases of posterior fossa neoplasms have been reported to show a pattern of nystagmus and vertigo[1,2] identical to that of benign paroxysmal positional vertigo. However, patients with posterior fossa lesions have been unresponsive to the therapy to which benign positional vertigo responds (see Case C9).

The presence of any symptoms or signs that are atypical for benign paroxysmal positional vertigo should suggest the possibility of a posterior fossa structural abnormality. Examples of such findings are a lack of spinning sensation with position change; a lack of latency after changing position; a prolonged time course of individual paroxysms; and a lack of fatigability of symptoms and signs, that is, reduction or absence of vertigo and nystagmus if the patient is repeatedly positioned with the Dix-Hallpike maneuver.

This patient was given the diagnosis of *benign positional nystagmus and vertigo,* also known as *benign positional vertigo (BPV).*

TREATMENT AND MANAGEMENT

The patient was treated with a particle-repositioning maneuver (see Case C9) and had a complete recovery.

SUMMARY

A 65-year-old woman presented with positional dizziness. History and physical examination revealed paroxysmal positional vertigo and nystagmus without other otologic or neurologic signs or symptoms. Based upon the characteristic response to the Dix-Hallpike maneuver, the patient was diagnosed as having benign positional vertigo. The diagnosis was reached primarily on the basis of the patient's history, which aided in localizing the problem to the peripheral vestibular system and guided the confirmatory physical examination. Treatment consisted of a particle-repositioning maneuver that completely relieved the patient's symptoms.

TEACHING POINTS

1. **Vertigo differs from dizziness:** Whereas *dizziness* may mean lightheadedness, a swimming sensation, a sense of giddiness, or imbalance, *vertigo* is an illusory sensation of motion of either self or surroundings. This illusory motion can be rotational (a sense of spinning), translational (a sense of rising), or static reorientation of the visual world (tilting of self or surroundings).
2. **Eliciting a history from the dizzy patient** is difficult because such patients are often unable to describe their symptoms accurately, possibly because of the meager and impure representation in the cerebral cortex for vestibular sensations. Nevertheless, an attempt should be made to understand what a patient means by suggesting several different subjective manifestations and descriptors of dizziness.
3. **The history of the dizzy patient** should include questions pertaining to (1) the characteristics of the dizziness, (2) the time course and aggravating factors, (3) associated otologic symptoms, and (4) associated symptoms suggesting central

nervous system disease. A "dizziness questionnaire" is a useful aid in eliciting the history. This questionnaire does *not* replace eliciting a history personally; rather, it focuses the patient's thinking and ensures that none of the essential elements of the history are omitted.

4. **Details of the first episode of dizziness may provide unique information:** If the dizziness is episodic, note the duration, severity, and frequency of the episodes. If the dizziness is constant, determine whether the symptoms are getting progressively worse, slowly improving, or remaining static.

5. **Vestibular and nonvestibular diseases often differ in terms of history:** Vestibular system abnormalities are often manifested by episodic vertigo, for example, a sensation of spinning, or by imbalance; symptoms may be exacerbated by changes in head position. Nonvestibular dizziness is more frequently described as a sensation of floating, swimming, dissociation, or lightheadedness.

6. **Peripheral and central vestibular diseases often differ in terms of history:** Central vestibular ailments are typically associated with neurologic symptoms and signs. Peripheral vestibular abnormalities, more often than central vestibular abnormalities, are accompanied by nausea with or without vomiting and by other otologic abnormalities such as hearing loss and tinnitus.

7. **A history of positional vertigo** is an indication that Dix-Hallpike maneuvers should be performed, preferably using Frenzel glasses, to search for paroxysmal positional nystagmus, which is discussed extensively in several other cases.

REFERENCES

1. Watson, P, et al: Positional vertigo and nystagmus of central origin. J Can Sci Neurol 8(2):133, 1981.
2. Watson, CP, and Terbrugge, K: Positional nystagmus of the benign paroxysmal type with posterior fossa medulloblastoma. Arch Neurol 39:601, 1982.

CASE

T2

Physical Examination of the Dizzy Patient

HISTORY

A 25-year-old male respiratory therapist complained of the acute onset of dizziness and disequilibrium one day before evaluation. The patient's symptoms included blurred vision and poor balance when standing and walking. There were no complaints of vertigo, hearing loss, or tinnitus. The patient's symptoms were more or less constant and unaffected by head movement. There was no significant past medical history. The patient used no medications and had no family history of neurologic or otologic disease.

Question 1: Based on the history, where is this patient's abnormality localized and what are the diagnostic possibilities?

Answer 1: This patient's complaints of dizziness, disequilibrium, blurred vision, and poor balance suggest a vestibular disorder that cannot be easily localized. Each of the patient's symptoms could be caused by either a peripheral or a central vestibular lesion. The patient's blurred vision could be a manifestation of either a vestibular imbalance causing nystagmus or abnormal ocular motor function. The absence of vertigo makes a central vestibular rather than a peripheral vestibular lesion somewhat more likely, although many patients with peripheral vestibular disorders do not necessarily describe vertigo, an illusory sensation of motion of self or surroundings. The absence of hearing loss and tinnitus also argues against a peripheral otologic disorder.

Diagnostic considerations include an acute peripheral vestibulopathy, such as vestibular neuritis (see Cases T5 and C1); a posterior fossa inflammatory or viral infectious process; demyelinating disease, which is the first episode of multiple sclerosis; a vascular abnormality, such as brainstem hemorrhage; or a structural abnormality, such as a tumor.

44

Question 2: What are the elements of the physical examination of a patient with dizziness and disequilibrium? Which of the aspects of the physical examination are likely to be particularly helpful in reaching a diagnosis for this patient?

Answer 2: Physical examination of the dizzy patient should include a general medical examination, an otologic examination, a neurologic examination, and selected aspects of the neurotologic examination, that is, a subset of several special examination tools. Neurologic examination should include the usual subcomponents, including evaluation of the cranial nerves, motor system, sensation, coordination, Romberg's test, and an assessment of gait including tandem walking. The otologic examination should include otoscopy, preferably using an operating microscope, and pneumatic otoscopy to allow an assessment of tympanic membrane mobility and sensitivity of the patient to abrupt fluctuations of external auditory canal pressure. Hearing should be assessed at the bedside using a tuning fork (512 Hz). The two most commonly used tuning fork tests are Weber's test and the Rinne test.

Weber's test is performed by placing the vibrating tuning fork on the vertex of the head (forehead) and noting whether the sound is heard in the midline ("Weber midline") or in one ear or the other "Weber right" or "Weber left"). With unilateral disease, Weber's test usually lateralizes toward the ear with a *conductive* hearing loss because of auditory masking in the normal ear or away from the ear with a *sensorineural* hearing loss.

The Rinne test is performed by first placing the stem of the vibrating tuning fork on the subject's mastoid bone (the bony prominence behind the pinna), and then placing the tines of the vibrating tuning fork ½ inch away from the external auditory canal without touching the patient. If the sound is perceived as louder during air conduction, which is normal, the result is called "Rinne positive." If the sound is perceived as louder during bone conduction, the result is called "Rinne negative."

Weber's test and the Rinne test are generally used together to help indicate whether an asymmetry of hearing is present and whether the hearing loss is conductive or sensorineural. Used in conjunction, these tests provide valuable information about the relative hearing between the patient's two ears and whether a hearing loss is primarily sensorineural or conductive.

The neurotologic examination (described in more detail below), which provides information regarding the vestibulo-ocular and vestibulospinal systems, includes (1) a search for nystagmus while the patient wears Frenzel glasses; (2) bedside vestibulo-ocular reflex testing; (3) position*al* and position*ing* (Dix-Hallpike maneuvers) tests to look for persistent and paroxysmal positional nystagmus, respectively; (4) head-fixed, body-turned maneuvers; (5) postural sway while standing on a compliant (foam) surface; and (6) the stepping test.

Nystagmus that increases in intensity or is seen only with Frenzel glasses (Fig. T2-1) is suggestive of a vestibular system imbalance, because Frenzel glasses reduce visual fixation.

Bedside vestibulo-ocular reflex testing can be accomplished in several ways, including (1) head shaking while observing the fundus of one eye with an ophthalmoscope while the other eye is occluded[1]; (2) observing eye movements following abrupt head movements[2]; (3) searching for post–head-shaking nystagmus[3,4]; and (4) assessing acuity during head shaking.[5]

To best accomplish head shaking during ophthalmoscopy, the patient should be asked to make high-frequency head rotations of very small amplitude. Normally, the fundus appears fixed in space. If the fundus appears to move, either an

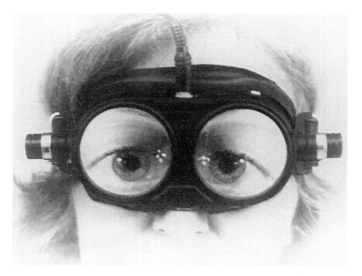

Figure T2–1
Patient's eyes illuminated by lights behind high plus lenses. Frenzel glasses significantly reduce visual fixation and at the same time magnify the patient's eyes so that the examiner may more easily observe vestibular nystagmus. (With permission from Baloh, RW: Dizziness, Hearing Loss, and Tinnitus: The Essentials of Neurotology. Philadelphia: FA Davis, 1984, p. 79.[13])

uncompensated vestibular loss or a bilateral vestibulopathy with decreased gain of the vestibulo-ocular reflex is suggested.[1]

The amount of eye movement required to refixate a visual target immediately on cessation of an abrupt 30-degree passive head movement is small and symmetric following head turning to the right versus turning to the left. Unilateral vestibular loss results in an asymmetry.[2]

Post–head-shaking nystagmus is observed using Frenzel glasses following about 5 to 10 seconds of brisk passive horizontal head movement.[3,4] With asymmetric central vestibular function (see Cases C11 and U9), patients will manifest a transitory nystagmus. Unfortunately, post–head-shaking nystagmus is not a specific test for vestibular abnormalities; that is, it has a relatively high false positive rate.[4]

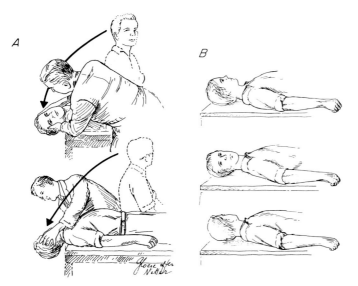

A

B

Figure T2–2
Techniques for performing positional testing. (*A*) The Dix-Hallpike maneuver for diagnosing benign positional vertigo. In the sitting position, the patient's head is turned 45 degrees to the right or left. Next, the patient is taken rapidly from the sitting to the supine position. The head is then gently moved to the final head-hanging position. (*B*) Head positions for observing static positional nystagmus. (With permission from Baloh, RW: Dizziness, Hearing Loss, and Tinnitus: The Essentials of Neurotology. Philadelphia: FA Davis, 1984, p. 81.[13])

The assessment of visual acuity during head shaking, also known as the "illegible E test,"[5,6] can uncover an abnormal vestibulo-ocular reflex. Loss of more than two lines of acuity usually indicates an abnormally low vestibulo-ocular reflex magnitude. Unfortunately, this type of testing is inexact because the head movement delivered to each patient differs. Nonetheless, this bedside maneuver can provide useful information.

Positional testing is performed by observing the patient's eyes through Frenzel glasses while the patient assumes the supine, head left, left lateral, head right, and right lateral positions (Fig. T2–2). The significance of persistent positional nystagmus is uncertain. However, a direction-*fixed* positional nystagmus (a nystagmus that beats in the same direction in all positions) is more likely to be related to a *peripheral* vestibular abnormality. A direction-*changing* positional nystagmus (a nystagmus whose direction changes when the patient changes from one ear down to the other ear down) can be caused by *either* peripheral *or* central vestibular lesions.

Paroxysmal positioning testing, the Dix-Hallpike maneuver (Fig. T2–2), is helpful in diagnosing *paroxysmal* positional nystagmus and vertigo, including both benign (paroxysmal) positional vertigo, which is discussed in Cases T1, C9, and C15, and nonbenign forms.

Head-fixed, body-turned maneuvers are performed to assess the cervico-ocular reflex by keeping the head fixed with eyes open in the dark, thereby eliminating visual and vestibular inputs. Nystagmus seen during head-fixed, body-turned maneuvers suggests an abnormal cervical ocular reflex and is called cervical nystagmus.

Romberg's testing of the patient with dizziness and disequilibrium should be modified to include the use of a compliant surface such as a wheelchair pad[7,8] (Fig. T2–3). Because movement at the ankle is greatly diminished while standing on foam, the somatosensory system provides an erroneous estimate of postural sway. Thus, if a patient stands on foam with the eyes closed, only the vestibular system remains to provide accurate information regarding orientation.

The stepping test is performed by asking patients to march in place with their eyes closed (Fig. T2–4).[9] This test should be performed using a standard number of steps such as 60 and a threshold of normality such as a rotational deviation greater than 45°. Forward movement is not pathologic.[10,11] Excessive rotation suggests a vestibulospinal imbalance.[11]

In this patient, a 25-year-old man with an acute onset of disequilibrium, each of the features of the examination described above is important. However, because of the patient's symptoms of imbalance, special emphasis should be given to an examination of eye movements and of his coordination and gait.

PHYSICAL EXAMINATION

The general and otologic examinations were normal. The neurologic examination was significant for a bilateral internuclear ophthalmoplegia, wherein the patient had difficulty with adduction bilaterally. That is, when the patient looked to the left, the right eye moved slowly and incompletely to the left, and when the patient looked to the right, the left eye moved slowly and incompletely to the right. Also, when he looked to the left, there was a dissociated nystagmus, so that the left eye had a left-beating nystagmus with no nystagmus visible in the right eye. Moreover, the patient had up-beating nystagmus on upgaze. Pursuit eye movements were performed poorly; the patient was noted to have multiple "catch-up" saccades (rapid eye movements) while

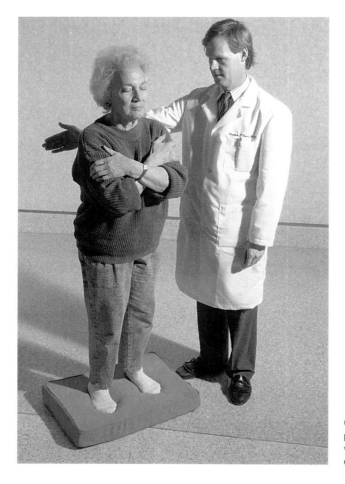

Figure T2–3
Clinical "foam" posturography. The
patient stands on a dense foam pad
with arms folded on the chest with
eyes open, then closed.

tracking a slowly moving object. Vergence, the ability to converge the eyes on a near
target, was normal. Coordination testing revealed mildly impaired finger-to-nose and
heel-knee-shin testing. The patient had normal strength and sensation. During Romberg's test, the patient could not stand without assistance even with his eyes open on
a stable floor. Evaluation of the patient's gait revealed a widened base. The patient
could not tandem walk. The stepping test revealed wide-based, ataxic stepping without
significant rotational deviation.

Question 3: Why is examination of the ocular motor system essential when
evaluating a patient with dizziness and disequilibrium? What are the component
features of the ocular motor examination?

Answer 3: Evaluation of the ocular motor system is essential because vestibular
system abnormalities, both peripheral and central, can alter eye movements in a
characteristic fashion. Moreover, central nervous system lesions that produce
imbalance may also affect various ocular motor subsystems independent of a
vestibular disorder and thus provide localizing information. The components of the
ocular motor examination include (1) an assessment of the *alignment* of the two
eyes, (2) *range* of eye movement, (3) the presence of any *instabilities* such as

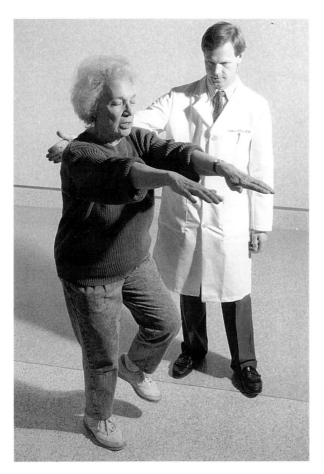

Figure T2–4
Unterberger (Fukuda) stepping test. The patient marches in place with eyes closed. Typically, the patient is asked to march 60 steps and the angle of deviation is observed. Up to 45 degrees of deviation are considered normal.

nystagmus or involuntary saccades, and (4) an assessment of each of the ocular motor *subsystems.* These subsystems include (1) saccades, (b) pursuit/optokinetic movements, (c) vergence, and (d) the vestibulo-ocular reflex. Although a complete discussion of each type of eye movement is beyond the scope of this book, elements of the ocular motor examination will be discussed in more detail as they arise in other case discussions. For an in-depth discussion of eye movement abnormalities, the reader is referred to Leigh and Zee's excellent work entitled *The Neurology of Eye Movements.*[12]

Question 4: Based on the additional information provided by the physical examination, does this patient have an otologic or a neurologic abnormality, and what is the localization of his problem?

Answer 4: The patient's bilateral internuclear ophthalmoplegia places his problem in the medial longitudinal fasciculus bilaterally. This fiber bundle travels from the pons to the midbrain and connects the abducens nucleus to the medial rectus subnucleus of the oculomotor nucleus (Fig. T2–5). A bilateral internuclear ophthalmoplegia accounts for both the bilateral adduction deficit and the upbeating nystagmus on up-gaze, which is a frequently observed sign of bilateral internuclear ophthalmoplegia,

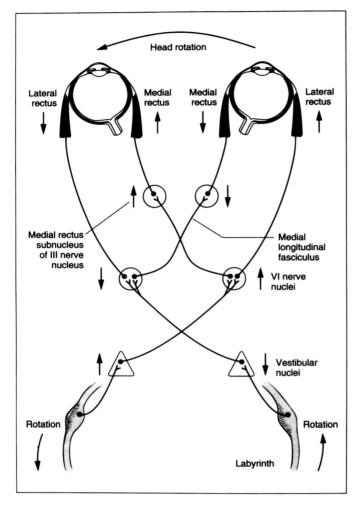

Figure T2–5
This diagram, which illustrates the pathways for the horizontal vestibulo-ocular reflex, includes the medial longitudinal fasciculus, which connects the sixth nerve nucleus to the medial rectus subnucleus of the third nerve nucleus. Note that the sixth nerve nucleus contains cell bodies for the lateral rectus motoneurons as well as cell bodies for the fibers that ascend in the medial longitudinal fasciculus to innervate the motoneurons for the medial rectus muscle. The medial longitudinal fasciculus coordinates the action of the two eyes so that horizontal eye movements are conjugate. Note that a lesion of the medial longitudinal fasciculus is associated with an abnormality of adduction that manifests itself as an internuclear ophthalmoplegia. (Adapted with permission from Furman, JM: Nystagmus and the vestibular system. In Podos, SM, and Yanoff, M (eds): Textbook of Ophthalmology. New York: Gower Medical Publishers, 1993.[14])

presumably as a result of poor vertical gaze-holding mechanisms.[12] Moreover, the patient's dissociated nystagmus on left gaze suggests that the right medial longitudinal fasciculus is more seriously affected than the left. The patient's blurred vision also is easily explained by his internuclear ophthalmoplegia. His incoordination and postural instability, however, suggest additional impairment of brainstem and/or cerebellar structures in addition to the medial longitudinal fasciculus lesion. Thus, the physical examination provides definitive evidence of a central nervous system lesion without any suggestion whatsoever of a peripheral vestibular or otologic abnormality.

Questions 5: Based on the physical examination, what is the differential diagnosis and the most likely diagnosis in this patient?

Answer 5: The most likely diagnosis is a demyelinating disorder, that is, multiple sclerosis. Less likely diagnoses include a brainstem/cerebellar abnormality caused by an inflammatory condition such as a viral infection, or a cerebrovascular abnormality such as a pontine or cerebellar hemorrhage. A mass lesion is extremely unlikely.

Question 6: What laboratory studies would be useful in establishing a diagnosis in this patient?

Answer 6: The most important study for establishing a diagnosis in this patient is a magnetic resonance imaging (MRI) scan of the brain with special attention to the posterior fossa. Blood studies should include an erythrocyte sedimentation rate, an FTA-ABS, Lyme titers, and HIV.

Laboratory Testing

Vestibular Laboratory Testing

ELECTRONYSTAGMOGRAPHY:	Not performed
ROTATION TESTING:	Not performed
POSTUROGRAPHY:	Not performed

Audiometric Testing: Not performed

Imaging: An MRI scan of the brain indicated multiple areas of bright signal intensity in the brainstem, cerebellum, and cerebral white matter, which was consistent with a demyelinating disorder.

Other: None

DIAGNOSIS/DIFFERENTIAL DIAGNOSIS

Based on the patient's history, physical examination, and MRI scan, the most likely diagnosis is a demyelinating disorder. Because this patient's dizziness and disequilibrium represent his first episode of neurologic dysfunction, the designation of *possible multiple sclerosis* is appropriate at this time. Less likely disorders include inflammatory and viral/postviral conditions.

TREATMENT/MANAGEMENT

The patient was treated with prednisone, 60 mg PO qd for 7 days. A follow-up evaluation was scheduled.

SUMMARY

A 25-year-old man presented with the acute onset of dizziness, disequilibrium, and blurred vision. The patient's examination revealed an internuclear ophthalmoplegia, suggesting the diagnosis of a demyelinating disease. An MRI scan supported this diagnosis. The patient was treated with a short course of steroids.

TEACHING POINTS

1. **The physical examination of the dizzy patient** should include a general medical, otologic, neurologic, and neurotologic assessment aimed at localizing the patient's abnormality to the peripheral or central vestibular system.

2. **Assessment of the ocular motor system** is a critical component of the examination of the patient with dizziness and disequilibrium. A thorough ocular motor system assessment may provide information regarding both the peripheral and central vestibular system and other central nervous system structures important for balance and spatial orientation.

3. **The neurotologic examination** consists of a group of several special bedside examination tools that provide information regarding the vestibulo-ocular and vestibulospinal systems. These include (1) a search for nystagmus while the patient wears Frenzel glasses, (2) bedside vestibulo-ocular reflex testing, (3) positional and positioning (Dix-Hallpike maneuvers) tests to look for persistent and paroxysmal positional nystagmus, respectively, (3) the stepping test, and (4) an assessment of postural sway while the patient is standing on a compliant foam surface.

4. **Bedside vestibulo-ocular reflex testing** can be accomplished in several ways including (1) head shaking while observing the fundus of one eye with an ophthalmoscope while the other eye is occluded, (2) observing eye movements following abrupt head movements, (3) searching for post–head-shaking nystagmus, and (4) assessing acuity during head shaking.

REFERENCES

1. Zee, D: Ophthalmoscopy in examination of patients with vestibular disorders. Ann Neurol 3(4):373–374, 1978.
2. Halmagyi, G, and Curthoys, I: A clinical sign of canal paresis. Arch Neurol 45:737–739, 1988.
3. Kamei, T, and Kornhuber, H: Spontaneous and head-shaking nystagmus in normals and in patients with central lesions. Can J Otolaryngol 3:372–380, 1974.
4. Hain, TC, Fetter, M, and Zee, DS: Head-shaking nystagmus in patients with unilateral peripheral vestibular lesions. Am J Otolaryngol 8:36–47, 1987.
5. Longridge, NS, and Mallinson, AI: A discussion of the dynamic illegible "E" test: A new method of screening for aminoglycoside vestibulotoxicity. Otolaryngol Head Neck Surg 92:671–677, 1984.
6. Longridge, NS, and Mallinson, AI: The dynamic illegible E-test. Acta Otolaryngol (Stockh) 103:273–279, 1987.
7. Shumway-Cook, A, and Horak, FB: Assessing the influence of sensory interaction of balance. Phys Ther 66:1548–1550, 1986.
8. Weber, PC, and Cass, SP: Clinical assessment of postural stability. Am J Otol 14(6):566–569, 1993.
9. Fukuda, T: The stepping test. Acta Otolaryngol 50:95–108, 1959.
10. Zilstorff-Pedersen, K, and Peitersen, E: Vestibulospinal reflexes. Arch Otolaryngol 77:237–245, 1963.
11. Peitersen, E: Vestibulospinal reflexes. Arch Otolaryngol 79:481–486, 1976.
12. Leigh, RJ, and Zee, D: The Neurology of Eye Movements, 2nd ed. Philadelphia: FA Davis, 1991.
13. Baloh, RW: Dizziness, Hearing Loss, and Tinnitus: The Essentials of Neurotology. Philadelphia: FA Davis, 1984.
14. Furman, JM: Nystagmus and the vestibular system. In Podos, SM, and Yanoff, M (eds): Textbook of Ophthalmology. New York: Gower Medical Publishers, 1993.

T3

Peripheral Vestibular Anatomy and Physiology

HISTORY

A 34-year-old woman who worked as a secretary complained of dizziness that had begun 18 months before evaluation. The patient's symptoms were severe vertigo and unilateral left-sided hearing loss, roaring tinnitus, and ear fullness on an episodic basis. She noted that symptoms could occur as often as several days each week with individual episodes lasting for several minutes or for as long as an hour. During the 18 months before evaluation, the patient was asymptomatic for several months. However, during the 2 weeks before evaluation, the patient's symptoms had been more frequent. She was unable to identify any activities that precipitated her dizziness attacks. Except for blurred vision and imbalance during her episodes, the patient had no weakness, numbness, or other neurologic complaints. She had no impairment of consciousness. Between episodes, the patient was asymptomatic except for a mild sensation of dizziness and disequilibrium that lasted for a few hours following the resolution of the vertigo associated with each acute episode. Between episodes, the patient also noted a slight decrease in hearing and a slight tinnitus on the left. She did not have positional sensitivity between episodes, but noted that rapid head movement of any sort during episodes exacerbated her symptoms. She had no family history of neurologic or otologic disease.

Question 1: Based on the patient's history, what is the most likely diagnosis?

Answer 1: This patient's history is consistent with a peripheral vestibular abnormality. There is little to suggest a neurologic disorder. Moreover, the patient's vertigo, which is associated with hearing loss, tinnitus, and ear fullness, suggests an otologic condition. The most likely diagnosis is endolymphatic hydrops.[1] Although other vestibular disorders may include one or more of the features of this patient's complaints, the simultaneous occurrence of episodic vertigo, unilateral hearing loss, tinnitus, and ear fullness, in the absence of neurologic complaints, renders any other diagnosis unlikely.

Question 2: Why is vertigo a manifestation of peripheral vestibular disease?

Answer 2: As discussed in the review of anatomy and physiology of the vestibular system (see Chap. 1), an imbalance in neural activity in the left and right eighth cranial nerves is interpreted by the central nervous system as head movement. For example, when the head is accelerated rotationally to the left, the left labyrinth is excited while the right is inhibited, thereby causing a difference in the left versus the right vestibular nerves. The central nervous system correctly interprets such a difference as movement of the head. Similarly, when a disease process, such as endolymphatic hydrops, causes an imbalance in the two vestibular nerves, the patient experiences an illusory sensation of motion, or vertigo. Depending on the particular nature of the vestibular imbalance caused by the attack, the patient may experience a sensation of rotating, translating, or being tilted with respect to gravity. Some patients experience a sensation of self-motion, others experience a sensation of motion of the world around them.

Question 3: What is the importance, if any, of the character of a patient's vertigo? That is, what is the significance of whether a patient feels as if *he* or *she* is moving or as if the *world* is moving about him or her? Does the direction of rotation provide lateralizing information?

Answer 3: Although a history of illusory motion of any type is highly suggestive of a vestibular system abnormality, particularly a peripheral vestibular system abnormality, the distinction between motion of self versus motion of surroundings is much less significant. A patient's perception regarding motion of self versus motion of surroundings is *not* a reliable indicator of peripheral versus central vestibular abnormalities. Moreover, the direction of motion perceived by a patient does *not* provide lateralizing information. Conversely, a complaint of an illustory persistent *tilt* of self or of the visual world does suggest a central rather than a peripheral vestibular abnormality.

PHYSICAL EXAMINATION

Physical examination revealed a normal general examination and a normal neurologic examination. Otologic examination revealed a normal appearance of the tympanic membrane and middle ear spaces. Tuning-fork examination revealed that Weber's test lateralized to the right and the Rinne test was positive bilaterally. This indicates a sensorineural hearing loss in the left ear.

Neurotologic examination revealed a low-amplitude nystagmus with Frenzel glasses that was not seen during visual fixation. The nystagmus was predominantly horizontal with the fast component beating to the right. There was a small torsional component with the upper poles of the eyes beating toward the right ear. The nystagmus was conjugate and increased when the patient was asked to gaze to the right and was absent upon leftward gaze even with Frenzel glasses. The patient has a negative Romberg's test and was able to stand on a compliant foam surface with her eyes open. However, while standing on a compliant foam surface with her eyes closed, the patient was unable to stand unaided. A stepping test revealed a slight ataxia with the eyes closed and rotation of the body 90 degress to the left.

Question 4: Why was this patient's nystagmus horizontal-torsional?

Answer 4: This patient was probably suffering from an incompletely resolved attack of endolymphatic hydrops (see Cases T9, C10, C14, C16) with an ablative lesion in the left ear. The patient's nystagmus, which was typical vestibular nystagmus because of its direction (horizonal-torsional) and its increase with loss of fixation, was a vestibulo-*ocular* manifestation of vestibular asymmetry. Presumably, the disorder affected each of the suborgans of the left vestibular labyrinth, including the three semicircular canals and the two otolith organs. The horizontal-torsional nystagmus was, therefore, a result of the unopposed combined action of all of the suborgans of the right vestibular labyrinth (see Chap. 1). The direction of the nystagmus can be explained as follows: the unopposed right *horizontal* semicircular canal activity drives the eyes horizontally to the left, and the combined activity of the two right *vertical* semicircular canals, that is, the right superior and right posterior semicircular canals, causes a torsional movement of the eyes with the upper poles moving toward the left. No vertical component is produced because the right superior semicircular canal tends to drive the eyes up, while the right posterior semicircular canal tends to drive the eyes down, thereby canceling the vertical influences.

Question 5: Why did the patient's nystagmus increase during gaze toward the right and decrease during gaze toward the left?

Answer 5: The alterations in the patient's nystagmus as a function of eye position in the orbit are typical of most types of nystagmus wherein the intensity of the nystagmus, including its frequency and amplitude, increases when a patient looks in the direction of the quick component. In this patient's case, as expected, right-beating nystagmus was increased when looking to the right and was absent when looking to the left. This phenomenon, whereby the magnitude of the nystagmus changes as a function of eye position, is known as *Alexander's law.* The physiologic basis for Alexander's law may relate to the elastic restoring forces of the eye.[2] For example, when a patient with a right-beating nystagmus looks to the right, both the elastic restoring forces of the eye and the vestibular imbalance cause leftward eye movement, thereby increasing the magnitude of the nystagmus. However, on left gaze, the vestibular imbalance and elastic restoring forces oppose one another, thereby decreasing the intensity of the nystagmus.

Laboratory Testing

*Vestibular Laboratory Testing**

ELECTRONYSTAGMOGRAPHY:	Ocular motor testing was normal with the exception of a right-beating spontaneous vestibular nystagmus in the dark. A left-reduced vestibular response was seen on caloric testing.
ROTATIONAL TESTING:	Rotational testing revealed a right directional preponderance.
POSTUROGRAPHY:	Posturography testing indicated excessive sway on conditions 5 and 6, that is, a vestibular pattern.

* Chapter 2 and Cases T7 and T8 discuss vestibular testing in detail.

Audiometric Testing:† Audiometric testing revealed a mild, low-tone sensorineural hearing loss in the left ear. Pure-tone thresholds in the right ear were normal, as was word recognition bilaterally.

Imaging: The patient had a normal MRI scan of the brain.

Other: None

Question 6: Why does this patient manifest both auditory and vestibular laboratory abnormalities?

Answer 6: Endolymphatic hydrops is thought to result from excess endolymph within the inner ear, caused by either excess production or inadequate reabsorption[3] (Fig. T3–1). The endolymphatic spaces of the cochlea and the vestibular labyrinth are continuous, thereby allowing the excess endolymph and/or elevated endolymphatic pressure to affect both the balance and the hearing organs.

Question 7: In addition to endolymphatic hydrops, what other disorders cause both auditory and vestibular symptoms?

Answer 7: Several other disorders, especially those that affect the eighth nerve such as acoustic tumors, viral-mediated inflammatory neuritis, or vascular insults to the inner ear, may also cause a combination of vestibular and auditory symptoms. Neoplasms located within the cerebellopontine angle, such as an acoustic tumor, characteristically cause hearing loss and tinnitus. Although an acoustic tumor rarely causes acute vertigo, patients often report mild to moderate unsteadiness and disequilibrium. The severity of these symptoms often depends partly on the size of the tumor and the age of the patient. The generally mild vestibular symptoms caused by acoustic tumors result from slow tumor growth that gradually reduces vestibular

---

† Audiometric testing is discussed in Chapter 3 and Case T9.

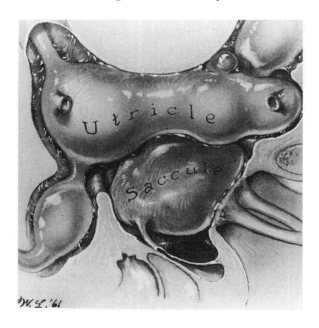

Figure T3–1
Dilated utricle and saccule in endolymphatic hydrops. (Reprinted by permission of the publisher from Schuknecht, HF: Pathology of the Ear. Cambridge, MA: Harvard University Press. Copyright 1974 by the President and Fellows of Harvard College.[4])

function in a way that enables gradual vestibular compensation to occur and thus limit vestibular symptoms.

DIAGNOSIS/DIFFERENTIAL DIAGNOSIS

This patient is suffering from *endolymphatic hydrops*. Her condition could also be termed *Meniere's disease* or *Meniere's syndrome*. The term *Meniere's disease* is most commonly used to describe the constellation of symptoms that characterizes endolymphatic hydrops when the cause of hydrops is idiopathic. A full description of terminology is provided in Case C10.

TREATMENT

Question 8: What are the treatment options for patients with endolymphatic hydrops?

Answer 8: Treatment modalities include dietary, pharmacologic, and surgical interventions. An extensive discussion of these treatment options for patients with endolymphatic hydrops can be found in Cases C10 and C14.

This patient was treated with dietary restriction of salt and a combination of hydrochlorothiazide and triamterene (Dyazide) once daily and had a marked reduction in symptoms.

SUMMARY

A 34-year-old woman complained of 18 months of episodic vertigo associated with hearing loss, tinnitus, and ear fullness. Examination revealed hearing loss in the left ear and a low-amplitude spontaneous right-beating vestibular nystagmus observed using Frenzel glasses. Laboratory evaluation suggested a peripheral otologic lesion on the left based on a reduced vestibular response to caloric irrigation and a low-tone sensorineural hearing loss. Rotational and posturography testing suggested an ongoing vestibulo-ocular and vestibulospinal asymmetry. The patient was diagnosed as having endolymphatic hydrops. She was placed on a low-salt diet and was treated with a combination of hydrochlorothiazide and triamterene.

TEACHING POINTS

1. **Endolymphatic hydrops** should be strongly considered when episodic vertigo, unilateral hearing loss, tinnitus, and ear fullness occur simultaneously and in the absence of neurologic complaints.
2. **Vertigo is a common manifestation of peripheral vestibular disease** because an imbalance in neural activity in the left and right eighth cranial nerves is interpreted by the central nervous system as head movement. Such an imbalance may occur when the head is accelerated rotationally and when a disease process, such as endolymphatic hydrops, causes an imbalance in the two vestibular nerves. De-

pending on the particular nature of the vestibular imbalance, the patient may experience a sensation of rotation, translation, or tilt with respect to gravity.

3. **Illusory motion** is highly suggestive of a vestibular system abnormality, particularly a peripheral vestibular system abnormality. The distinction between motion of self versus motion of surroundings is not a reliable indicator of peripheral versus central vestibular abnormalities. Moreover, the direction of motion perceived by a patient does not provide lateralizing information. However, an illusory tilt of self or of the visual world suggests a central rather than peripheral vestibular abnormality.

4. **Typical vestibular nystagmus** is horizontal-tortional and increases with loss of fixation. This horizontal-torsional direction is a result of the unopposed combined action of all of the suborgans of one of the two labyrinths: the unopposed horizontal semicircular canal activity drives the eyes horizontally, while the combined activity of the two vertical semicircular canals causes a torsional eye movement. No vertical component is produced because the superior semicircular canal tends to drive the eyes up, while the posterior semicircular canal tends to drive the eyes down, thereby canceling the vertical influences.

5. **Alexander's law,** wherein the intensity of nystagmus (including its frequency and amplitude) increases when a patient looks in the direction of the quick component, is typical of most types of nystagmus. The physiologic basis for Alexander's law may be related to the elastic restoring forces of the eye.

6. **The endolymphatic spaces** of the cochlea and the vestibular labyrinth are continuous, thereby allowing excess endolymph and/or elevated endolymphatic pressure to affect both the balance and the hearing organs at the same time.

7. **Disorders that affect the eighth cranial nerve,** such as acoustic tumors or viral-mediated inflammatory neuritis or vascular insults to the inner ear, may cause a combination of vestibular and auditory symptoms.

REFERENCES

1. Rauch, SD, Merchant, SN, and Thedinger, BA: Meniere's syndrome and endolymphatic hydrops: Double-blind temporal bone study. Ann Otol Rhinol Laryngol 98:873–882, 1989.
2. Robinson, DA, et al: Alexander's law: Its behavior and origin in the human vestibulo-ocular reflex. Ann Neurol 16:714–722, 1984.
3. Paparella, MM: The cause (multifactorial inheritance) and pathogenesis (endolymphatic malabsorption) of Meniere's disease and its symptoms (mechanical and chemical). Acta Otolaryngol (Stockh) 99:445–451, 1985.
4. Schuknecht, HF: Pathology of the Ear. Cambridge, MA: Harvard University Press, 1974.

Central Vestibular Anatomy and Physiology

HISTORY

A 55-year-old male high school teacher presented with an acute onset of severe disequilibrium 1 week before evaluation that was characterized by a sensation of being pushed to the ground from the left. The patient also complained of vertigo, nausea, blurred vision, and an inability to stand without assistance. His symptoms were constant. There was no associated hearing loss or tinnitus. His past medical history was significant for hypertension. The family history was significant for cerebrovascular disease.

Question 1: Based on the patient's history, what is the likely diagnosis?

Answer 1: The patient's history suggests a vestibular system abnormality. The presence of an illusionary sensation of movement, visual impairment, and postural instability are all suggestive of a vestibular system problem, but do not allow localization to either the central or peripheral vestibular system. The patient's complaint of being pushed to the ground, so-called lateropulsion, and persistent symptoms for 1 week suggest a central rather than periperhal vestibular abnormality. Moreover, the patient's history of hypertension suggests that he may have cerebrovascular disease. Thus, the patient's most likely diagnosis is an acute vascular insult of central vestibular structures. However, the differential diagnosis is very broad and includes both peripheral and central vestibular disorders.

PHYSICAL EXAMINATION

The patient had a normal general examination except for mildly elevated blood pressure. He was awake and alert. A right gaze preference was observed when the patient was distracted, but when he was encouraged to look straight ahead or to the left, he could do so. When asked to look side to side, the patient exhibited *saccadic lateropulsion,* a condition characterized by excessively large saccades in one direction (known as overshoot dysmetria or saccadic hypermetria) and excessively small saccades in the other direction (known as undershoot dysmetria or saccadic hypometria). In this patient's case, the saccadic overshoots were seen when looking from left to right, and the undershoots were seen when he looked from right to left. The patient had asymmetrically impaired ocular pursuit, although there was more difficulty pursuing targets moving to the left. He had a low-amplitude primary-position left-beating nystagmus that increased on left gaze. On right gaze, however, the nystagmus became right-beating and was coarse, that is, low frequency with a large position amplitude. It was clearly different from the nystagmus seen in the primary position, which was fine, that is, high frequency with a small position amplitude. The patient was noted to have diminished sensation to all modalities on the right side of the face. He had no asymmetry of facial movement. The gag reflex was diminished. Strength was normal. Dysmetria was seen in the right upper extremity on finger-to-nose testing. Sensation to pain and temperature was diminished on the left side of the body, including the left arm and left leg. The patient was unable to stand without assistance, and when walking, which he could do only with assistance, he had a wide-based gait. Otologic examination was normal.

Question 2: Based on the patient's physical examination, what physiologic mechanisms have been disrupted, and what is the most likely localization of this patient's lesion?

Answer 2: The patient's right gaze preference suggests that tonic drive to the medial and lateral rectus muscles is unequal. Such an imbalance could be the result of an acute lesion affecting mechanisms that drive the eyes to the left, for example, an abnormality in the right "frontal eye fields," or in the left pontine "gaze center," which includes the paramedian pontine reticular formation. This patient's history and physical examination suggest a brainstem abnormality because of the combination of a dissociated sensory loss, incoordination, abnormal eye movements, and subjective as well as objective lateropulsion. The patient's left-beating primary-position nystagmus, which increased on left lateral gaze, suggests a vestibular system abnormality characterized by diminution of the drive coming from the right vestibular system.[1] The patient's coarse nystagmus on right gaze is probably gaze-evoked nystagmus resulting from cerebellar system involvement (see Case C3 for a discussion of gaze-evoked nystagmus). Given the other features of this patient's condition, it is likely that central vestibular structures, including the vestibular nuclei in the right medulla, have been damaged.

Question 3: What are the central nervous system structures important for processing vestibular information? How can this patient's signs and symptoms be explained by damage to central vestibular pathways?

Answer 3: The central vestibular system is composed of the vestibular nuclei, vestibulo-ocular pathways, vestibulospinal pathways, vestibuloautonomic pathways, vestibulocortical pathways, the vestibulocerebellum, and other associated structures, such as the perihypoglossal nuclei. As noted in Chapter 1, the vestibular nuclei also receive information from several nonvestibular sensory modalities, especially vision and proprioception. The vestibular nuclei are thus sensory integration nuclei (Fig. T4–1).

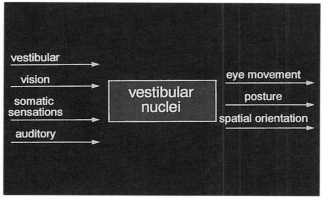

Figure T4–1

Schematic diagram of the vestibular nuclei. The vestibular nuclei comprise at least four anatomical subdivisions named the superior, medial, lateral, and inferior vestibular nuclei. The vestibular nuclei receive inputs from the vestibular labyrinth and, in addition, receive powerful input from other sensory modalities including vision, somatic sensation, and audition. As a result of these varied sensory inputs, naming these structures *vestibular* nuclei is somewhat misleading. These "vestibular" nuclei are, in fact, sensory integration nuclei whose outputs have profound influences on eye movements, truncal stability, and spatial orientation.

This patient's right gaze preference suggests that the tonic balance between the left and right vestibular nuclei has been disrupted so that the eyes are being driven slowly to the right. The left-beating nystagmus is a result of this tonic imbalance interrupted by rapid eye movements to the left. An acute vestibular imbalance with resulting vestibulospinal difficulties can also account for the patient's inability to stand or walk without assistance. The patient's complaints of nausea are probably related to a vestibuloautonomic imbalance. The complaint of being pushed to the ground may be related to erroneous signals to the cerebral cortex via vestibulocortical projections.

Laboratory Testing

Vestibular Laboratory Testing

ELECTRONYSTAGMOGRAPHY: Not performed

ROTATIONAL TESTING: Not performed

POSTUROGRAPHY: Not performed

Audiometric Testing: Not performed

Imaging: An MRI scan of the brain revealed increased signal intensity in the right lateral medulla with no other abnormality seen.

Other: None

DIAGNOSIS/DIFFERENTIAL DIAGNOSIS

Question 4: What is this patient's diagnosis? What other lesions present similarly?

Answer 4: It is likely that this patient suffered an ischemic infarction in the territory of the posterior-inferior cerebellar artery, that is, a lateral medullary infarction also known as Wallenberg's syndrome. Other conditions that can present similarly include the anterior-inferior cerebellar artery syndrome (see Case U4). Distinguishing between the lateral medullary syndrome and the syndrome of the anterior-inferior cerebellar artery can be difficult. However, the character of the patient's nystagmus, the lack of hearing loss, and the location of the abnormality as seen on focal MRI scan make lateral medullary syndrome the most likely diagnosis.[2] Although other lesions such as demyelination and neoplasia can rarely present with a syndrome similar to Wallenberg's syndrome, these diagnoses are most unlikely because of the acute onset of this patient's symptoms and signs.

The patient was diagnosed as having *Wallenberg's syndrome.*

TREATMENT/MANAGEMENT

This patient was treated with antihypertensive agents and aspirin, one tablet per day.

SUMMARY

A 55-year-old hypertensive man presented with the acute onset of vertigo, nausea, disequilibrium, and blurred vision. Examination revealed signs characteristic of the lateral medullary syndrome, including nystagmus, limb dysmetria, and contralateral impairment of pain and temperature. An MRI scan confirmed a lateral medullary infarction. Treatment consisted of blood pressure control and an antiplatelet agent.

TEACHING POINTS

1. **The central vestibular system** is composed of the vestibular nuclei, vestibulo-ocular pathways, vestibulospinal pathways, vestibuloautonomic pathways, vestibulocortical pathways, vestibulocerebellum, and other associated structures, such as the perihypoglossal nuclei.
2. **An illusory sensation of movement** suggests a vestibular system problem but does not allow localization to either the central or peripheral vestibular system.
3. **Lateropulsion,** a feeling of being pushed or pulled to the ground, suggests a central vestibular abnormality.
4. **An acute central vestibular imbalance** can cause: (1) nystagmus, because of an abnormal vestibulo-ocular reflex; (2) an inability to stand or walk without assistance because of vestibulospinal difficulties; (3) nausea, because of vestibuloautonomic imbalance; and (4) vertigo, for example, the sensation of being pushed to ground, because of erroneous signals in vestibulocortical projections.
5. **Wallenberg's syndrome** is characterized by the acute onset of a vestibular imbalance in the presence of unequivocal central nervous sytem symptoms or signs suggestive of lateral medullary infarction. Another condition that can present similarly is the anterior-inferior cerebellar artery syndrome, although certain clinical findings, such as hearing loss, allow a distinction to be made between the lateral medullary syndrome and the syndrome of the anterior-inferior cerebellar artery (see Case U4).

REFERENCES

1. Baloh, RW, Yee, RD, and Honrubia, V: Eye movements in patients with Wallenberg's syndrome. Ann NY Acad Sci 374:600–614, 1981.
2. Amarenco, P, et al: Anterior inferior cerebellar artery infarcts. Arch Neurol 50:154–161, 1993.

C A S E
T5

Acute Unilateral Vestibular Loss and Vestibular Compensation

HISTORY

A 25-year-old woman who worked as a registered nurse presented with the chief complaint of acute vertigo that began 3 days before evaluation. The patient's vertigo was associated with nausea and vomiting for several hours. Following this episode, the patient had disequilibrium, gait instability, and a severe complaint of poor vision for 2 days. She had no associated complaints of hearing loss or tinnitus and no fullness or stuffiness in the ears. There were no complaints of changes in strength or sensation. The patient had experienced a flulike illness that had begun approximately 2 weeks before the onset of the vertigo. At the time of evaluation, she noticed imbalance in the dark and spatial disorientation, especially after large head movements. She had no significant past medical history, and the family history was noncontributory.

Question 1: Based on the patient's history, what is the most likely diagnosis?

Answer 1: This patient's history is consistent with an acute vestibular syndrome characterized by vertigo, nausea, vomiting, blurred vision, and disequilibrium. The absence of auditory symptoms and the prior flulike illness suggest the possibility of vestibular neuritis. Other, less likely conditions include endolymphatic hydrops and a demyelinating disorder. The absence of other otologic symptoms argues against endolymphatic hydrops (see Cases T3, T9, C10, C14, C16). A demyelinating lesion would have to be located at the root entry zone of the eighth nerve to present in this way (see Case C26). Also, the absence of nonvestibular neurologic symptoms and the absence of previous neurologic deficits make a demyelinating lesion much less likely.

PHYSICAL EXAMINATION

The patient's general examination was normal. Neurologic examination revealed a left-beating horizontal-torsional nystagmus on leftward gaze with the upper poles of the eyes beating to the left. The remainder of the cranial nerve examination was normal. Strength, sensation, and coordination were normal. The patient had a negative Romberg's test. Gait was wide based, and the patient could not tandem walk. On the stepping test, the patient rotated almost 180 degrees to the right. She was unable to stand on a compliant foam surface with her eyes closed. With Frenzel glasses, the patient's nystagmus increased in intensity; it was now observed in the primary position, and both the frequency and amplitude of the nystagmus were higher. The otologic examination was normal.

Question 2: What is the pathophysiology of the patient's symptoms and signs?

Answer 2: The patient is suffering from an acute vestibular syndrome almost certainly caused by an acute profound imbalance between the afferent activity from the left and right labyrinths. Because a large difference in neural activity normally occurs only on intense acceleration of head movement, the central nervous system interprets an acute loss of vestibular activity on one side as the head rotating briskly toward the intact ear. Patients thus experience vertigo. Vegetative symptoms of nausea, vomiting, and diaphoresis result from activity in the pathways from the vestibular system to the autonomic nervous system. The purpose of these vestibuloautonomic connections and the reason for vestibular stimulation causing vegetative symptoms are not known.

Question 3: Why is the direction of the patient's nystagmus horizontal-torsional?

Answer 3: The patient's nystagmus is caused by the imbalance in afferent activity from the left and right labyrinth and is primarily the result of imbalanced semicircular canal activity rather than imbalance of otolith activity. Because of the orientation of the three semicircular canal pairs, the afferent activity from the intact side combines in such a way that the horizontal semicircular canal activity is unopposed, leading to the predominantly *horizontal* direction of the nystagmus; the torsional drive from the two vertical semicircular canals sum with one another so that the upper pole of the eye drifts toward the lesioned ear; the vertical eye movement drives of the two vertical semicircular canals cancel one another. Thus, the net effect of the three unopposed semicircular canals of the patient's left ear combines to produce a predominantly horizontal-torsional nystagmus whose slow component is toward the lesioned ear and whose quick component (for which the nystagmus direction is named) beats toward the intact ear.

Question 4: Why is the patient's nystagmus increased in magnitude when she is wearing Frenzel glasses?

Answer 4: Vestibular nystagmus, whether physiologic or pathologic, can be significantly inhibited by visual fixation when vision and visual fixation and visual tracking mechanisms are intact. Frenzel glasses allow the patient's eyes to be observed while they significantly reduce visual fixation. Thus, an increase in a patient's nystagmus on wearing Frenzel glasses supports the idea that the patient's nystagmus originates from a vestibular imbalance. In clinical parlance, a horizontal-torsional nystagmus that increases in magnitude with loss of visual fixation is called *vestibular nystagmus.*

Laboratory Testing

Vestibular Laboratory Testing

ELECTRONYSTAGMOGRAPHY:*	Ocular motor testing was normal. Testing confirmed the presence of a left-beating spontaneous vestibular nystagmus that increased with loss of visual fixation. Caloric testing revealed absent responses in the right ear, including absent responses to ice-water irrigation.
ROTATIONAL TESTING:	Not performed
POSTUROGRAPHY:	Not performed

Audiometric Testing: Normal

Imaging: Not performed

Other: None

---

* Chapter 2 and Cases T7 and T8 discuss vestibular testing in detail.

Question 5: How do results from laboratory testing influence the diagnostic considerations for this case?

Answer 5: The most significant finding on vestibular laboratory testing is the reduced vestibular response in the right ear on caloric testing. Although a unilateral caloric weakness was suspected from the clinical evaluation, laboratory testing provides objective evidence of a severe loss of sensitivity of the right labyrinth, confirming the clinical suspicion.

    The normal audiometric testing suggests that the patient is suffering from a pure vestibular syndrome such as vestibular neuritis as opposed to a more generalized "labyrinthitis" or from endolymphatic hydrops, which is often associated with a low-tone sensorineural hearing loss.

DIAGNOSIS/DIFFERENTIAL DIAGNOSIS

As noted, this patient is almost certainly suffering from *vestibular neuritis.*[1-3] Other names for this condition include labyrinthitis, vestibular neuronitis, and acute vesti-bulopathy of uncertain etiology. These terms are used interchangeably. It should be realized that a "peripheral" vestibular lesion could actually be affecting the hair cells, the eighth nerve afferents, or the eighth nerve root entry zone. From the vestibular signs and symptoms alone, a distinction cannot be made among these three localizations. Other entities that should be considered include labyrinthine infarction (see Case U4). It would be extremely rare for a mass lesion such as an acoustic neuroma to present soley with an acute vestibular syndrome without hearing loss, tinnitus, or other neu-rologic signs or symptoms.

TREATMENT/MANAGEMENT

A short (10- to 14-day) course of corticosteroids, for example, prednisone, 20 mg PO bid, decreases the duration of vestibular symptoms and may also reduce the chance of future recurrent episodes of acute vertigo.[4] Corticosteroids also have been shown experimentally to speed vestibular compensation.[5] This patient was treated with a 2-week course of corticosteroids. Vestibular suppressants and antinausea agents were also prescribed on an as-needed basis for symptomatic relief (see Case C18).

FOLLOW-UP

The patient was seen in follow-up 1 month after the initial presentation. At that time, she was very much improved and experienced symptoms only during rapid head movement, which caused transitory dizziness and lightheadedness, and during walking in dimly lit or dark environments. The patient also noted some difficulty with driving, especially immediately after rapid head movements just before changing lanes.

Physical examination at the 1-month follow-up visit revealed no nystagmus with visual fixation. However, with Frenzel glasses, a low-amplitude left-beating horizontal-torsional nystagmus was observed. The patient's gait had a normal base, but there was some difficulty during tandem walking. Her rotation on the stepping test improved, rotating only 45 degress right. The patient was able to stand on a compliant foam pad even with her eyes closed with minimal difficulty. She was referred for a course of vestibular rehabilitation (see Chap. 4).

Question 6: By what process did this patient's symptoms and signs almost completely resolve?

Answer 6: Despite the fact that the patient's vestibular loss in the right ear almost certainly persists, vestibular "compensation" (see Chap. 1), a process that invovles rebalancing of the activity in central vestibular structures, has occurred. Through this mechanism, the perceptual, vestibulo-ocular, vestibulospinal, and autonomic symptoms and signs largely resolve. Vestibular compensation occurs automatically in individuals with a normal central nervous system, normal vision and proprioception, and adequate physical activity. This patient's recovery is typical even for individuals who have suffered complete unilateral peripheral vestibular loss. The process of vestibular compensation is thought to involve brainstem and cerebellar structures, so that resting activity in the left and right vestibular nuclei becomes more or less balanced despite unilaterally reduced or absent vestibular nerve activity.

SUMMARY

A 25-year-old woman presented with the acute onset of a vestibular syndrome indicative of an acute unilateral peripheral vestibular loss. The patient's history suggested a viral/postviral affliction of the vestibular labyrinth or nerve. Examination revealed typical spontaneous vestibular nystagmus, an inability to stand on a foam surface with the eyes closed, and poor tandem walking. Laboratory testing revealed a right reduced vestibular response. The patient was treated with a 2-week course of corticosteroids. Vestibular suppressant agents and antinausea agents were used only on an as-needed basis. Through the process of vestibular compensation, the patient's symptoms decreased dramatically. At a 1-month follow-up evaluation, nystagmus was present only while the patient was wearing Frenzel glasses, and she could stand on a compliant surface and tandem walk.

TEACHING POINTS

1. **An acute vestibular syndrome** is characterized by vertigo, nausea, vomiting, blurred vision, and disequilibrium.
2. **An acute loss of vestibular activity on one side** provokes symptoms that result from an imbalance between the afferent activity from the left and right labyrinths. The central nervous system interprets this imbalance as a brisk head rotation toward the intact ear. Patients thus experience vertigo.
3. **Vegetative symptoms of nausea, vomiting, and diaphoresis** are caused by activity in the pathways from the vestibular system to the autonomic nervous system. The purpose of these vestibuloautonomic connections and the reason why vestibular stimulation causes vegetative symptoms are not known.
4. **The direction of acute vestibular nystagmus** results primarily from the unopposed horizontal semicircular canal afferent activity from the intact side that produces a *horizontal* direction of nystagmus. The torsional drives from the two intact vertical semicircular canals sum with one another such that the upper pole of the eye drifts toward the lesioned ear. The vertical eye movement drives of the two vertical semicircular canals cancel one another. The net effect of the three unopposed semicircular canals of the intact ear thus combines to produce a predominantly horizontal-torsional nystagmus whose slow component is toward the lesioned ear and whose quick component (for which the nystagmus direction is named) beats toward the intact ear.
5. **Visual fixation can inhibit vestibular nystagmus** when vision and visual-fixation/visual tracking mechanisms are intact. Frenzel glasses allow the patient's eyes to be observed while they significantly reduce visual fixation. Thus, an increase in a patient's nystagmus on wearing Frenzel glasses supports the idea that the patient's nystagmus originates from a vestibular imbalance. In clinical parlance, a horizontal-torsional nystagmus that increases in magnitude with loss of visual fixation is called *vestibular nystagmus.*
6. **Vestibular compensation** rebalances the neural activity in central vestibular structures. This process causes a reduction of the symptoms and signs of an acute vestibular syndrome. Through compensation, the perceptual, vestibulo-ocular, vestibulospinal, and autonomic symptoms and signs of the acute vestibular syndrome largely resolve. Vestibular compensation occurs automatically in individuals with a normal central nervous system, normal vision and proprioception, and adequate physical activity. The process of vestibular compensation is thought to involve brainstem and cerebellar structures, so that resting activity in the left and right vestibular nuclei becomes more or less balanced despite unilaterally reduced or absent vestibular nerve activity.
7. **Vestibular neuritis** is an acute vestibular syndrome that occurs without auditory or neurologic signs or symptoms. Other conditions that can cause an acute vestibular syndrome include endolymphatic hydrops, a demyelinating disorder, and infarction involving the labyrinth or brainstem/cerebellum.
8. **Treatment of vestibular neuritis** with a short (10- to 14-day) course of corticosteroids may decrease the duration of vestibular symptoms and may improve long-term recovery.

REFERENCES

1. Dix, MR, and Hallpike, CS: The pathology, symptomology and diagnosis of certain common disorders of the vestibular system. Proc R Soc Med 45:341–354, 1952.
2. Coats, AC: Vestibular neuronitis. Acta Laryngol (suppl) 251:5–28, 1969.
3. Schuknecht, HF, and Kitamura, K: Vestibular neuritis. Ann Otol Rhinol Laryngol (suppl) 78(90):1–19, 1981.
4. Ariyasu, L, et al: The beneficial effect of methylprednisolone in acute vestibular vertigo. Arch Otolaryngol Head Neck Surg 116:700–703, 1990.
5. Flohr, H, and Luneburg, U: Effects of ACTH on vestibular compensation. Brain Res 248:169–173, 1982.

Mixed Peripheral and Central Vestibular Impairment

HISTORY

A 65-year-old woman had a chief complaint of dizziness that had been worsening during the past 6 months. The patient's major symptom was disequilibrium without vertigo, which was present daily, occurred with head movement, and was particularly bothersome when walking. She noted veering of her gait both to the right and to the left. There also was a complaint of tinnitus in the left ear that was worsening gradually. She had no significant past medical history, and the family history was noncontributory.

Question 1: Based on the patient's history, what diagnoses should be considered?

Answer 1: The patient's history is consistent with both vestibular and auditory abnormalities. Moreover, her disequilibrium without vertigo and the gradually worsening course suggest the possibility of a central vestibular abnormality. Diagnostic considerations that can account for both the patient's tinnitus and the imbalance include a cerebellopontine angle mass or, less likely, a peripheral otologic condition of uncertain etiology. The differential diagnosis for the patient's balance symptoms independent of tinnitus is quite broad.

PHYSICAL EXAMINATION

General examination was normal. Neurologic examination indicated Brun's nystagmus, which is a coarse, gaze-evoked nystagmus during leftward horizontal gaze and a fine vestibular (horizontal-torsional) nystagmus on rightward gaze. With Frenzel glasses, the patient was noted to have a primary-position, right-beating, horizontal-torsional nystagmus of small amplitude. There was no alteration of strength or sensation, or incoordination of the limbs. The patient had an ataxic gait. Romberg's test was negative.

Bedside evaluation of the patient's hearing indicated that Weber's test lateralized to the right and the Rinne test was positive bilaterally, indicating a sensorineural hearing loss on the left.

Question 2: What is the mechanism of this patient's nystagmus?

Answer 2: Brun's nystagmus is a combination of a gaze-evoked nystagmus in one direction and a vestibular nystagmus that beats in the opposite direction. The gaze-evoked nystagmus is based on a cerebellar lesion ipsilateral to the direction of the gaze-evoked nystagmus. The vestibular nystagmus is based on a vestibular lesion contralateral to the direction of the vestibular nystagmus. In this patient's case, the gaze-evoked nystagmus is left-beating on left gaze and suggests a left-sided cerebellar lesion. The vestibular nystagmus is right-beating on right gaze and suggests a *left-sided* vestibular lesion. Thus, this patient is likely to have a left-sided cerebellar lesion *and* a left-sided vestibular lesion.[1,2] Right-beating vestibular nystagmus observed in the primary position with Frenzel glasses can often be seen only on right lateral gaze when the patient is examined in the light (see Case T3 for a discussion of Alexander's law).

Question 3: Based on the patient's history and physical examination, what is the most likely abnormality and what diagnostic test(s) should be performed?

Answer 3: This patient is likely to have a left cerebellopontine angle neoplasm. Diagnostic considerations include a large acoustic neuroma, or meningioma, of the posterior fossa; an aneurysm acting as a mass lesion; one of a number of uncommon posterior fossa neoplasms, such as an epidermoid tumor, chordoma, or lipoma; or, rarely, a metastatic tumor. The patient should undergo magnetic resonance imaging (MRI) of the brain with special attention to the cerebellopontine angle. Auditory and vestibular testing would also be helpful to delineate the patient's functional abnormalities.

Laboratory Testing

Vestibular Laboratory Testing*

ELECTRONYSTAGMOGRAPHY:	Ocular motor testing revealed overshoot saccades to the left, an asymmetric impairment of ocular pursuit with difficulty pursuing targets moving to the left, and normal optokinetic nystagmus. A right-beating spontaneous vestibular nystagmus was seen in the dark. Caloric testing revealed a reduced vestibular response of moderate degree on the left.
ROTATIONAL TESTING:	Rotational testing revealed asymmetric responses with more right-beating nystagmus than left-beating nystagmus.
POSTUROGRAPHY:	Posturography testing indicated excessive sway on conditions 5 and 6, that is, a vestibular pattern.

Audiometric Testing:† Testing revealed a moderate to severe sensorineural hearing loss on the left with a word recognition score of 30 percent. Hearing was normal on the right.

Imaging: An MRI scan of the brain revealed a 4-cm mass in the left cerebellopontine angle that

---

* Chapter 2 and Cases T7 and T8 discuss vestibular testing in detail.
† Audiometric testing is discussed in Chapter 3 and Case T9.

filled the porus of the left internal auditory canal. There was a shift of the cerebellum and brainstem by mass effect of the tumor (Fig. T6–1).

Other: None

Question 4: What additional information was provided by the laboratory testing?

Answer 4: The MRI scan confirms the clinical suspicion of a cerebellopontine angle tumor. The MRI scan is most suggestive of an acoustic neuroma. Audiometric testing suggests that the patient has little functional hearing remaining in the left ear. Vestibular laboratory testing confirms the presence of both peripheral vestibular and central nervous system abnormalities. The patient's caloric reduction suggests impairment of afferent vestibular activity. The abnormal saccades and pursuit suggest impairment of cerebellar/brainstem function. The patient's spontaneous nystagmus and directional preponderance on rotational testing indicate an ongoing vestibulo-ocular asymmetry. Posturography suggests that some of the patient's imbalance is a result of vestibular influences.

DIAGNOSIS/DIFFERENTIAL DIAGNOSIS

This patient's history, physical examination, and laboratory studies indicate a *cerebellopontine angle lesion* with a mixed central and peripheral vestibular disorder.

Question 5: In what way do combined peripheral and central vestibular abnormalities interact to cause a synergistic adverse effect on a patient's balance?

Answer 5: As noted in Case T5, with a normal central nervous system, patients can compensate for a peripheral vestibular lesion and become nearly symptom free. Vestibular compensation requires changes in brainstem and cerebellar structures including the vestibulocerebellum. This patient's cerebellopontine angle lesion has caused a left-right vestibular asymmetry and, in addition, as evidence by the patient's neurologic signs, has impaired the function of some of the central nervous system

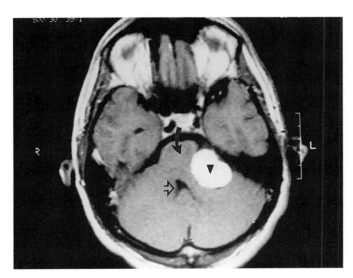

Figure T6–1
Axial magnetic resonance imaging of the brain demonstrating a 4-cm cerebellopontine angle neoplasm consistent with an acoustic neuroma. Note compression and shift of the brainstem and distortion of the fourth ventricle. Arrowhead = neoplasm; curved arrow = brainstem; open arrow = fourth ventricle.

structures important for vestibular compensation. Thus, despite a gradual vestibular loss rather than an acute vestibular loss and a partial rather than a complete vestibular loss, this patient has symptoms of dizziness and imbalance suggesting that compensation has not occurred.

Question 6: What are the causes of combined peripheral and central vestibular dysfunction?

Answer 6: The causes of combined peripheral and central vestibular lesions include large cerebellopontine angle lesions, as in this case; anterior inferior cerebellar artery territory infarction (see Case U4); trauma (see Cases T7, C8, and C22); and multisystem degenerations (see Case C11), for example, Friedreich's ataxia. Also, some patients with peripheral vestibular lesions have pre-existing central nervous system abnormalities that prevent normal compensation from occurring (see Case C16).

TREATMENT/MANAGEMENT

The patient was treated surgically using a translabyrinthine approach. The diagnosis of an acoustic neuroma was confirmed on pathologic analysis. Complete tumor resection was accomplished with preservation of all cranial nerves except the eighth nerve, which was resected with the tumor. Postoperatively, the patient had no complications and was referred for vestibular rehabilitation therapy (see Chap. 4).

FOLLOW-UP

The patient recovered uneventfully from the surgery. Three months after surgery, she reported tiring easily and continued mild to moderate unsteadiness and disequilibrium. She was reassured and encouraged to keep up with her home vestibular rehabilitation program.

SUMMARY

A 65-year-old woman presented with a gradual onset of imbalance and unilateral hearing loss over 6 months. Physical examination suggested a mixed central and peripheral vestibular lesion. MRI scanning confirmed the presence of a cerebellopontine angle tumor. Vestibular studies documented peripheral and central vestibular abnormalities, and abnormalities of ocular motor control. The patient thus demonstrated poor compensation for her peripheral vestibular abnormality. Treatment consisted of surgical resection of the tumor. Follow-up evaluation showed mild to moderate residual unsteadiness, but the patient reported no significant disability caused by her balance dysfunction.

TEACHING POINTS

1. **A cerebellopontine angle lesion** should be suspected in the setting of unilateral or asymmetric hearing loss or tinnitus. Diagnostic considerations should include a large acoustic neuroma or meningioma involving the posterior fossa. Several un-

common tumors may also affect the posterior fossa, including epidermoid tumor, chordoma, lipoma, or (rarely) metastatic tumor. A vertebrobasilar aneurysm acting as a mass lesion may also present with similar symptoms. The patient should undergo MRI of the brain with special attention to the cerebellopontine angle.

2. **Large cerebellopontine angle tumors** may produce a combination of peripheral and central vestibular abnormalities. Both vestibular nerve and cerebellar function may be impaired. These impairments may be manifested by abnormal ocular motor testing, spontaneous nystagmus, a reduced vestibular response on caloric testing, a directional preponderance on rotational testing, and abnormal posturography.

3. **Combined peripheral and central vestibular abnormalities** interact to cause a synergistic adverse effect on a patient's balance. With a normal central nervous system, patients can compensate for a peripheral vestibular lesion and become nearly symptom free. However, if central nervous system abnormalities involve the structures that are critical for vestibular compensation, a peripheral vestibular lesion may produce persistent symptoms resulting from impaired compensation. Combined peripheral and central vestibular dysfunction may be caused by large cerebellopontine angle lesions, anterior inferior cerebellar artery territory infarction, trauma, and multisystem degenerations. Also, some patients with peripheral vestibular lesions have pre-existing central nervous system abnormalities that prevent normal compensation from occurring.

4. **Brun's nystagmus** represents a manifestation of a combined peripheral and central vestibular abnormality. It is a combination of a gaze-evoked nystagmus in one direction, presumably based on an ipsilateral cerebellar lesion, and a vestibular nystagmus in the opposite direction.

REFERENCES

1. Lundborg, T: Diagnostic problems concerning acoustic tumors. Acta Otolaryngol (suppl) 99:1–111, 1950.
2. Nedzelski, JM: Cerebellopontine angle tumors: Bilateral flocculus compression as cause of associated oculomotor abnormalities. Laryngoscope 93:1251–1260, 1983.

C A S E
T7

Electronystagmography

HISTORY

A 35-year-old woman who worked as a real estate agent presented with a chief complaint of dizziness that had begun 6 months before evaluation. The patient said that her symptoms had started after a motor vehicle accident in which the car she was driving was struck on the passenger's side by another vehicle, causing her head to strike the inside of the driver's door. She had not lost consciousness, but had experienced disequilibrium at the time of the accident. For the past 6 months, she had experienced chronic headache and a constant sense of lightheadedness and disequilibrium during rapid head movements. The patient did not complain of positional dizziness, even when turning in bed. She had no complaints of hearing loss, tinnitus, or fullness or stuffiness in the ears. She had some instability of gait, veering more toward the left than toward the right, which was more noticeable when walking in dimly lit environments. The patient also experienced a feeling of unsteadiness while in the shower. Other than her dizziness, she had no significant past medical history. The family history was noncontributory.

A CT scan of the brain performed shortly after the motor vehicle accident was normal.

Question 1: Based on the history, what is the most likely diagnosis?

Answer 1: This patient's history suggests a labyrinthine concussion (see Cases T7, C8, and C22). The abnormalities appear to be limited to the vestibular system because there are no complaints of hearing loss or tinnitus. Other than a complaint of recurrent headaches, the patient's history contains nothing to suggest a central nervous system abnormality.

PHYSICAL EXAMINATION

The patient's physical examination was entirely normal including general, neurologic, otologic, and neurotologic examinations, with the exception of poor tandem walking, unsteadiness during Romberg's test, and inability to stand on a compliant foam pad with her eyes closed.

Question 2: What information from laboratory studies would help define and objectify this patient's abnormalities? What laboratory studies should be ordered?

Answer 2: Vestibular laboratory testing, especially electronystagmography, which includes caloric testing, can provide information beyond that available from the history and physical examination. Specifically, caloric testing provides an objective measure of the sensitivity of each labyrinth. Additionally, electronystagmography (ENG) may provide information regarding an ongoing vestibulo-ocular asymmetry, that is, a directional preponderance. The ocular motor battery of the ENG is useful for assessing possible brainstem or cerebellar dysfunction[1] (see Chap. 2).

Rotational testing provides information regarding the status of vestibular compensation for peripheral vestibular injury.[2] Also, abnormalities in the timing of vestibulo-ocular responses provide definitive evidence of a vestibular system abnormality (see Chap. 2).

Posturography testing provides information regarding vestibular compensation in terms of upright postural stability[3] (see Chap. 2). Thus, this patient should undergo electronystagmography to document a vestibular system abnormality. Additionally, rotational and posturography testing, if available, would provide additional useful information regarding the presence of ongoing vestibular imbalance.

An audiometric evaluation would also be useful. Despite the fact that the patient has no complaint of hearing loss, an audiometric evaluation is important to document the extent, if any, of traumatic chochlear injury and to provide a baseline should the patient subsequently develop a delayed post-traumatic otologic disorder, such as delayed endolymphatic hydrops.

Question 3: What abnormalities would you expect to find on ENG if the initial impression of labyrinthine concussion was correct?

Answer 3: Based on the patient's history of head trauma followed by dizziness, it is suspected that she has a peripheral vestibular injury and will have a reduced vestibular response on electronystagmography testing. Although the history suggests that the patient struck the left side of her head, it is difficult to predict on which side the vestibular reduction might be. The physical examination does not provide any further clue in this regard. Additionally, the patient's lightheadedness and disequilibrium during head movements and instability of gait suggest that she will have a directional preponderance on rotational testing and a vestibular pattern on posturography testing. Abnormalities on the ocular motor battery could raise the possibility of post-traumatic brainstem or cerebellar dysfunction.

Laboratory Testing

Vestibular Laboratory Testing*

ELECTRONYSTAGMOGRAPHY: Ocular motor testing was normal. Positional testing revealed a nystagmus that was right-beating in all positions including the

---

* Chapter 2 and Case T8 discuss vestibular testing in detail.

	supine, head-right, head-left, right-lateral, and left-lateral positions. This type of positional nystagmus is called "direction fixed" because it is in the same direction in all positions. Caloric testing indicated a 50 percent reduced vestibular response on the left.
ROTATIONAL TESTING:	Rotational testing revealed responses of normal magnitude and timing. However, there was a significant right directional preponderance.
POSTUROGRAPHY:	Posturography testing indicated excessive sway on conditions 5 and 6, that is, a vestibular pattern.

Audiometric Testing:† Audiometric testing indicated a mild high-frequency sensorineural hearing loss on the left and normal hearing on the right. Word recognition was excellent bilaterally.

Imaging: Not performed

Other: Not performed

Question 4: How does the additional information provided by laboratory studies influence the diagnostic considerations in this case?

Answer 4: Laboratory studies confirm a peripheral vestibular lesion with incomplete compensation. Although baseline information regarding the patient's otologic status before the motor vehicle accident is not available, her history, coupled with laboratory testing, significantly increases the likelihood of labyrinthine concussion. Moreover, the patient has evidence of trauma to both the vestibular and auditory portions of the inner ear.

DIAGNOSIS/DIFFERENTIAL DIAGNOSIS

Question 5: Based on the history, physical examination, and laboratory testing, what is this patient's diagnosis and what is the status of her vestibular system function?

Answer 5: The patient has suffered a labyrinthine concussion on the left. The persistent complaints of dizziness and disequilibrium, especially with rapid head movement and abnormal rotational and posturography testing, suggest incomplete vestibular compensation. Some patients experience symptoms even when compensation is complete, suggesting a persistent impairment during challenging activities such as high-velocity head movements and walking in low-light environments.

The patient was diagnosed as having a *labyrinthine concussion* on the left with incomplete compensation by the central nervous system.

TREATMENT/MANAGEMENT

The patient was treated with a mild vestibular suppressant, diazepam, 2 mg PO bid on an as-needed basis, and a course of vestibular rehabilitation therapy (see Case C18 for

† (Audiometric testing is discussed in Chap. 3 and Case T9.)

a discussion of symptomatic treatment of vestibulopathy and Chapter 4 for a discussion of vestibular rehabilitation therapy).

Question 6: What are the indications for ordering ENG testing?

Answer 6: ENG testing is appropriate for the assessment of patients suspected of having disorders that affect the vestibular system. Because ENG allows measurement of eye movements during caloric stimulation of each ear, with and without visual fixation, caloric testing provides the most useful information available regarding peripheral vestibular function and allows the possibility of identifying the involved ear. Another component of ENG, positional testing, is also valuable because of its ability to objectively record nystagmus both with and without visual fixation while a patient's orientation with respect to gravity is changed.[4]

FOLLOW-UP

During the 3 months after evaluation, the patient's symptoms improved dramatically. She was discharged from balance rehabilitation, and she used diazepam infrequently.

SUMMARY

A 35-year-old woman complained of dizziness and disequilibrium following a motor vehicle accident in which she struck the side of her head without loss of consciousness. Physical examination was normal. Vestibular laboratory testing revealed a moderate vestibular reduction on the left. Rotational testing and posturography were abnormal. Audiometric testing revealed a high-frequency sensorineural hearing loss on the left. The patient was diagnosed as having a labyrinthine concussion. Treatment consisted of a brief course (several weeks) of low-dose diazepam on an as-needed basis and a course of vestibular rehabilitation therapy.

TEACHING POINTS

1. **Electronystagmography,** which includes caloric testing, positional testing, and an ocular motor function test battery, can provide information beyond that available from the history and physical examination. Thus, ENG testing is often appropriate for the assessment of patients suspected of having disorders that affect the vestibular system.
2. **Caloric testing** provides an objective measure of the sensitivity of each labyrinth and thus allows the possibility of identifying the involved ear. Caloric testing may also provide information regarding an ongoing vestibulo-ocular asymmetry, that is, a directional preponderance. Other vestibular tests such as rotational testing or posturography are nonlateralizing.
3. **Positional testing** allows objective recording of nystagmus both with and without visual fixation while a patient's orientation with respect to gravity is changed. An inability to suppress nystagmus with vision suggests a central nervous system abnormality.

REFERENCES

1. Stockwell, CW: Vestibular function testing: Four year update. In Cummings, CW, et al (eds): Otolaryngology—Head and Neck Surgery. St. Louis: Mosby, 1990, p 39.
2. Baloh, RW, et al: Quantitative vestibular testing. Otolaryngol Head Neck Surg 92:145–150, 1984.
3. Voorhees, RL: Dynamic posturography findings in central nervous system disorders. Otolaryngol Head Neck Surg 103:96–101, 1990.
4. Barber, HO, and Wright, G: Positional nystagmus in normals. Adv Otolaryngol 19:276, 1973.

T8

Rotational and Posturography Testing

HISTORY

A 74-year-old woman complained of dizziness that had been more or less constant for about 12 months. The patient had difficulty identifying the precise onset of her symptoms but noted that recently she had experienced dizziness with rapid head movements and disequilibrium especially when walking in dimly lit environments. The patient did not complain of positional symptoms. There were no neurologic complaints including no changes in vision, strength, sensation, or limb coordination. The patient's past medical history was significant because she had had cardiac bypass surgery 2 years before evaluation and is being treated for chronic hypertension with a diuretic and a beta blocker. Family history was noncontributory.

The patient recently underwent a thorough evaluation by her primary care physician, which included magnetic resonance imaging (MRI) of the brain that failed to reveal a cause for her dizziness.

Question 1: Based on the patient's history, what are the diagnostic considerations in this case?

Answer 1: This patient has nonspecific balance system complaints. The complaint of dizziness with rapid head movement and worsening of symptoms when vision was not available suggests a vestibular abnormality. The negative evaluation by the patient's primary care physician ruled out many nonvestibular disorders such as diabetes, hypothyroidism, and severe anemia. Based on the history alone, the patient may have either a peripheral or a central vestibular system abnormality or both. It is unlikely that the patient is suffering from one of the common and easily recognized vestibular syndromes, such as benign positional vertigo (see Cases T1, C9, and C15) or endolymphatic hydrops (see Cases T3, T9, C10, C14, and C16).

PHYSICAL EXAMINATION

The patient's general examination was normal. Neurologic examination revealed a low-amplitude downbeating nystagmus with downgaze and nystagmus with an oblique-torsional quick component with down and lateral gaze. Otherwise, the patient's neurologic examination was normal except that she had a slightly wide-based gait and could not tandem walk. Otologic examination was normal. During neuro-otologic examination, the patient fell while trying to stand on a compliant foam surface, but otherwise no abnormalities, including spontaneous nystagmus, were seen.

Question 2: Based on the history and physical examination, what is the likely diagnosis?

Answer 2: This patient has symptoms that suggest a vestibular system abnormality and an abnormality (down-beating nystagmus) on physical examination that suggests a central nervous system abnormality, specifically a cerebellar abnormality (see Case C3). The patient's history suggests the possibility of a peripheral vestibular ailment in addition to a central nervous system abnormality. Both the patient's central nervous system abnormality and possible peripheral abnormality are of uncertain etiology. Possibly, considering the patient's hypertension and history of coronary artery disease, the patient's abnormalities have a vascular basis.

Laboratory Testing

Vestibular Laboratory Testing

ELECTRONYSTAGMOGRAPHY:	On caloric testing, the patient was found to have a 30 percent left-reduced vestibular response. Ocular motor testing revealed symmetric impairment of ocular pursuit. There was no positional nystagmus.
ROTATIONAL TESTING:	Rotational testing revealed a right directional preponderance, that is, an excessive amount of right-beating nystagmus during rotational vestibular stimulation (Fig. T8–1) (see Chapt. 2).
POSTUROGRAPHY	Posturography testing indicated a "vestibular pattern" (see Chapt. 2) wherein the patient had excessive sway when standing on a sway-referenced platform either with eyes closed or while viewing sway-referenced visual surroundings, that is, conditions 5 and 6.

Audiometric Testing: Not performed

Imaging: Not performed

Other: None

Question 3: What is the significance of the laboratory test results? How do the results influence the diagnostic considerations?

Answer 3: The patient's caloric reduction suggests a left-reduced vestibular response. Because the patient's history did not include an acute vestibular syndrome, the caloric reduction is probably long-standing. The rotational and posturography abnormalities suggest an ongoing abnormality in both the vestibulo-ocular and vestibulospinal systems, respectively. Symmetric impairment of ocular pursuit is a

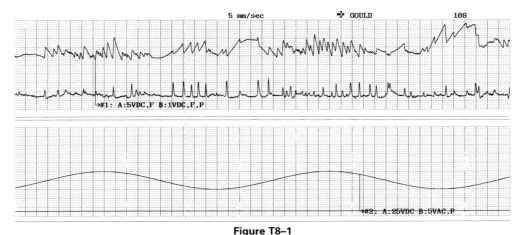

Figure T8–1
The electro-oculographic record indicates horizontal (top trace) eye position and vertical (middle trace) eye position using the standard convention of upward pen deflection indicating a rightward or an upward movement. The record shows nystagmus induced by earth-vertical axis rotation. The lowest trace indicates turntable velocity, which in this case, is varying sinusoidally at 0.05 Hz. Note that there is much more right-beating nystagmus than left-beating nystagmus.

nonspecific finding that is likely to be related to abnormal cerebellar function. Thus, this patient appears to have a chronic vestibular imbalance on the basis of a peripheral vestibular abnormality of uncertain age and cause and central vestibular abnormalities to such an extent that the normal compensation process has not occurred.

Question 4: What is the role of rotational testing in the evaluation of the patient with dizziness and disequilibrium? Why is rotational testing appropriate in the evaluation of this patient?

Answer 4: As discussed in Chapter 2, rotational testing is a physiologic stimulus that can provide information regarding the status of compensation for unilateral peripheral vestibular loss. An asymmetry of response, especially at low frequency, indicates that the patient has an ongoing vestibulo-ocular asymmetry. As is discussed in other case descriptions, rotational testing is also appropriate for the assessment of bilateral vestibular loss (Cases C6 and C21) and for assessing visual-vestibular interaction (see Case C11). The primary limitation of rotational testing is that both labyrinths are stimulated simultaneously, which precludes rotational testing from providing lateralizing peripheral vestibular information. However, rotational testing can provide information regarding central nervous system processing of vestibular information.

In this patient's case, rotational testing provided objective evidence of a vestibular system imbalance. In this manner, rotational testing confirmed the presence of a vestibular system disorder. Additionally, rotational testing indicated a failure of the process of compensation.

Question 5: What is the role of posturography testing in the evaluation of the patient with dizziness and disequilibrium? Was such testing appropriate in this case?

Answer 5: Posturography testing can provide objective evidence regarding upright balance and vestibulospinal function (see Chap. 2). Thus, posturography can add additional information beyond that provided by electronystagmography and rotational testing. Several patterns of response have been recognized for dynamic posturography testing. This patient's posturography abnormality suggested a vestibular deficit pattern. Such a finding indicates that some of the patient's disequilibrium is probably caused by a vestibular system abnormality rather than a nonvestibular central nervous system disorder. Because no clear diagnosis could be reached and the patient had a mixture of peripheral and central signs, posturography was appropriate.

Question 6: When is it appropriate to order rotational testing?

Answer 6: Rotational testing should *not* be ordered for every patient with dizziness and disequilibrium. Indeed, rotational testing is not available in many communities. Rotational testing is appropriate in the following instances: (1) for patients in whom a detailed objective assessment is needed regarding the status of vestibular compensation, (2) to assess the status of bilateral vestibular loss, and (3) in challenging cases wherein it is important to determine the dynamic characteristics of the vestibulo-ocular reflex or assess visual-vestibular interaction (see Chap. 2).

Question 7: Should posturography be ordered in all patients with dizziness and disequilibrium? Is posturography a screening tool?

Answer 7: Posturography should *not* be ordered in every patient with dizziness and disequilibrium. It should be reserved for patients in whom there is a strong suspicion of a vestibular abnormality wherein information regarding upright balance is critical. Posturography testing can (1) suggest a vestibular system abnormality, (2) suggest excessive reliance upon somatosensory inputs, (3) provide information regarding the status of vestibular compensation, and (4) provide information regarding how patients will function in environments that challenge the balance control system. Posturography is not useful for localizing lesions but may be useful in management of the patient with disequilibrium. Particular patterns of abnormality may be useful in designing vestibular rehabilitation programs (see Chap. 4).[1] Moreover, for patients with occupations that require balance for safety, posturography can provide an objective and quantitative assessment of balance control in several different sensory environments.

DIAGNOSIS/DIFFERENTIAL DIAGNOSIS

This patient is probably suffering from a *chronic peripheral vestibular loss with poor compensation.* The cause of the vestibular loss is uncertain, but may be related to cerebrovascular disease. The patient's central nervous system abnormalities are also nonspecific and of uncertain cause, but probably include dysfunction of the vestibulo-cerebellum.

TREATMENT/MANAGEMENT

The patient was treated with a course of balance rehabilitation therapy. She was advised not to use vestibular suppressant medications (see Case C1).

SUMMARY

A 74-year-old woman had a history of at least 1 year of almost constant dizziness. She described disequilibrium without vertigo or hearing loss. Physical examination revealed down-beating nystagmus, difficulty standing on a compliant surface, and an inability to tandem walk. Laboratory testing suggested a left-sided peripheral vestibular loss accompanied by both vestibulo-ocular and vestibulospinal system abnormalities. The patient was treated with vestibular rehabilitation therapy and discontinuation of vestibular suppressant medications.

TEACHING POINTS

1. **Rotational testing is a physiologic vestibular stimulus** that is useful for assessing the status of compensation for unilateral peripheral vestibular loss. An asymmetry of response, especially at low frequency, indicates that a patient has an ongoing vestibulo-ocular asymmetry.
2. **Bilateral vestibular loss** can be evaluated with rotational testing. Absent responses on caloric testing are not sufficient to diagnose bilateral vestibular loss. Rotational testing can be used to confirm the presence or absence of vestibular responses in a patient who demonstrates absent responses on caloric testing.
3. **The primary limitation of rotational testing** is that both labyrinths are stimulated simultaneously, so that rotational testing does not provide lateralizing peripheral vestibular information. However, rotational testing can provide information regarding central nervous system processing of vestibular information.
4. **Rotational testing is appropriate** (1) for patients in whom a detailed objective assessment is needed regarding the status of vestibular compensation, (2) to assess the status of bilateral vestibular loss, (3) in patients with absent caloric responses to confirm the presence or absence of vestibular function, and (4) in challenging cases wherein it is important to determine the dynamic characteristics of the vestibulo-ocular reflex or assess visual-vestibular interaction.
5. **Posturography testing** can provide objective evidence regarding upright balance and vestibulospinal function. Thus, posturography can provide additional information beyond that provided by electronystagmography and rotational testing.
6. **Posturography should be reserved** for patients in whom there is a strong suspicion of a vestibular abnormality wherein information regarding upright balance is critical. Posturography testing can (1) suggest a vestibular system abnormality, (2) suggest excessive reliance upon somatosensory inputs, (3) provide information regarding the status of vestibular compensation, (4) suggest poor patient effort, and (5) provide information regarding how patients will function in environments that challenge the balance control system.
7. **Posturography is not a localizing test** but may be useful in the management of patients with disequilibrium. Particular patterns of abnormality may be of particular use in designing physical therapy programs. Moreover, for patients with occupations that require balance for safety, posturography can provide an objective and quantitative assessment of balance control in several different sensory environments.

REFERENCES

1. Furman, JM: Posturography: Uses and limitations. Bailliere's Clin Neurol 3(3):501–513, 1994.

C A S E
T9

Audiometry

HISTORY

A 63-year-old male electrician complained of progressively worsening unsteadiness and disequilibrium. The patient reported a 20-year history of unilateral Meniere's disease but stated that his current complaints were very different from the recurrent vertigo from which he had suffered during the preceding 20 years. He noted that he had a new gait instability with veering to both the right and the left, which was worse in the dark or while walking on soft (compliant) or uneven surfaces. No true vertigo was noted. In addition to unsteadiness, the patient reported difficulty with his vision, especially when attempting to focus on traffic signals while walking or driving in a car. He volunteered that the world seemed to jiggle up and down while he walked. He felt disabled and was unable to work.

In addition to these balance complaints, the patient reported worsening of his hearing. He had first noted episodic loss of hearing in his right ear approximately 20 years ago at about the time when he first began having attacks of vertigo. At first this loss resolved between spells of vertigo and acute hearing loss, but over time, the loss of hearing became permanent. The patient's hearing had seemed quite stable during the preceding 3 years. However, during the last few months, he had noticed increasing difficulty with communication, especially in understanding speech in the presence of background noise. He found that he had become increasingly reliant on lip reading.

PHYSICAL EXAMINATION

The general and neurologic examinations, including evaluation of eye movements, were normal. The patient had increased sway on Romberg's test and a wide-based ataxic gait. He was unable to maintain balance while standing on a compliant foam pad with his eyes either open or closed. The stepping test revealed no definite rotation but was wide-based and ataxic. Examination of the fundus with the ophthalmoscope while the patient's head was actively oscillated in the horizontal plane revealed significant movement of the optic disk, suggesting a decreased vestibulo-ocular reflex gain (see Case T2). Dix-Hallpike maneuvers were negative.

Question 1: A notable absence of vertigo is reported by the patient. Instead, unsteadiness, disequilibrium while moving, and difficulty focusing while walking and riding in a car are the main complaints. What do these symptoms suggest?

Answer 1: Unsteadiness, disequilibrium, and visual dysfunction typical of oscillopsia in the absence of vertigo are suggestive of bilateral vestibular dysfunction.[1] In this patient with a long history of unilateral Meniere's disease, the possibility of *bilateral* Meniere's disease with accompanying bilateral audiovestibular dysfunction should be considered. The two principal symptoms of bilateral vestibular dysfunction are oscillopsia and ataxia (see Cases C6 and C21), not vertigo. Oscillopsia represents an illusory movement of the visual surroundings that manifests itself as a bobbing or jiggling during high-frequency head movement such as that experienced while walking or while riding in a car. Oscillopsia prevents patients from focusing clearly on the visual surroundings while the head is moving.[2]

Causes of bilateral vestibulopathy include bacterial meningitis; syphilitic labyrinthitis; chemical ototoxicity (see Case C6); bilateral Meniere's disease (bilateral endolymphatic hydrops); autoimmune inner ear disease (see Case C24); neurofibromatosis type II (bilateral acoustic neuromas); neurodegenerative syndromes such as Friedreich's ataxia (see Case C11); and idiopathic causes.[3]

Question 2: What is the value of assessing hearing in the evaluation of the dizzy patient?

Answer 2: Because the vestibular and auditory periphery share common inner-ear fluid homeostasis, blood supply, nerves, and location within the temporal bone (see Chap. 1), disorders that affect the peripheral vestibular apparatus often affect hearing as well. An evaluation of hearing can help localize a vestibular system disorder to the periphery and often can help to lateralize an abnormality.[4] In addition, certain vertigo syndromes have characteristic types of associated hearing loss, for example, endolymphatic hydrops, which is frequently associated with a low-tone sensorineural hearing loss with good word recognition, whereas vestibular neuritis is characterized by normal hearing. Compression of the eighth cranial nerve bundles within the internal auditory canal and/or cerebellopontine angle by a tumor can also produce symptoms of unsteadiness and disequilibrium as well as hearing loss. In this situation, the hearing loss is usually primarily in the high frequencies and word recognition is relatively poor.

ADDITIONAL PHYSICAL EXAMINATION INFORMATION

Examination of the tympanic membrane and middle ear space revealed no abnormalities. Pneumatic otoscopy produced no dizziness or nystagmus. Tuning-fork testing revealed a positive Rinne test bilaterally. Weber's test was midline.

Question 3: How is hearing tested in the laboratory, and how can it add to the information provided by bedside evaluation?

Answer 3: The mainstay of hearing assessment is pure tone and speech audiometry, which constitute a basic audiogram. Additional tests that are commonly performed include tympanometry and acoustic reflex testing (see Chap. 3). Brainstem auditory-evoked potential testing, electrocochleography, and otoacoustic emissions are advanced audiologic tests that can be used to help evaluate and localize disorders affecting the auditory system.

Brainstem auditory-evoked potential testing can be used to evaluate the integrity of the auditory pathway from the level of the cochlea through the brainstem auditory relay centers. Mass lesions of the cerebellopontine angle, such as a meningioma or an acoustic neuroma, often interfere with transmission through the auditory nerve and can be detected by auditory brainstem auditory-evoked potential testing. Lesions intrinsic to the brainstem, such as metastases, glioma, or focal demyelination, interfere with transmission through the auditory relay areas and thus also may be detected by brainstem auditory-evoked potential testing.

Electrocochleography is a modification of brainstem auditory response audiometry in which the first portion (wave I) of the brainstem auditory-evoked potential is amplified to reveal its fine structure. Electrocochleography can be helpful in diagnosing endolymphatic hydrops as the underlying cause of a balance disorder, especially in cases where the symptoms are not clearly defined as in some cases of Meniere's disease and in complex cases such as this one, where both ears are affected.

Otoacoustic emission testing provides a sensitive and objective measurement of hearing that specifically assesses function of cochlear hair cells and is thus capable of distinguishing between sensory (hair cell) and neural (eighth nerve) dysfunction. Otoacoustic emission testing has become valuable for detecting the monitoring drug-related ototoxicity and for use in infant hearing screening programs. Even though otoacoustic emission testing does not directly assess vestibular function, the ability to distinguish sensory versus neural dysfunction within the inner ear cannot be achieved otherwise and should help to provide unique insights into vestibular dysfunction in the future.

Laboratory Testing

Vestibular Laboratory Testing:

ELECTRONYSTAGMOGRAPHY:	Ocular motor testing, positional testing, and caloric testing were normal.
ROTATIONAL TESTING:	Rotational testing demonstrated a mild left directional preponderance.
POSTUROGRAPHY:	Posturography indicated excessive sway on conditions 5 and 6, that is, a vestibular pattern.

Audiometric Testing: The audiogram showed a bilateral hearing loss that was worse in the right ear (Fig. T9–1). The hearing loss in the left ear was primarily in the low frequencies, whereas the right ear had a "flat" hearing loss across all frequencies. A brainstem auditory-evoked potential test was performed and was normal. Electrocochleography was performed and showed a normal summating potential to action potential ratio (SP/AP) on the right and an abnormally elevated SP/AP ratio of 60 percent on the left.

Imaging: Not performed

Other: A metabolic blood screen was performed to rule out thyroid disease, autoimmune disorders, blood dyscrasias, and syphilis, and no abnormalities were detected.

Question 4: Based on the history, physical examination, and laboratory testing, what is this patient's most likely diagnosis?

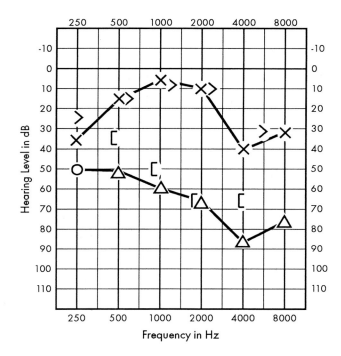

Figure T9–1
Audiogram.

Word Recognition Score		
Right : 92%		
Left : 100%		

		Right	Left
Air	unmasked	o——o	x——x
	masked	△——△	□——□
Bone	unmasked	◄---◄	►---►
	masked	⊢---[	]---⊣

Answer 4: This patient has a history of unilateral Meniere's disease with complaints of a recent onset of increased hearing loss and worsening balance. The audiogram demonstrated bilateral hearing loss suggestive of bilateral endolymphatic hydrops. Because of the previous history of right-sided Meniere's disease, it is not clear whether both ears or only the newly affected left ear is responsible for the current vestibular symptoms. Vestibular function testing could not localize the abnormality because caloric testing was normal and the other abnormalities noted on testing cannot be used to localize the offending ear.

The electrocochleography was helpful because it showed active endolymphatic hydrops in the left ear and was normal in the right ear. These findings suggest that the right ear is not in an active phase of endolymphatic hydrops, and that the left ear is actively affected by endolymphatic hydrops and is the source of the patient's current symptoms. The negative metabolic screen suggests that the cause of the bilateral endolymphatic hydrops is unknown and can be labeled Meniere's disease.

DIAGNOSIS/DIFFERENTIAL DIAGNOSIS

This patient was diagnosed as having *bilateral Meniere's disease* with active endolymphatic hydrops in the left ear.

TREATMENT/MANAGEMENT

Treatment of bilateral Meniere's disease is difficult and should be conservative. Surgery is rarely indicated because the success of surgery depends on an intact contralateral ear (see Case C14). Another trial of medical treatment using a diuretic and a salt-restricted diet or a trial of a steroid medication such as prednisone should be instituted. If these medical measures fail, then repeated intramuscular streptomycin injections may be used in a titration fashion to slowly reduce vestibular function in both ears. Intramuscular streptomycin titration can be highly effective in controlling vestibular symptoms in bilateral Meniere's disease and is usually used when both ears are active or when it is not clear which ear is active.[5-7] Finally, in cases of bilateral Meniere's disease in which one ear is clearly identified as the active ear, middle-ear injection of an aminoglycoside such as gentamicin may be considered[8] (see Case C14). Extreme caution must be exercised when using either intramuscular injections of streptomycin or middle-ear injections of gentamicin because a severe bilateral loss of vestibular function may quickly ensue that may worsen the patient's symptoms.

In this patient's case, treatment with a diuretic and salt restriction and then with a brief course of steroids failed. Eight intramuscular streptomycin injections were given over a 6-week period to reduce vestibular function in both ears. The patient enjoyed significant improvement in his vestibular symptoms and was able to return to work for 2 additional years until his planned retirement.

SUMMARY

A 63-year-old man with a 20-year history of Meniere's disease developed new symptoms of imbalance. Evaluation revealed bilateral Meniere's disease. The diagnosis was confirmed using results of an audiogram and electrocochleography, which indicated that the newly involved ear had active endolymphatic hydrops. Treatment consisted of a trial of a diuretic and salt restriction and then a brief course of steroids, both of which failed. Then the patient underwent intramuscular streptomycin therapy, which markedly reduced his symptoms.

TEACHING POINTS

1. **Hearing assessment** is a fundamental part of the evaluation of the dizzy patient. Because the vestibular and auditory periphery share common inner-ear fluid homeostasis, blood supply, nerves, and location within the temporal bone, disorders that affect the peripheral vestibular apparatus often affect hearing as well. An evaluation of hearing can help localize a vestibular system disorder to the periphery and can often help to lateralize an abnormality.
2. **The type of hearing loss** can help to diagnose vestibulopathy. Several vertigo syndromes have characteristic types of associated hearing loss. For example, endolymphatic hydrops is frequently associated with a low-tone sensorineural hearing loss with good word recognition, whereas vestibular neuritis is characterized by normal hearing. Compression of the eighth cranial nerve bundles within the internal auditory canal and/or cerebellopontine angle by a tumor can produce hearing loss as well as symptoms of unsteadiness and disequilibrium. In this situation, the hear-

ing loss is usually worse in the high frequencies and word recognition is relatively poor.

3. **A basic audiogram,** the mainstay of hearing assessment, consists of pure tone and speech audiometry. Additional tests that are commonly performed include tympanometry and acoustic reflex testing. Brainstem auditory-evoked potential testing, electrocochleography, and otoacoustic emissions are advanced audiological tests that can be used to help evaluate and localize disorders affecting the auditory system.

4. **Brainstem auditory-evoked potential testing** can be used to evaluate the integrity of the auditory pathway and is most commonly used to detect mass lesions of the cerebellopontine angle such as a meningioma or an acoustic neuroma, or lesions intrinsic to the brainstem such as metastases, glioma, or focal demyelination.

5. **Electrocochleography** is a modification of brainstem auditory-evoked potential audiometry and can be helpful in diagnosing endolymphatic hydrops. Electrocochleography is especially valuable in cases in which the symptoms are not clearly defined, such as some cases of Meniere's disease and complex cases in which both ears are affected.

6. **Treatment of bilateral Meniere's disease** is difficult and should be conservative. Surgery is rarely indicated because the success of surgery depends on an intact contralateral ear and vestibular compensation. Treatment options include use of a diuretic and salt-restricted diet, a diagnostic and therapeutic trial of a steroid medication such as prednisone, titrated reduction of vestibular function using intramuscular streptomycin injections, and chemical labyrinthectomy using middle-ear injection of an aminoglycoside such as gentamicin. Extreme caution must be exercised when using either intramuscular injections of streptomycin or middle-ear injections of gentamicin because a severe bilateral loss of vestibular function may quickly ensue and may worsen the patient's symptoms.

REFERENCES

1. "JC": Living without a balancing mechanism. N Engl J Med 246:458–460, 1952.
2. Wist, ER, Brandt, TH, and Krafczyk, S: Oscillopsia and retinal slip. Brain 106:153–168, 1983.
3. Baloh, R, Jacobson, K, and Honrubia, V: Idiopathic bilateral vestibulopathy. Neurology 32:272–275, 1989.
4. Shone, G, Kemink, JL, and Telian, SA: Prognostic significance of hearing loss as a lateralizing indicator in the surgical treatment of vertigo. J Laryngol Otol 105:618–620, 1991.
5. Wilson, WR, and Schuknecht, HF: Update on the use of streptomycin therapy for Meniere's disease. Am J Otol 2(2):108–111, 1980.
6. Silverstein, H: Streptomycin treatment for Meniere's disease. Ann Otol Rhinol Laryngol (suppl 112, part 2) 93:44–47, 1984.
7. Langman, AW, Kemink, JL, and Graham, MD: Titration streptomycin therapy for bilateral Meniere's disease. Ann Otol Rhinol Laryngol 99:923–926, 1990.
8. Pyykko, I, et al: Intratympanic gentamicin in bilateral Meniere's disease. Otolaryngol Head Neck Surg 110:162–167, 1994.

PART

III

Common Disease
Case Studies

C1

Poor Vestibular Compensation

HISTORY

A 65-year-old woman presented with a complaint of 6 months of dizziness and disequilibrium. Her symptoms were characterized by nearly constant imbalance when walking or standing and lightheadedness even when seated. The patient's dizziness was exacerbated by head movement, especially rapid head movement, associated with blurred vision. She did not complain of any positional symptoms. Specifically, there were no complaints of dizziness when rolling over in bed. The patient noted no recent change in hearing and no tinnitus or aural fullness. She was essentially asymptomatic when lying still.

The patient dated her symptoms to an acute episode of vertigo associated with nausea, vomiting, and severe disequilibrium lasting for several hours 6 months before evaluation. She had not complained of dizziness before that episode. She was evaluated by her primary care physician and was felt to have a peripheral vestibular ailment. The patient was treated with meclizine, 25 mg orally, three times daily. This provided her with some relief but was not entirely successful in alleviating her symptoms. The patient had to decrease her activity level to such a degree that she no longer drove an automobile or took her morning walk and discontinued gardening. Despite these changes in her activities, she continued to experience daily dizziness, and her physician increased the dosage of her meclizine to 25 mg, four times daily. Other than dizziness, the patient had no significant past medical history. The family history was noncontributory.

Question 1: Based on the patient's history, what is the most likely diagnosis? Why is the patient experiencing dizziness?

Answer 1: This patient's most likely diagnosis is vestibular neuritis (see Case T5). Acute vertigo unaccompanied by associated hearing loss, tinnitus, and aural fullness is unlikely to be caused by Meniere's disease. Other possibilities include a labyrinthine infarction or some other nonspecific vestibulopathy. In any case, the patient's history is consistent with an acute peripheral vestibular ailment 6 months before evaluation.

The patient's persistent dizziness suggests that she has not compensated for her presumed peripheral vestibular loss. Her continued symptoms of instability during standing and walking suggest an ongoing vestibulospinal abnormality. The patient's blurred vision immediately following head movement suggests a vestibulo-ocular abnormality. Meclizine does not appear to be a successful treatment. Possibly, this medication is actually worsening the patient's symptoms by suppressing needed vestibular input.

PHYSICAL EXAMINATION

General examination revealed an elderly-appearing woman who made minimal spontaneous head movements. Neurologic examination revealed a few beats of right-beating nystagmus on right-lateral gaze that were unsustained. Otherwise, the patient's cranial nerve examination was normal. There were no changes in strength or sensation. There was no incoordination. The patient's gait was slow with a short stride length. Her head was held rigidly during walking. The patient could tandem walk only with assistance. Romberg's test was negative. However, the patient could not stand on a compliant foam surface with eyes open or closed. On the stepping test, the patient's stepping was tentative and wide-based, and she rotated almost 180 degrees to the left. There was no nystagmus seen with Frenzel glasses. Dix-Hallpike maneuvers were negative. Otologic examination was normal.

Question 2: What additional information regarding the cause of this patient's dizziness was provided by the physical examination?

Answer 2: The patient's examination suggests that she is avoiding vestibular stimulation by severely limiting head movement. Moreover, the patient's nystagmus, although minimal, suggests an ongoing vestibulo-ocular asymmetry or a vestibular compensation abnormality. It is likely that the patient has not compensated for her presumed peripheral vestibular deficit. Moreover, one reason for the patient's failure to compensate may be inadequate vestibular stimulation because she limits head movement so severely.

Laboratory Testing

Vestibular Laboratory Testing:

ELECTRONYSTAGMOGRAPHY: Ocular motor function was normal. A very low amplitude right-beating nystagmus was seen with eyes open in the dark. This nystagmus increased with rightward gaze. Caloric testing revealed a 50 percent reduced vestibular response on the left.

ROTATIONAL TESTING: Rotational testing revealed responses of normal amplitude and timing. However, there was a right-directional preponderance.

POSTUROGRAPHY: Posturography indicated a "surface dependence" pattern wherein the patient had excessive postural sway whenever she was standing on a "sway-referenced" platform regardless of the visual condition, that is, on conditions 4, 5, and 6. She was able to maintain her balance only when the support surface was fixed.

Audiometric Testing: An audiogram showed a mild high-frequency sensorineural hearing loss that was symmetrical in both ears. Word recognition scores were 100 percent bilaterally.

Imaging: An MRI of the brain performed before evaluation was normal.

Other: None.

Question 3: What additional information does laboratory testing provide?

Answer 3: Laboratory testing indicates that the patient has both a unilateral peripheral vestibular loss and an ongoing vestibulo-ocular and vestibulospinal asymmetry. Moreover, the patient's posturography abnormalities suggest that she has become dependent on a rigid surface for maintaining balance. Taken together, the findings suggest poor vestibular compensation for a unilateral peripheral vestibular insult despite the passage of 6 months since the patient's acute vestibular syndrome.

Question 4: What are the causes of poor vestibular compensation for peripheral vestibular injury? Which of these causes may be underlying this patient's persistent symptoms?

Answer 4: Vestibular compensation depends upon consistent peripheral vestibular activity, even if reduced or only from one labyrinth, in combination with other sensory inputs such as that from vision and somatosensation, and normal function of central vestibular structures.[1,2] Thus, failure to compensate for a peripheral vestibular lesion can be on the basis of fluctuating or unusual peripheral vestibular activity, a vestibular compensation abnormality, clinical or subclinical involvement of the contralateral ear, multiple sensory deficits, or a sedentary lifestyle. Vestibular compensation abnormalities that impair compensation include both structural abnormalities and dysfunction caused by certain drugs such as benzodiazepines.

This patient's failure to compensate for a peripheral vestibular lesion is probably the result of a combination of a sedentary lifestyle and overmedication with vestibular suppressant medications that together caused inadequate vestibular stimulation and impaired vestibular compensation, especially cerebellar function. Nothing in the history or physical examination suggests fluctuating or unusual vestibular input from the involved ear, although this cannot be ruled out entirely. Also, there is nothing to suggest abnormalities in other sensory systems.

DIAGNOSIS/DIFFERENTIAL DIAGNOSIS

This patient's history, physical examination, and laboratory studies suggest *left-sided vestibular neuritis and impaired compensation*; that is, the patient has failed to undergo normal vestibular compensation for her peripheral vestibular ailment.

TREATMENT/MANAGEMENT

This patient was treated by tapering off the medicines that were prescribed for vestibular suppression. Additionally, she was scheduled for a course of vestibular rehabilitation therapy in hope of potentiating compensation for her peripheral vestibular deficit. Physical therapy was recommended with the intent of reducing the patient's symptoms of dizziness and improving her balance by expediting vestibular compensation and reducing her dependence upon somatosensation, that is, reducing her "surface dependence."

SUMMARY

A 65-year-old woman presented with a history of an episode of acute vertigo, nausea, and vomiting 6 months prior to evaluation. The patient's symptoms evolved into constant disequilibrium. Physical examination suggested an ongoing vestibular imbalance. This was confirmed by laboratory testing, which indicated a reduced vestibular response and both vestibulo-ocular and vestibulospinal asymmetry. The patient was felt to have a peripheral vestibular ailment with poor compensation centrally. Her vestibular suppressant medication dosage was reduced significantly and she was enrolled in a course of balance rehabilitation therapy.

TEACHING POINTS

1. **Persistent dizziness** that continues following an acute peripheral vestibular ailment may be the result of poor vestibular compensation for a peripheral vestibular injury. Typical symptoms of poor compensation include instability during standing and walking and blurred vision associated with quick head movements.
2. **Patients with poor vestibular compensation** for a peripheral vestibular injury often avoid vestibular stimulation by severely limiting head movements. Their gait is often slow with a short stride length and the head is held rigidly during walking. Although limiting head movements reduces vestibular stimulation and thus sensations of dizziness, this strategy is maladaptive because vestibular stimulation is necessary to stimulate the process of vestibular compensation.
3. **Failure to compensate** for a peripheral vestibular lesion can be related to fluctuating or unusual peripheral vestibular activity; a vestibular compensation abnormality; clinical or subclinical involvement of the contralateral ear; the presence of other sensory deficits, especially involving vision and somatosensation; or a sedentary lifestyle. Vestibular compensation abnormalities that impair compensation include both structural abnormalities and dysfunction caused by certain drugs such as benzodiazepines.
4. **Vestibular laboratory test** results that are consistent with poor vestibular compensation include the presence of a spontaneous nystagmus, a directional preponderance on rotational testing, and abnormal platform posturography testing.
5. **Treatment of patients with poor vestibular compensation** includes tapering off any vestibular suppressant medications and a course of vestibular rehabilitation to stimulate central compensation for the peripheral vestibular deficit.

REFERENCES

1. Hart, C, McKinley, P, and Peterson, B: Compensation following acute unilateral total loss of peripheral vestibular function. In Graham, M., and Kemink, J (eds): The Vestibular System: Neurophysiologic and Clinical Research. New York: Raven Press, 1987, pp 187–192.
2. Lacour, M, et al (eds): Vestibular Compensation: Facts, Theories and Clinical Perspectives. Proceedings of the International Symposium. Paris: Elsevier Publishing Company, 1988.

C2

Anxiety and Psychogenic Dizziness

HISTORY

A 43-year-old woman who worked as an accountant presented with the chief complaint of dizziness for the previous several years. Her symptoms were described as a sense of lightheadedness and disequilibrium without true vertigo, present at a low level constantly. The patient suffered periodic exacerbations. She was particularly bothered by certain environments, such as shopping malls, grocery stores, and driving on winding roads. Additionally, she occasionally experienced tingling of the fingers and toes associated with her dizziness. There was no positional sensitivity, hearing loss, or tinnitus.

Question 1: Based on the history, what are the diagnostic possibilities for this patient?

Answer 1: This patient has nonspecific complaints that are difficult to localize entirely to the vestibular system. Moreover, her history suggests a symptom complex that has been labeled *space and motion discomfort*.[1] Space and motion discomfort refers to symptoms elicited by a specific stimulus pattern in some patients with vestibular dysfunction and some with panic disorder. Space and motion discomfort occurs in situations characterized by inadequate visual or kinesthetic information for normal spatial orientation. Space and motion discomfort coupled with intermittent paresthesias strongly suggests an anxiety component to the patient's problem. Thus, this patient may have a vestibular disorder, an anxiety disorder, or both.

PHYSICAL EXAMINATION

The patient's general examination was normal. Neurologic examination revealed square-wave jerks, that is, small involuntary to-and-fro saccades on and off the point of visual regard. The patient was unaware of these movements. Examination of her motor system, sensation, and coordination were normal. The patient was able to tandem walk without difficulty. Romberg's test was negative. Otologic and neuro-otologic examinations were normal, including no difficulty standing on a foam pad with the eyes closed.

Laboratory Testing

Vestibular Laboratory Testing

ELECTRONYSTAGMOGRAPHY: Ocular motor, positional, and caloric testing were normal.

ROTATIONAL TESTING: Rotational testing revealed responses of normal amplitude and timing with a significant right directional preponderance.

POSTUROGRAPHY: Posturography was normal.

Audiometric Testing: Not performed

Imaging: Not performed

Other: Not performed

Question 2: In what way does the additional information from the physical examination and vestibular laboratory testing influence the diagnostic considerations?

Answer 2: The patient's square-wave jerks are a nonspecific finding often seen in the elderly where they are of no clinical significance. In young adults, however, square-wave jerks are considered abnormal and may indicate a brainstem or cerebellar abnormality (see Cases U2 and U3), but often are seen with anxiety without other neurologic abnormalities. The combination of normal caloric responses and a directional preponderance on rotational testing suggests an ongoing vestibulo-ocular asymmetry without peripheral vestibular disease. Thus, the patient may have a central nervous system abnormality. Taken together, the patient's history, physical examination, and laboratory abnormalities suggest an anxiety disorder and a central vestibular abnormality as well.

Question 3: What is psychogenic dizziness?

Answer 3: Psychogenic dizziness is a term used by many physicians synonymously with psychic dizziness, psychiatric dizziness, psychophysiologic dizziness, and functional dizziness.[2] The diagnosis of psychogenic dizziness is commonly based on the nature of the dizziness; lightheadedness or giddiness is said to be more likely to be psychogenic.[3] Moreover, dizziness is often diagnosed as psychogenic when it occurs in anxious or phobic individuals. This use of the term psychogenic dizziness can be criticized for several reasons. A large number of patients who fulfill diagnostic criteria for a psychiatric disorder may also have vestibular dysfunction. Indeed, there is a definite association between anxiety disorders and vestibular disorders.[4] The term psychogenic dizziness should be used only for those patients in whom dizziness occurs exclusively in combination with other symptoms as part of a recognized psychiatric symptom cluster.[2] For example, dizziness that occurs as a component of the symptom cluster of panic attacks should be called psychogenic.

Question 4: What is the role of hyperventilation as part of the evaluation of patients with suspected anxiety disorders?

Answer 4: The hyperventilation test has been described by Drachman and Hart (1972) and Nedzelski and colleagues (1986).[5,6] They described dizziness related to 3 minutes of hyperventilation. It is common practice to consider dizziness "psychogenic" if a patient's sensations can be replicated by hyperventilation. Such a practice is questionable, however, in that Herr and associates (1989) found that the hyperventilation test was positive in approximately 20 percent of patients who had diagnoses other than that of vestibular dysfunction, thereby indicating a lack of specificity of the hyperventilation test.[7] The sensitivity of the hyperventilation test is also unknown. Thus, although the hyperventilation test can provide the clinician with useful information, the results of such testing should be interpreted with great caution.

DIAGNOSIS/DIFFERENTIAL DIAGNOSIS

The patient's symptoms of dizziness with rapid head movement coupled with abnormal vestibular laboratory studies suggest a vestibular system abnormality. Her history of space and motion discomfort, parasthesias, and square-wave jerks suggests an anxiety disorder. Thus, this patient has both a *vestibular disorder of uncertain etiology and an anxiety disorder.*

Question 5: What is the cause-and-effect relationship, if any, between vestibular disorders and anxiety disorders?

Answer 5: Three functional mechanisms that are not necessarily exclusive might account for the association between vestibular abnormalities and anxiety disorders: the somatopsychic, psychosomatic, and neurologic linkage mechanisms. The *somatopsychic model* postulates that vestibular sensations are catastrophically reinterpreted by the panic patient as signifying immediate danger, resulting in panic attacks.[4] Agoraphobic avoidance develops as a result of this situational specificity of vestibular symptoms, for example, space and motion discomfort.[8] The *psychosomatic model* postulates that vestibular dysfunction occurs as a result of anxiety or hyperventilation, perhaps by altering central vestibular processing. In favor of this mechanism are the observations that increases in vestibular responses occur with heightened arousal and hyperventilation alters vestibular responses on the rotational test and the positional test.[9–11] The *neurologic linkage model* postulates that panic disorder, along with vestibular and audiologic dysfunction, involves abnormal activity in overlapping or interconnected areas in the brainstem, such as the locus coeruleus.[2]

Question 6: What is the appropriate treatment for this patient, who is believed to have a combination of a vestibular system abnormality and an anxiety disorder?

Answer 6: Treatment approaches to patients with anxiety that may be related to vestibular dysfunction are currently under development. No controlled outcome studies have been conducted. However, the vestibular disorder and the anxiety disorder should be treated simultaneously. The vestibular disorder should be treated in the same manner as a nonspecific vestibulopathy (see Case C18). The treatment of anxiety disorder includes pharmacotherapy and behavioral therapy.[12] Pharmacotherapy could include antianxiety agents (Table C2–1). Note that benzodiazapines act as both a vestibular suppressant and an anxiolytic and thus are an excellent first choice of treatment for such patients.

TABLE C2–1
Medications for Anxiety Associated with Dizziness

Medication	Trade Name	Class	Dosage	Side Effects
Diazepam	Valium	Benzodiazepine	2–10 mg orally, IM, or IV every 4 to 6 hours	Lethargy
Chlordiazepoxide	Librium	Benzodiazepine	5–10 mg orally every 6–8 hours	Drowsiness
Hydroxyzine	Vistaril, Atarax	Piperazine derivative	50–100 mg orally every 6 hours	Drowsiness, dry mouth
Imipramine	Imavate, Janimine, Presamine, SK-Pramine, Tofranil	Tricyclic	25–100 mg orally daily	Anticholinergic effects, drowsiness
Desipramine	Norpramin, Pertofrane	Tricyclic	25–100 mg orally daily	Anticholinergic effects, drowsiness
Amitriptyline	Amitril, Elavil, Endep	Tricyclic	25–100 mg orally daily	Anticholinergic effects, drowsiness
Buspirone	BuSpar	Arylpiperazine	5 mg orally every 8 hours	Drowsiness, nausea

Question 7: Should this patient be referred to a psychiatrist for further evaluation?

Answer 7: Controlled studies are necessary to evaluate the role of psychiatric treatment for patients with a combination of a balance disorder and a psychiatric disorder. However, psychiatric referral is certainly warranted for patients who are suffering from a severe anxiety disorder, patients with frequent panic attacks, and patients suffering from panic disorder with agoraphobia.[13] This patient was treated with a combination of vestibular rehabilitation therapy and diazepam 2 mg by mouth, twice daily.

SUMMARY

A 43-year-old woman presented with symptoms consistent with both a vestibular system abnormality and an anxiety disorder. Physical examination and laboratory testing further suggested the absence of significant neurologic disease but did suggest a vestibular imbalance and the presence of objective evidence of anxiety (square-wave jerks). The patient was treated with low-dose benzodiazepines and balance rehabilitation therapy.

TEACHING POINTS

1. **Anxiety frequently accompanies dizziness** and symptoms of a vestibular disorder. The cause-and-effect relationship between anxiety and dizziness is uncertain but may be related to a somatopsychic, psychosomatic, or a common neurologic mechanism.
2. **Space and motion discomfort**, that is, symptoms elicited by situations characterized by inadequate visual or kinesthetic information necessary for normal spatial orientation, is often seen in patients who are both anxious and dizzy.

3. **Square-wave jerks,** that is, small saccades that briefly take the eye off target, are a nonspecific sign often seen in normal elderly persons. In young adults, however, square-wave jerks are considered abnormal and may indicate a brainstem or cerebellar abnormality, but are often seen with anxiety without other neurologic abnormalities.

4. **The term psychogenic dizziness** should be used only for patients in whom dizziness occurs exclusively in combination with other symptoms as part of a recognized psychiatric symptom cluster. For example, dizziness that occurs as a component of the symptom cluster of panic attacks should be called psychogenic. However, the term psychogenic dizziness should not be used to describe patients who have anxiety as a component of a balance disorder.

5. **Hyperventilation** is a maneuver that is commonly used to determine whether dizziness is ''psychogenic.'' The test is actually quite nonspecific, and the results of such testing should be interpreted with great caution.

6. **Treatment of patients with a combined anxiety and vestibular disorder** should include measures aimed at both conditions simultaneously. The vestibular disorder should be treated in whatever manner is appropriate. The treatment of anxiety disorders includes pharmacotherapy and behavioral therapy. A psychiatric referral is warranted for patients who are suffering from frequent panic attacks or from panic disorder with agoraphobia.

REFERENCES

1. Jacob, RG, Woody, SR, and Clark, DB, et al: Discomfort with space and motion: A possible marker of vestibular dysfunction assessed by the Situational Characteristics Questionnaire. J Psychopathol Behav Assessment 15:299–324, 1993.
2. Jacob, RG, Furman, JM, and Balaban, CD: Psychiatric aspects of vestibular disorders. In Baloh, RW, and Halmagyi, M (eds): Handbook of Neurotology/Vestibular System. New York: Oxford University Press (in press).
3. Moore, BE, and Atkinson M: Psychogenic vertigo. Arch Otolaryngol 67:347–353, 1958.
4. Jacob, RG: Panic disorder and the vestibular system. Psychiatric Clin North Am 11:361–374, 1988.
5. Drachman, DA, and Hart CW: An approach to the dizzy patient. Neurology 22:323–334, 1972.
6. Nedzelski, JM, Barber, HO, and McIlmoyl L: Diagnoses in a dizziness unit. J Otolaryngol 15(2):101–104, 1986.
7. Herr, RD, Zun, L, and Matthews, JJ: A directed approach to the dizzy patient. Ann Emerg Med 18(6):664/101-672/109, 1989.
8. Jacob, RG, Furman, JM, Clark, DB, et al: Psychogenic dizziness. In Barber, HO and Sharpe, JA (eds): The Vestibular Ocular Reflex, Nystagmus, and Vertigo. New York: Raven Press (in press).
9. Collins, WE: Arousal and vestibular habituation. In Kornhuber, HH (ed): Vestibular System Part 2: Psychophysics, Applied Aspects and General Interpretations. Berlin: Springer-Verlag, 1974.
10. Theunissen, EJM, Huygen, PLM, and Folgering, HTH: Vestibular hyperreactivity and hyperventilation. Clin Otolaryngol 11:161–169, 1986.
11. Monday, LA, and Tetrault, L: Hyperventilation and vertigo. Laryngoscope 109:1003–1010, 1980.
12. Reid, WH: The treatment of psychologic disorders (Revised for the DSM-III-R). New York: Brunner/Mazel, 1945.
13. American Psychiatric Association: Diagnostic and Statistical Manual of Mental Disorders, Fourth Edition. Washington, DC: American Psychiatric Association, 1994.

C A S E
C3

Central Vestibular Nystagmus

HISTORY

A 19-year-old female college student complained of constant dizziness and disequilibrium for several years. The patient noted that she had gait instability with veering to both the right and the left. There was no true vertigo. Rather, she experienced light-headedness and disequilibrium, especially when tipping her head back, even while seated. The patient was not particularly bothered by rapid head movements and had no complaints of hearing loss or tinnitus. There was no significant past medical history. The family history was noncontributory.

Question 1: Based on the patient's history, what are the diagnostic considerations?

Answer 1: This patient's history is extremely nonspecific but does suggest a balance system disorder. The symptoms cannot be definitively localized to either the central or peripheral vestibular system. However, the absence of vertigo and the absence of symptoms with rapid head movements suggest a central rather than a peripheral vestibular system abnormality. The worsening of the patient's symptoms when tipping her head back suggests the possibility of a posterior fossa abnormality such as a posterior (vertebrobasilar) circulation abnormality or a cervical abnormality (see Case C7).

PHYSICAL EXAMINATION

General examination was normal. Neurologic examination revealed gaze-evoked nystagmus on left gaze, right gaze, and upward gaze. Oblique down and lateral gaze revealed an oblique torsional nystagmus (downbeating nystagmus). The patient also had saccadic overshoot dysmetria when looking both to the right and to the left and abnormal ocular pursuit with "catch-up" saccades. She had no nystagmus in the primary position, but with Frenzel glasses demonstrated a spontaneous right-beating nystagmus. The remainder of the patient's cranial nerve examination was normal. Strength and sensation were normal. Coordination testing was normal. The patient had a widened base of gait. Romberg's test was negative. Otologic examination was normal. The patient had difficulty standing on a compliant foam surface.

Question 2: Based on the physical examination, what is the most likely localization of this patient's lesion and what are the likely diagnostic possibilities?

Answer 2: The patient's downbeating nystagmus is suggestive of a craniocervical junction abnormality. In combination with the patient's gaze-evoked nystagmus, saccadic dysmetria, and abnormal ocular pursuit, the patient appears to have a lesion of the caudal midline cerebellum. Diagnostic considerations include a Chiari malformation, that is, caudally positioned cerebellar tonsils, a mass lesion, such as a foramen magnum meningioma, or demyelinating disease. Given the patient's gradual worsening and relatively benign history, less likely etiologies include an infectious process such as a viral or postviral syndrome, inflammatory disease, and olivocerebellar degeneration syndrome.

Laboratory Testing

Vestibular Laboratory Testing

ELECTRONYSTAGMOGRAPHY:	Not performed
ROTATIONAL TESTING:	Not performed
POSTUROGRAPHY:	Not performed

Audiometric Testing

Imaging: An MRI scan revealed a Chiari malformation with the cerebellar tonsils approximately 5 mm below the foramen magnum with an obliterated ambient cistern (Fig. C3-1).

Other: None

Question 3: What is the role, if any, for vestibular laboratory testing in Chiari malformation? Should vestibular laboratory testing be ordered for this patient?

Answer 3: Although vestibular laboratory testing is not required to confirm the diagnosis of Chiari malformation, such information may be helpful in planning management, for example, whether to request a neurosurgical consultation, and in following the patient's progress following posterior fossa decompression surgery if the patient undergoes such a procedure. Vestibular laboratory testing provides a quantitative assessment of the extent of a patient's vestibular system abnormalities, including documentation of any vestibular nystagmus suspected on physical examination. Moreover, some patients with Chiari malformation manifest peripheral vestibular signs, for example, a caloric reduction. Such information may aid in management.

Despite the fact that vestibular laboratory testing may have confirmed some of the abnormalities seen on physical examination, this patient's Chiari malformation is already thought to be "symptomatic" on the basis of the clinical evaluation, thereby justifying a referral to a neurosurgeon. Thus, vestibular laboratory testing was not obtained.

Question 4: What is the pathophysiologic basis for this patient's nystagmus?

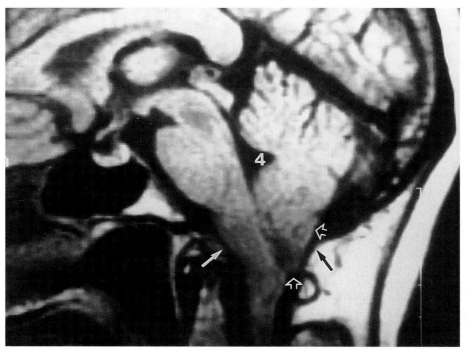

Figure C3-1

Sagittal MRI scan demonstrating a Chiari malformation. The cerebellar tonsils extend into the vertebral canal with no displacement of the fourth ventricle (4). The foramen magnum is seen between white and black solid arrows. The cerebellar tonsil is outlined by open arrowheads. (With permission from Weber, PC, and Cass, SP: Neurotologic manifestations of Chiari 1 malformation. St. Louis: Mosby-Year Book, Inc., Otolaryngol Head Neck Surg 109:853–860, 1993.[1])

Answer 4: This patient had three types of nystagmus: (1) gaze-evoked nystagmus, (2) downbeating nystagmus, and (3) spontaneous vestibular nystagmus. It is important to note that, by convention, gaze-evoked nystagmus is left-beating on left lateral gaze, right-beating on right lateral gaze, and upbeating on upward gaze. Gaze-evoked nystagmus is typically conjugate, that is, both eyes move equally. Nystagmus that beats down, even when seen only with downgaze, is considered "downbeating nystagmus," not gaze-evoked nystagmus.

Gaze-evoked nystagmus is thought to be a result of poor gaze holding caused by an abnormal "neural integrator,"[2] that is, a central nervous system circuit that converts (integrates in the mathematical sense) an eye velocity command to an eye position signal. The mechanism of gaze-evoked nystagmus is as follows: The viscoelastic restoring forces of the globe tend to bring the eye toward the primary, that is, straight-ahead position. In order to keep the eye on a target placed away from the primary position, a tonic level of neural activity is required to overcome these restoring forces. This required tonic level of activity during gaze away from the primary position declines quickly in patients with abnormalities of the neural integrator. With this decline of tonic activity, the eye gradually drifts back toward the primary position. This slow drift of the eyes during attempted gaze deviation is interrupted by quick (saccadic) eye movements that bring the eyes back toward the target, away from the primary position. This alternation of slow drift (as a result of a slowly declining tonic drive to the eye muscles) and the rapid repositioning movements constitute gaze-evoked nystagmus. Because the rapid repositioning movements are always in the direction of gaze, gaze-evoked nystagmus, by definition, always beats in the same direction as that of the gaze that evoked it.

There are multiple causes of gaze-evoked nystagmus. The most common causes are the effect of drugs such as anticonvulsants and structural abnormalities in the posterior fossa especially those affecting the cerebellum. The precise location of the gaze-holding mechanism (i.e., the "neural integrator") is unknown, but the nucleus prepositus hypoglossi, which is located in the medulla oblongata near the hypoglossal (twelfth cranial nerve) nucleus, is a likely candidate.[3] However, the integrity of the neural integrator probably also depends on the cerebellum because cerebellar lesions are so frequently associated with gaze-evoked nystagmus.

Downbeating nystagmus is, by definition, a nystagmus wherein the quick component is down or obliquely down and lateral (Fig. C3–2). Often, with oblique downbeating nystagmus on down and lateral gaze, there is a torsional component with the upper pole of the eye beating in the direction of lateral gaze. Downbeating nystagmus is thought to be caused by an imbalance of up versus down tonic drive to the eyes. This up-down imbalance may be a result of unequal central *vestibular* pathways so that there is a stronger tonic drive to move the eyes up as opposed to the drive to move the eyes down,[4] resulting in a slow drift up and resetting quick movements down. An alternative hypothesis is that downbeating nystagmus is caused by a vertical ocular *pursuit* asymmetry so that the eyes drift up.[5] In any case, the slow drifts up are interrupted by quick resets down, leading to downbeating nystagmus. Downbeating nystagmus is most often seen with lesions of the craniocervical junction.

This patient's spontaneous vestibular nystagmus is likely to be caused by a central vestibular imbalance arising from an impairment of vestibular nuclear

Figure C3-2
Shown are the direction and magnitude of nystagmus in each of the nine cardinal positions of gaze. Note that the nystagmus is oblique-torsional on downgaze and lateral gaze and that it is abolished by upgaze. Although it is common for patients with downbeating nystagmus to have nystagmus in only downgaze and lateral gaze, others have nystagmus that persists even with upward gaze. (With permission from Furman, JM: Nystagmus and the vestibular system. In Podos, SM, and Yanoff, M (eds): Textbook of Ophthalmology. New York: Gower Medical Publishers, 1993.[7])

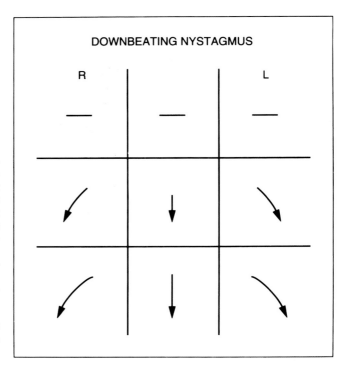

DOWNBEATING NYSTAGMUS

R   L

structures. As discussed in Chapter 1, spontaneous vestibular nystagmus usually results from a *peripheral* vestibular lesion. However, as in Case T4, medullary lesions involving the vestibular nuclei can also result in a tonic vestibular imbalance and cause spontaneous vestibular nystagmus on a *central* basis. The fact that this patient's spontaneous primary position nystagmus is seen only with a loss of fixation suggests that her fixational abilities allowed her to suppress her vestibular nystagmus. This ability to suppress vestibular nystagmus is somewhat surprising because the patient demonstrated impairment of ocular pursuit, which is considered to be very important for visual-vestibular interaction (see Case C11). In some patients, however, there can be a discrepancy between pursuit and vestibulo-ocular reflex fixations.[6]

DIAGNOSIS/DIFFERENTIAL DIAGNOSIS

This patient had a symptomatic *Chiari malformation* with associated ocular motor abnormalities and imbalance.

TREATMENT/MANAGEMENT

This patient was treated with a suboccipital craniectomy and decompression of her Chiari malformation. Following this treatment, the patient was symptomatically much improved with a resolution of her spontaneous vestibular nystagmus. Abnormal ocular pursuit, gaze-evoked nystagmus, and downbeating nystagmus persisted.

SUMMARY

A 19-year-old woman with a complaint of several years of dizziness and disequilibrium had signs of a posterior fossa abnormality. An MRI scan disclosed a Chiari malformation. The patient was treated with a suboccipital craniectomy and decompression. Symptoms of dizziness and disequilibrium were markedly reduced. The spontaneous vestibular nystagmus disappeared, but gaze-evoked and downbeating nystagmus persisted.

TEACHING POINTS

1. **Downbeating nystagmus** is, by definition, a nystagmus wherein the quick component is down or obliquely down and lateral. Downbeating nystagmus is thought to be caused by an imbalance of up versus down tonic drive to the eyes. Downbeating nystagmus is most often seen with lesions of the craniocervical junction.
2. **Downbeating nystagmus localizes the lesion** to the craniocervical junction. Causes include: (1) a Chiari malformation; (2) a mass lesion, such as a foramen magnum meningioma; or (3) demyelinating disease. Less likely causes include: (4) an infectious process such as a viral or postviral syndrome, (5) inflammatory disease, and (6) olivocerebellar degeneration syndrome.
3. **Gaze-evoked nystagmus** refers to a nystagmus that is left-beating on left lateral gaze, right-beating on right lateral gaze, and upbeating on upward gaze. Gaze-evoked nystagmus is typically conjugate. Nystagmus that beats down, even when seen only with downgaze, is considered "downbeating nystagmus" (see above),

not gaze-evoked nystagmus. Gaze-evoked nystagmus is thought to result from poor gaze holding arising from an abnormal "neural integrator," a central nervous system circuit that converts (integrates in the mathematical sense) an eye *velocity* command into an eye *position* signal. The most common causes of gaze-evoked nystagmus are the effect of drugs such as anticonvulsants and structural abnormalities in the posterior fossa, especially those affecting the cerebellum.

REFERENCES

1. Weber, PC, and Cass, SP: Neurotologic manifestations of Chiari 1 malformation. St. Louis: Mosby-Year Book, Inc., Otolaryngol Head Neck Surg 109:853–860, 1993.
2. Leigh, RJ, and Zee, DS (eds): The Neurology of Eye Movements, ed 2. Philadelphia: FA Davis, 1991.
3. Cannon, SC, and Robinson, DA: The final common integrator is in the prepositus and vestibular nuclei. In Keller, EL, and Zee, DS (eds): Adaptive Processes in Visual and Oculomotor Systems. Oxford: Pergamon Press, 1986.
4. Baloh, RW, and Spooner, JW: Downbeat nystagmus: A type of central vestibular nystagmus. Neurology 31:304–310, 1981.
5. Zee, DS, Friendlich AL, and Robinson, DA: The mechanism of downbeat nystagmus. Arch Neurol 30:227–237, 1974.
6. Chambers, B, and Gresty, M: The relationship between disordered pursuit and vestibulo-ocular reflex suppression. J Neurol Neurosurg Psychiatry 46:61–66, 1983.
7. Furman, JM: Nystagmus and the vestibular system. In Podos, SM, and Yanoff, M (eds): Textbook of Ophthalmology. New York: Gower Medical Publishers, 1993.

CASE

C4

Migraine

HISTORY

A 30-year-old man who worked as a bank teller presented with the chief complaint of dizziness for 6 weeks. The patient dated his symptoms to discontinuation of amitriptyline, which was being used for depression. He stated that he had discontinued his amitriptyline "to see if he could do without his antidepressant medication." The patient characterized his symptoms as a constant sense of lightheadedness and disequilibrium that was exacerbated by head movements and certain visual environments such as flickering lights and checkerboard patterns. He had no complaints of hearing loss; tinnitus; aural fullness; or abnormal vision, strength, sensation, or coordination. The patient related that before he had started amitriptyline 2 years before evaluation, he had also suffered from similar dizziness complaints, although they were less severe. These previous symptoms included episodic exacerbations, occasionally associated with headache.

Question 1: What are the diagnostic considerations in this case and what further history would be helpful?

Answer 1: This patient's dizziness and disequilibrium are nonspecific and not particularly suggestive of a peripheral vestibular disorder, given their character and time course. Myriad diagnostic considerations cannot be ruled out at this point in the evaluation. However, clues to the patient's diagnosis include the association with discontinuation of a tricyclic antidepressant, exacerbation by certain visual environments, and a previous history of headache. Further history should be obtained regarding precipitating factors and details of the past history of headaches and their association with dizziness. Also, any family history of a migrainous disorder would be helpful.

ADDITIONAL HISTORY

When asked about the association between his dizziness and headache, the patient volunteered that during the previous 2 years he had suffered three or four episodes of severe unilateral throbbing headache associated with nausea, lightheadedness, and disequilibrium that were more severe than his symptoms now but similar in character. He noted that headaches were more frequent before his treatment with a tricyclic antidepressant and that most of his headaches were associated with dizziness and disequilibrium. The patient's family history was significant for his mother and his paternal aunt, who suffered from "migraine headaches."

Question 2: How does this additional history affect this patient's diagnosis?

Answer 2: The characteristics of the patient's headaches, coupled with the positive family history, make migraine-associated dizziness the most likely diagnosis.[1] A vestibulopathy unrelated to headaches is possible. Much less likely are vertebrobasilar insufficiency or a craniovertebral junction abnormality. A thorough examination and appropriate laboratory testing may aid the diagnosis.

PHYSICAL EXAMINATION

The patient had normal general, neurologic, otologic, and neurotologic examinations.

Question 3: What laboratory testing, if any, would be helpful in establishing this patient's diagnosis?

Answer 3: There is no definitive laboratory test to diagnose migraine-associated dizziness, which is a diagnosis of exclusion. The patient has nothing in the history or the physical examination to suggest a structural neurologic abnormality, and thus brain imaging is not indicated at this point in the evaluation. Vestibular laboratory testing might suggest an alternative diagnosis as well as provide information regarding the status of the patient's balance system.

Audiometric testing should be obtained to screen for asymmetric hearing loss that may indicate the presence of a cerebellopontine angle or brainstem neoplasm or hearing loss suggestive of endolymphatic hydrops.

Laboratory Testing

Vestibular Laboratory Testing

ELECTRONYSTAGMOGRAPHY:	Ocular motor testing, positional testing, and caloric testing were normal.
ROTATIONAL TESTING:	Rotational testing revealed a right directional preponderance.
POSTUROGRAPHY:	Posturography was normal.

Audiometric Testing: Normal

Imaging: Not performed

Other: None

Question 4: In what ways can migraine manifest itself as dizziness and disequilibrium?

Answer 4: Migraine-associated dizziness can present as a vertiginous aura *preceding* a migraine headache in much the same way as positive visual phenomena or auras such as scintillating scotomata and fortification spectra. Dizziness, disequilibrium, and vertigo can occur *during* a migraine headache. Some patients with migraine-associated dizziness have "migraine without headache," also known as migraine equivalent, or dizziness separate from or instead of headaches. Some patients, like this one, may experience disequilibrium *between* episodes, that is, more or less constantly.[2] This patient's symptoms are typical of migraine-associated dizziness, which often includes dizziness and disequilibrium exacerbated by certain visual environments.

Question 5: What vestibular laboratory abnormalities have been described in patients with migraine and how can they be explained pathophysiologically?

Answer 5: The vestibular abnormalities that have been described in patients with migraine include abnormalities on electronystagmography, rotational testing, and posturography.[3,4] Table C4–1 indicates the percentage of patients with migraine who have abnormal vestibular laboratory testing.[3,5] By far the most common abnormality noted was a directional preponderance on rotational testing. The abnormalities in Table C4–1 suggest a peripheral vestibular component in some patients, such as those with a reduced vestibular response, and a central vestibular abnormality in others, such as those with a directional preponderance. A smaller but not insignificant number of patients with migraine-related dizziness show either a spontaneous or a positional nystagmus or both. Posturography abnormalities that can be ascribed to the vestibular system in patients with migraine or related dizziness are uncommon.

The pathophysiology of the vestibular abnormalities in migraine-related dizziness is uncertain. Cutrer and Baloh[1] have proposed an asymmetry in neuropeptide release at the efferent vestibular terminals. Whether such a phenomenon actually occurs is unknown. Moreover, how such a mechanism accounts for vestibular abnormalities *between* episodes is also uncertain. Cass and colleagues[5] have suggested that serotonin may play a role in the vestibular abnormalities seen with migraine either through direct effects or through release of neuropeptides. Such activation of serotonergic or peptidergic pathways could be asymmetric, thereby producing asymmetric activation of central vestibular pathways. Alternately, even symmetric activation of serotonergic or peptidergic pathways might produce vestibular imbalance

TABLE C4–1
Most Common Patterns of Abnormalities on Vestibular Tests Including Electronystagmography, Rotational Testing, and Posturography in Migraine-Related Vestibulopathy (N = 100)

Pattern	Percent
Normal	27
Isolated directional preponderance on rotation	22
Directional preponderance on rotation + reduced vestibular response	12
Directional preponderance on rotation + abnormal posturography	9
Directional preponderance on rotation + reduced vestibular response + abnormal posturography	6
Isolated reduced vestibular response	5
Isolated abnormal posturography	4

Source: Cass, SP, et al: Migraine-related vestibulopathy. Ann Otol Rhinol Laryngol (in press), with permission.[5]

by unmasking latent asymmetries that may be inherent in an individual's balance system.

DIAGNOSIS/DIFFERENTIAL DIAGNOSIS

This patient's diagnosis was *migraine-associated dizziness*. His condition was exacerbated by discontinuation of amitriptyline, which was evidently acting as an antimigrainous agent.

TREATMENT/MANAGEMENT

Question 6: What are the treatment options for a patient with migraine-associated dizziness and what factors should be considered?

Answer 6: The treatment options for patients with migraine-associated dizziness are outlined in Table C4–2. First, it is necessary to educate the patient regarding the association of dizziness with the underlying migrainous condition and the importance of avoiding of dietary triggers such as tyramine-containing foods, alcohol, and caffeine; and avoiding stress and fatigue. Second, the underlying migrainous condition should be treated with prophylactic medications, even if headaches are not currently prominent. Our experience is that a third to half of patients respond favorably to each of the types of medications listed in Table C4–2. If the initial medication is unsuccessful, the other classes of agents should be tried in turn. Third, if the most prominent vestibular symptoms are movement-associated disequilibrium, vestibular rehabilitation therapy is recommended. Fourth, if the patient reports severe space and motion discomfort, we use anti–motion-sickness medications, such as a combination of phenergan and pseudoephedrine or a mild vestibular suppressant agent such as low-dose diazepam. Finally, in patients with panic attacks or agoraphobia we obtain

TABLE C4–2
Treatment Options for Migraine-Related Vestibulopathy

1. Avoid dietary triggers
2. Treat underlying migraine phenomenon
   - Tricyclic antidepressants (e.g., amitriptyline 50–100 mg/day)
   - Beta blockers (e.g., propranolol 80–320 mg/day)
   - Calcium channel blockers (e.g., verapamil 80–120 mg/day)
3. Treat movement-associated disequilibrium
   - Vestibular rehabilitation therapy
4. Treat space and motion discomfort
   - Phenergan/pseudoephedrine (25 mg/60 mg BID)
5. Treat associated anxiety or panic disorder
   - Behavioral therapy
   - Pharmacotherapy
       Tricyclic antidepressants
       Anxiolytic, e.g., benzodiazepine

Source: Cass, SP et al: Migraine-related vestibulopathy. Ann Otol Rhinol Laryngol (in press), with permission.[5]

psychiatric consultation and rely on both behavioral therapy as well as specific medical therapy using tricyclic antidepressants or anxiolytic medications.

This patient was restarted on amitriptyline and advised regarding dietary restriction. His symptoms of dizziness resolved.

SUMMARY

A 30-year-old man presented with dizziness and disequilibrium after discontinuation of a tricyclic anticyclic antidepressant. There was a past history of headache, and the patient's complaints were consistent with migraine-associated dizziness. This diagnosis was further supported by a positive family history of migraine. The patient was treated with reintroduction of amitriptyline 50 mg before sleep. This significantly reduced his daily symptoms, although he continued to have migraine headaches associated with dizziness approximately once every 6 months.

TEACHING POINTS

1. **Migraine-associated dizziness** should be suspected in patients with nonspecific dizziness or vertigo associated with headache, a significant past history of headaches, or positive family history of a migrainous disorder. Patients with migraine-associated dizziness almost invariably report exacerbation of symptoms by viewing certain moving visual environments or significant motion sickness sensitivity.

2. **Migraine can manifest itself as dizziness and disequilibrium** in a number of different ways. Migraine-associated dizziness can present as a vertiginous aura *preceding* a migraine headache in much the same way as positive visual phenomena or auras, such as scintillating scotomata and fortification spectra. Dizziness, disequilibrium, and vertigo can occur *during* a migraine headache. Some patients with migraine-associated dizziness have "migraine without headache," also known as migraine equivalent, that is, dizziness separate from or instead of headaches. Some patients, like this patient, may experience disequilibrium *between* episodes, that is, more or less constantly. This patient's symptoms are typical of migraine-associated dizziness, which often includes dizziness and disequilibrium exacerbated by certain visual environments.

3. **Vestibular laboratory abnormalities in migraine-associated dizziness** include a directional preponderance on rotational testing, and less often, a unilateral caloric weakness, positional nystagmus, or spontaneous nystagmus. Commonly, vestibulospinal dysfunction is found on posturography testing.

4. **Treatment options for patients with migraine-associated dizziness** are summarized in Table C4–2. First, the patient should be informed about the association of dizziness with the underlying migrainous condition and the importance of avoiding of dietary triggers such as tyramine-containing foods, alcohol, and caffeine; and avoiding stress and fatigue. Second, the underlying migrainous condition should be treated with prophylactic antimigrainous medications even if headaches are not currently prominent. Third, if the most prominent vestibular symptom is movement-associated disequilibrium or unsteadiness, vestibular rehabilitation therapy is recommended. Fourth, if the patient reports severe space and motion discomfort, anti–motion-sickness medications such as the combination of phenergan and pseudoephedrine or a mild vestibular suppressant agent such as low-dose diaze-

pam should be used. Finally, in patients with panic attacks or agoraphobia, psychiatric consultation should be obtained and both behavioral therapy as well as specific medical therapy using tricyclic antidepressants or anxiolytic medications should be relied on.

REFERENCES

1. Cutrer, FW, and Baloh, RW: Migraine-associated dizziness. Headache 32:300–304, 1992.
2. Kayan, A, and Hood, JD: Neuro-otological manifestations of migraine. Brain 107:1123–1142, 1984.
3. Eviatar, L: Vestibular testing in basilar artery migraine. Ann Neurol 9:126–130, 1980.
4. Olsson, J: Neurotologic findings in basilar migraine. Laryngoscope 101:1–41, 1991.
5. Cass, SP, et al: Migraine-related vestibulopathy. Ann Otol Rhinol Laryngol (in press).

C A S E
C5

Vascular Supply of the Central Vestibular System

HISTORY

A 70-year-old man presented with episodic dizziness. The patient's symptoms had been particularly troublesome during the last 6 weeks. He described spontaneous episodes occurring about twice a week, characterized by the acute onset of vertigo and a tendency to fall to the right, lasting for seconds to a few minutes. There were no clear precipitating factors such as changes in head position. The patient had no complaints of hearing loss or tinnitus. Past history was significant for hypertension and peptic ulcer disease. Current medications included an angiotensin converting enzyme inhibitor and an H_2 blocking agent.

Question 1: What are the diagnostic considerations in this case and what further historic information would be helpful in establishing a diagnosis?

Answer 1: This patient's symptoms are suggestive of an episodic dysfunction of peripheral vestibular function such as recurrent vestibulopathy, endolymphatic hydrops, or benign positional vertigo. The absence of symptoms related to changes in head position makes benign positional vertigo less likely. The frequency of vertigo attacks without associated otologic symptoms, coupled with the patient's age and history of hypertension, suggest the possibility of vertebrobasilar insufficiency. A structural abnormality of the posterior fossa is another diagnostic possibility. A thorough history regarding associated neurologic complaints would be helpful in establishing a diagnosis. A family history would also be helpful.

ADDITIONAL HISTORY

Upon careful questioning, the patient noted that with several of his vertiginous episodes he had experienced circumoral paresthesias and, on one occasion, double vision. His family related that during some of the patient's episodes his speech was often difficult

114

TABLE C5–1
Initial Symptoms of Vertebrobasilar Insufficiency

Symptoms	Percentage
Vertigo	48
Visual hallucinations	10
Drop attacks or weakness	10
Visceral sensations	8
Visual field defects	6
Diplopia	5
Headaches	3
Other	8

Source: Adapted from Baloh, RW, and Honrubia, V: Clinical Neurophysiology of the Vestibular System, 2d ed. Philadelphia: FA Davis, 1990, p 221.[4]

to understand and he walked "like he was drunk." The patient had no family history of neurologic or otologic disease.

Question 2: What are the characteristic features of vertebrobasilar insufficiency and what information would be helpful in establishing this as the patient's diagnosis?

Answer 2: It has been stated[1] that vertigo alone is rarely a symptom of vertebrobasilar insufficiency especially if the vertigo is chronic. However, this clinical dictum is controversial because Grad and Baloh[2] have indicated that vertigo alone can be the presenting sign of vertebrobasilar insufficiency. Table C5–1 indicates the initial symptoms of vertebrobasilar insufficiency in 65 patients. Note that vertigo appears in this list. Patients with vertebrobasilar insufficiency can experience vertigo in isolation for up to 1.5 years.[2] Table C5–2 indicates associated symptoms in patients with vertebrobasilar insufficiency.

A complete physical examination and brain imaging are likely to add additional diagnostic information to this case.

TABLE C5–2
Symptoms Associated with Vertebrobasilar Insufficiency

Symptoms	Percentage
Visual dysfunction	69
Drop attacks	33
Unsteadiness, incoordination	21
Extremity weakness	21
Confusion	17
Headache	14
Hearing loss	14
Loss of consciousness	10
Extremity numbness	10
Dysarthria	10
Tinnitus	10
Perioral numbness	5

Source: Adapted from Grad, A, and Baloh, RW: Vertigo of vascular origin. Arch Neurol 46:281–284, 1989.[2]

PHYSICAL EXAMINATION

The patient had an entirely normal general, neurologic, otologic, and neuro-otologic examination with the exception of several "soft" neurologic signs, including a very mild left pronator drift and an equivocal Babinski sign on the left. The patient had a slightly widened base to his gait and had difficulty tandem walking. He had difficulty standing on a compliant foam surface with his eyes closed. Dix-Hallpike maneuvers were negative.

Laboratory Testing

Vestibular Laboratory Testing

ELECTRONYSTAGMOGRAPHY: Not performed

ROTATIONAL TESTING: Not performed

POSTUROGRAPHY: Not performed

Audiometric Testing: Not performed

Imaging: An MRI scan of the head revealed an old infarction of the right frontal lobe, a right internal carotid artery occlusion, and bilateral white matter hyperintensities in the periventricular white matter. There were no obvious abnormalities in the brainstem or cerebellum.

Other: None

DIAGNOSIS/DIFFERENTIAL DIAGNOSIS

Question 3: Based on the history, physical examination, and laboratory studies, what is this patient's most likely diagnosis and why?

Answer 3: The patient's episodes are not typical of benign positional vertigo and Dix-Hallpike maneuvers were negative. There was no acute syndrome to suggest vestibular neuritis. A "vestibular-only" form of Meniere's disease (see Cases T3, T9, C10, C14, and C16) is possible, but the patient's episodes are brief compared to typical symptoms seen with endolymphatic hydrops, and some of the patient's episodes are associated with neurologic deficits. Migraine-associated dizziness (see Cases C4, C12, U12, and U16) is also a diagnostic possibility, but there is no prior history of headache or family history of migraine. Thus, the patient is probably suffering from vertebrobasilar insufficiency, considering the combination of symptoms that characterize his attacks, his history of hypertension, and evidence of cerebrovascular disease on brain imaging. However, this diagnosis is not certain.

The patient was given a diagnosis of *vertebrobasilar insufficiency*.

TREATMENT/MANAGEMENT

This patient was treated with an antiplatelet agent. The frequency of his vertiginous episodes decreased markedly, but dizziness episodes still occurred.

Question 4: What is the vascular supply of the vestibular system? What is the pathophysiologic basis for this patient's vertiginous episodes?

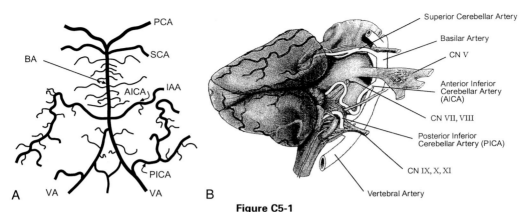

Figure C5-1

Blood supply to the brainstem and cerebellum. (*A*) Schematic drawing of the vertebral-basilar arterial tree. PCA = posterior cerebral artery; SCA = superior cerebellar artery; AICA = anterior inferior cerebellar artery; IAA = internal auditory canal artery; PICA = posterior inferior cerebellar artery; VA = vertebral artery; BA = basilar artery. (*B*) Drawing highlighting each of the three neurovascular complexes of the posterior fossa. The upper complex is related to the superior cerebellar artery; the middle complex is related to the anterior inferior cerebellar artery; the lower complex is related to the posterior inferior cerebellar artery. [(*A*) Modified with permission from Oas, JG, and Baloh, RW: Vertigo and the anterior inferior cerebellar artery syndrome. Neurology 42:2274–2279, 1992.[5] (*B*) With permission from Rhoton, AL: Microsurgical anatomy of posterior fossa cranial nerves. In Barrow, DL (ed): Surgery of the Cranial Nerves of the Posterior Fossa. American Associations of Neurological Surgeons, 1993.[6])

Answer 4: Figure C5–1A is a schematic diagram of the blood supply to the vestibular system including the vertebral arteries and the basilar artery. Note that the posterior-inferior cerebellar artery, which arises from the vertebral artery, supplies the vestibular nuclei, while the anterior-inferior cerebellar artery, which arises from the basilar artery, supplies the vestibulocerebellum and gives rise to the internal auditory artery (labyrinthine artery), which, in turn, gives rise to the anterior vestibular artery.

Ischemia in the vertebrobasilar artery system can cause vestibular symptoms on the basis of either peripheral vestibular dysfunction, central vestibular dysfunction, or both (Fig. C5–1B). Because the vestibular nuclei are supplied by the posterior-inferior cerebellar artery, a brief interruption of the vertebral artery or of the posterior-inferior cerebellar artery itself can cause transient symptoms similar to those experienced in Wallenberg's syndrome (see Case T4). Because the anterior-inferior cerebellar artery supplies the labyrinth and the vestibulocerebellum, a brief interruption of this artery can also lead to episodic vestibular symptoms (see also Case U4). It has been hypothesized by Baloh[3] that the vertigo seen with vertebrobasilar insufficiency is probably related to labyrinthine ischemia. For much of the blood supply to the vestibular system, the arteries are end-arterial and therefore the opportunity for collateral circulation is limited. This is especially true for the blood supply to the peripheral vestibular system, as well as for the small perforating arteries that arise from the vertebrobasilar system. The patient-to-patient variability in the vertebrobasilar system leads to variability in presentation, so that it may be difficult to ascribe particular symptoms to specific arterial territories.

SUMMARY

A 70-year-old man presented with episodic vertigo lasting for minutes and occasionally associated with double vision, slurred speech, and ataxic gait. The patient had a past history of hypertension. Examination revealed "soft" neurologic signs, and brain imaging revealed evidence of cerebrovascular disease. The patient was given the diagnosis of vertebrobasilar insufficiency and treated with an antiplatelet agent.

TEACHING POINTS

1. **The blood supply of the vestibular system** includes: (1) the posterior-inferior cerebellar artery, which arises from the vertebral artery and supplies the vestibular nuclei; (2) the anterior-inferior cerebellar artery, which arises from the basilar artery and supplies the vestibulocerebellum; and (3) the internal auditory artery, which arises from the anterior-inferior cerebellar artery and gives rise to the anterior vestibular artery, which supplies the vestibular apparatus.
2. **Ischemia in the vertebrobasilar artery** system can cause vestibular symptoms on the basis of either peripheral vestibular dysfunction, central vestibular dysfunction, or both. For much of the blood supply to the vestibular system, the arteries are end-arterial and therefore the opportunity for collateral circulation is limited, especially for the blood supply to the peripheral vestibular system.
3. **A diagnosis of vertebrobasilar insufficiency** should be reserved for patients who have clearly defined episodes of transient neurologic symptoms and signs that can be localized to the posterior circulation. Vertebrobasilar insufficiency can present with many different neurologic symptoms. Even if vertigo is not the presenting complaint of vertebrobasilar insufficiency, eventually most patients with vertebrobasilar insufficiency experience vertigo on one or more occasions.
4. **Isolated vertigo** is rarely a symptom of vertebrobasilar insufficiency. However, vertigo associated with definitive neurologic symptoms, especially in a patient with risk factors for cerebrovascular disease, should lead to a consideration of vertebrobasilar insufficiency.

REFERENCES

1. Fisher, CM: Vertigo in cerebrovascular disease. Arch Otolaryngol 85:529–534, 1967.
2. Grad, A, and Baloh, RW: Vertigo of vascular origin. Arch Neurol 46:281–284, 1989.
3. Baloh, RW: Otological aspects of cerebrovascular disease. In Tool, JF (ed): Handbook of Clinical Neurology, Vol. 11: Vascular Diseases, Part III. New York: Elsevier Science Publishers, 1989.
4. Baloh, RW, and Honrubia, V: Clinical Neurophysiology of the Vestibular System, 2nd ed. Philadelphia: FA Davis, 1990.
5. Oas, JG, and Baloh, RW: Vertigo and the anterior inferior cerebellar artery syndrome. Neurology 42: 2274–2279, 1992.
6. Rhoton, AL: Microsurgical anatomy of posterior fossa cranial nerves. In Barrow, DL (ed): Surgery of the Cranial Nerves of the Posterior Fossa. American Association of Neurological Surgeons, 1993.

C6

Bilateral Vestibular Loss

HISTORY

A 59-year-old woman who did not work outside the home presented with a complaint of dizziness, difficulty with vision, and instability while walking, especially in dimly lit environments or when the floor was uneven. The patient's complaints were constant during the previous 6 months. The patient was asymptomatic when sitting or lying still. Visual complaints were most noticeable when she was moving her head rapidly or riding in a motor vehicle, during which she experienced jumbling of the visual surroundings. Meclizine provided no relief from the patient's symptoms, but was still being used on an as-needed basis. There was no complaint of hearing loss, tinnitus, or aural fullness. The patient also had no complaints of double vision, loss of vision, weakness, loss of sensation, or incoordination aside from difficulty walking.

Question 1: Based on this portion of the patient's history, what are the diagnostic considerations?

Answer 1: The patient's complaints do not suggest a peripheral vestibular ailment because of the constant imbalance, absence of vertigo, and the absence of associated complaints of hearing loss or tinnitus. The patient may be suffering from a central nervous system abnormality affecting the balance system, such as a cerebellar abnormality. However, the fact that the patient's ambulation is worse in dimly lit environments suggests a vestibular component. Also, the patient's poor vision when the head is moving, particularly in motor vehicles, suggests an impaired vestibulo-ocular reflex.

ADDITIONAL HISTORY

Upon further questioning, the patient related that she had noted the onset of her symptoms approximately 1 week after discharge from the hospital where she had been admitted because of cholecystitis. She had been treated with intravenous gentamicin for

119

2 weeks before evaluation. The patient stated that, to the best of her knowledge, her gentamicin was given at an appropriate dose, with drug levels obtained regularly. The patient also indicated she had a past history of Sjögren's syndrome that was in remission for approximately 2 years. There was no significant family history.

PHYSICAL EXAMINATION

General examination was normal. Neurologic examination revealed full extraocular movements without nystagmus. The patient's visual symptoms could be reproduced by applying a gentle vibration just lateral to the outer canthus of the eye while the opposite eye was occluded. During ophthalmoscopy, the patient was asked to move her head back and forth at a high frequency with very small excursions.[1] The optic disc was noted to move with the patient's head movements rather than remain stable in space (see Case T2). The remainder of the neurologic examination was normal, except that the patient had gait ataxia with a widened base. The patient was unable to stand on a compliant foam surface with her eyes closed without falling. There was no nystagmus with Frenzel glasses. Otologic examination was normal.

Question 2: Based upon the additional historical information and the physical examination, what is the patient's likely diagnosis?

Answer 2: This patient is probably suffering from bilateral vestibular loss as a result of aminoglycoside ototoxicity, which causes hair cell damage. Compare Figure C6–1B to Figure C6–1A. The patient is manifesting Dandy's syndrome, that is, the combination of oscillopsia (a jumbling of the visual surround) and gait ataxia[2] caused by the bilateral loss of vestibular function. Dandy introduced vestibular nerve section as a treatment for Meniere's disease in 1928.[3] Many of Dandy's patients underwent bilateral vestibular nerve sections that resulted in the symptoms of oscillopsia and gait ataxia, a symptom complex that now bears his name. The motion of the fundus during head movement indicates a reduced vestibulo-ocular reflex. The past history of Sjögren's syndrome is of uncertain significance. Because Sjögren's syndrome is an autoimmune disorder that may be associated with vestibular loss (see Case C24), the patient may have had a combination of autoimmune inner ear disease and ototoxicity. By some unknown mechanism, the patient may have been more susceptible to ototoxicity because of her Sjögren's syndrome.

Question 3: What are the causes of bilateral vestibular loss? What laboratory tests should be requested?

Answer 3: Bilateral vestibular loss is most commonly a result of ototoxicity from aminoglycosides, including gentamicin, tobramycin, and streptomycin. Commonly used medications that are ototoxic are listed in Table C6–1. Other pharmaceutical agents, such as cisplatinum, can cause bilateral vestibular loss. Other diagnostic considerations for bilateral vestibular loss besides ototoxicity include autoimmune inner ear disease and syphilis. Thus, further laboratory testing should include rheumatologic parameters, such as an erythrocyte sedimentation rate and antinuclear antibody measurement, and a serum fluorescent treponemal antibody absorption test (FTA-ABS). Audiometry should be performed to determine whether or not there is a hearing loss associated with the patient's ototoxic drug exposure. Quantitative

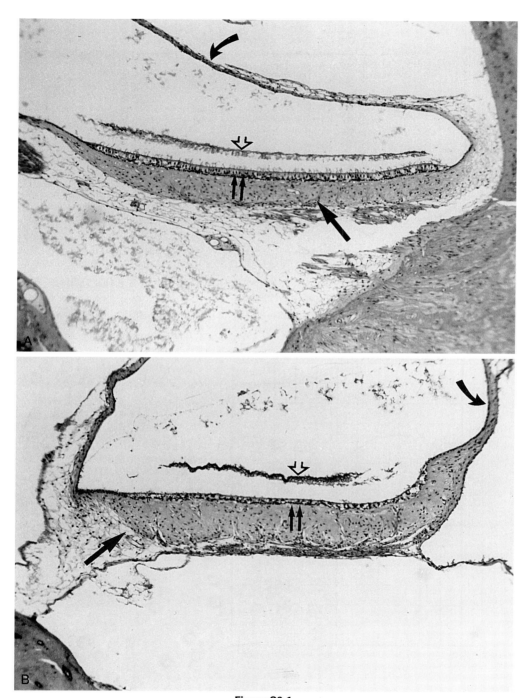

Figure C6-1

Histopathology of aminoglycoside ototoxicity. (*A*) Normal utricular macula. (*B*) Utricular macula following aminoglycoside-induced ototoxicity. Note flattening of the sensory epithelium and loss of stereocilia, denoting destruction of the utricular hair cells. Thick straight arrow = utricular macula; double arrows = sensory epithelium (hair cells) with stereocilia extending from their upper surface (panel A); otolithic membrane (cupula); curved arrow = endolymphatic membrane surrounding the utricle.

TABLE C6–1
Commonly Used Ototoxic Medications

Aminoglycoside antibiotics
  Streptomycin
  Gentamicin
  Tobramycin
Chemotherapeutic/Anticancer Agents
  Cisplatinum
Diuretics
  Furosemide
  Ethacrynic acid
Erythromycin
Salicylates

vestibular laboratory testing, including rotational testing, should be requested to confirm the extent of vestibular loss.

Note that in the case of bilateral vestibular loss in the presence of bilateral hearing loss, the patient should have an MRI scan to rule out the unlikely occurrence of bilateral mass lesions such as acoustic neuroma or cerebellopontine angle tumors.

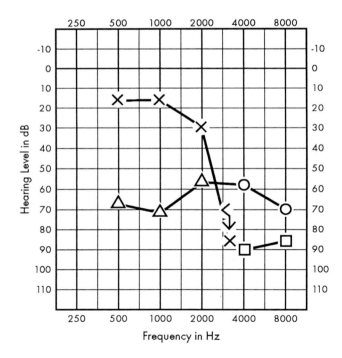

Word Recognition Score				Right	Left
Right : 40%	Air	unmasked		O—O	X—X
		masked		△—△	□—□
Left : 76%	Bone	unmasked		◄- - -◄	►- - -►
		masked		E- - -[	]- - -]

Figure C6-2
Audiogram.

Laboratory Testing

Vestibular Laboratory Testing

ELECTRONYSTAGMOGRAPHY: Ocular motor testing was normal. There was no static positional nystagmus. Caloric testing revealed absent responses even to ice water irrigation.

ROTATIONAL TESTING: Rotational testing revealed markedly reduced responses such that there were no eye movements generated at frequencies below 0.5 Hz and there were only a few beats of nystagmus following deceleration from a constant velocity rotation of 90 degrees per second.

POSTUROGRAPHY: Posturography indicated excessive sway on conditions 5 and 6, that is, a vestibular pattern.

Audiometric Testing: Audiometric testing indicated a bilateral asymmetric sensorineural hearing loss (Fig. C6–2). The left ear had primarily a high-frequency hearing loss. The right ear had a flat hearing loss.

Imaging: The patient had a normal erythrocyte sedimentation rate and negative antinuclear antibody and FTA-ABS measurements.

Other: None

DIAGNOSIS/DIFFERENTIAL DIAGNOSIS

This patient is manifesting bilateral vestibular loss as a result of aminoglycoside *ototoxicity*.

TREATMENT/MANAGEMENT

Question 4: Prevention is the best management for ototoxicity. What factors should alert the physician to the possible occurrence of ototoxicity?

Answer 4: The major risk factors for the occurrence of bilateral vestibulopathy when using ototoxic drugs include impaired renal function, age greater than 65, prior use of ototoxic drugs, high serum levels, pre-existing sensorineural hearing loss, and medical course greater than 14 days. Symptoms of bilateral vestibular loss can be progressive and also delayed from weeks to months even after the drug has been stopped.[4]

Question 5: Based on the patient's diagnosis and laboratory tests, what are the appropriate strategies for managing this patient's disequilibrium?

Answer 5: This patient is suffering from bilateral vestibular loss. Treatment should include discontinuation of all vestibular-suppressant medications. Also, the patient should be referred for a course of balance rehabilitation therapy to encourage the use of sensory input other than that from the vestibular system, such as from vision and proprioception. A properly fitted cane can provide increased proprioceptive input. The patient should also be cautioned to remove all loose rugs from the home, install night lights, and install hand rails on stairways and in the bathroom.

Question 6: Aside from discontinuing vestibular suppressants and encouraging the use of alternative sensory inputs, what other modalities are available to patients with

TABLE C6–2
Strategies for Patients with Bilateral Vestibular Loss

Sensory substitution
Altered patterns of head motion
Preprogramming of slow components in anticipation of head
  movements
Potentiation of cervico-ocular reflex
Saccadic substitution
Perceptual adjustments to decrease oscillopsia

bilateral vestibular loss to develop spatial orientation and stable vision while the head
is moving?

Answer 6: Possible strategies for patients with bilateral vestibular loss are listed in
Table C6–2. The use of nonvestibular sensory input such as vision and proprioception
is the primary means of partially overcoming the effects of bilateral vestibular loss.
During head movements, stabilization of vision can be achieved, in part, by alterations
of patterns of head movement such that the head is moved more slowly. Some
patients can learn to "preprogram" slow compensatory movements in anticipation of
head movements. Also, the cervico-ocular reflex can be potentiated in such patients[5]
(see Case C7). Saccadic eye movements can be substituted for slow eye
movements. There can be a perceptual adjustment to decrease the effect of
oscillopsia.[6] These behavioral adjustments may occur spontaneously to a greater or
lesser extent in an individual patient. However, by working with a physical therapist,
patients with bilateral vestibular loss can be helped to achieve optimal ocular motor
and balance function while decreasing symptoms.[7]

The patient was treated with discontinuation of vestibular suppressant medications
and a course of vestibular rehabilitation therapy.

FOLLOW-UP

The patient improved somewhat, especially in regard to her symptoms of dizziness
while still. Unfortunately, although improved, the patient still had oscillopsia and gait
instability in poorly lighted environments and poor balance when walking on uneven
flooring.

SUMMARY

A 59-year-old woman presented with oscillopsia and ataxia that began following treatment with an aminoglycoside antibiotic for cholecystitis. The patient had a past history
of Sjögren's syndrome that may have predisposed the patient to ototoxicity. Laboratory
testing confirmed the presence of bilateral vestibular loss and did not reveal any evidence of autoimmune disease. The patient was treated with discontinuation of vestibular-suppressant medications, a cane, and a course of balance rehabilitation therapy
designed to train the patient to use other sensory modalities and to adopt other behav-
iors to substitute for her vestibular function. Following treatment, the patient had decreased symptoms and was functionally improved but still impaired.

TEACHING POINTS

1. **The combination of oscillopsia and ataxia** (Dandy's syndrome) is pathognomonic for bilateral vestibular loss.

2. **Bilateral vestibular loss** most commonly occurs as a result of aminoglycoside-induced ototoxicity. Other pharmaceutical agents such as cisplatinum can also cause bilateral vestibular loss. Bilateral vestibular loss may also be caused by bilateral Meniere's disease, autoimmune inner ear disease, otosyphilis, or may be idiopathic. Patients with bilateral acoustic neuromas (neurofibromatosis type 2) also manifest bilateral vestibular loss.

3. **Laboratory testing of patients with bilateral vestibular loss** should include rheumatologic parameters, such as an erythrocyte sedimentation rate and antinuclear antibody and serum FTA-ABS measurements. Audiometry should be performed to evaluate the pattern of any associated hearing loss. Quantitative vestibular laboratory testing should be requested to confirm the extent of vestibular loss. Rotational testing is particularly helpful in this regard. MR imaging should be performed in cases of suspected neurofibromatosis type 2.

4. **Prevention is the best management for ototoxicity.** The major risk factors for the occurrence of bilateral vestibulopathy when using ototoxic drugs include impaired renal function, age greater than 65, prior use of ototoxic drugs, high serum levels, pre-existing sensorineural hearing loss, and an ototoxic drug exposure longer than 14 days. Symptoms of bilateral vestibular loss can be progressive and also can be delayed for weeks to months following discontinuation of the ototoxic medication.

5. **Treatment for bilateral vestibular loss** should include discontinuation of all vestibular suppressant medications and referral for a course of balance rehabilitation therapy to encourage the use of sensory input other than that from the vestibular system, such as from vision and proprioception. A properly fitted cane can provide increased proprioceptive input. The patient should also be cautioned to remove all loose rugs from the home, install night lights, and install hand rails on stairways and in the bathroom. If possible, the patient should not receive further ototoxic medications.

REFERENCES

1. Zee, DS: Ophthalmoscopy in examination of patients with vestibular disorders. Ann Neurol 3:373–374, 1978.
2. "JC": Living without a balancing mechanism. N Engl J Med 246:458–460, 1952.
3. Dandy, WE: Meniere's disease: Its diagnosis and methods of treatment. Arch Surg 16:1127, 1928.
4. Rybak, LP, and Matz, GJ: Auditory and vestibular effects of toxins. Manifestations of Systemic Disease. In Cummings, W (ed): Otolaryngology—Head and Neck Surgery, Vol. 4. St Louis: CV Mosby, 1986, pp 3161–3172.
5. Kasai, T, and Zee, DS: Eye-head coordination in labyrinthine-defective human beings. Brain Res 144:123–141, 1978.
6. Wist, ER, Brandt, T, and Krafczyk, S: Oscillopsia and retinal slip. Brain 106:153–168, 1983.
7. Herdman, SJ (ed): Vestibular Rehabilitation. Philadelphia: FA Davis, 1994.

C A S E
C7

Cervical Vertigo

HISTORY

A 49-year-old man who worked as a delivery van driver presented with the chief complaint of dizziness and lightheadedness during the previous 5 months. The patient had symptoms that fluctuated daily. Symptoms were exacerbated by head movements. The patient had no complaints of hearing loss or tinnitus and no neurologic complaints. He dated the onset of symptoms to an automobile accident in which he was struck from the rear, causing him to experience a flexion-extension "whiplash" injury of the neck. The patient did not strike his head or lose consciousness during the accident. His symptoms were worse on those days when he experienced neck pain or neck muscle spasm. There was no significant past medical history. The family history was noncontributory.

Question 1: Based on the patient's history, what is the likely diagnosis?

Answer 1: Exacerbation of the patient's symptoms with head movement suggests a balance abnormality, possibly vestibular in origin. However, the close association of symptoms with *neck* pain and the onset following a neck injury suggests that this patient's complaints are likely to be a result of *cervical vertigo*.[1,2] Cervical vertigo is a poorly defined term associated with dizziness and disequilibrium thought to be caused by abnormal afferent activity from the neck. Other diagnostic considerations include benign positional vertigo, post-traumatic endolymphatic hydrops, peripheral vestibulopathy of uncertain etiology, or a central nervous system abnormality, structural or otherwise, that is now manifesting as dizziness either independent of or exacerbated by the motor vehicle accident.

PHYSICAL EXAMINATION

General, neurologic, and otologic examinations were normal, with the exception of a decreased range of motion at the neck and a complaint of feelings of disequilibrium when turning the head, especially when attempting to bring the chin to the shoulder in either direction. Head-fixed body-turned maneuvers (Fig. C7–1) were performed with Frenzel glasses with the head held still and the body turned while the patient sat

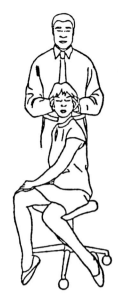 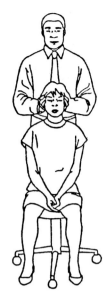 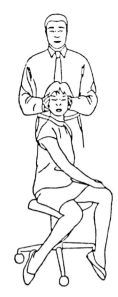

Figure C7-1
Head-fixed body-turned maneuvers. With the patient on a swivel chair, the examiner stabilizes the head while the patient turns the body in such a way that there is a rotation of the torso with respect to the head, thereby stimulating the neck without stimulating the labyrinth. (With permission from Fitz-Ritson, D: Assessment of cervicogenic vertigo. J Manipulative Physiol Ther 14(3):193–198, 1991, p 195.[9])

on a swivel chair (see Case T2). He experienced dizziness and was noted to have several beats of right-beating nystagmus during rotation of the body to the left while he was looking straight ahead.

Question 2: Based on the history and physical examination, what is this patient's likely diagnosis? What laboratory tests would be helpful in establishing a diagnosis?

Answer 2: This patient's history and physical examination are suggestive of cervical vertigo with a hyperactive cervico-ocular reflex. Given the uncertainty of this diagnosis and the controversial nature of cervical vertigo, both brain imaging and quantitative vestibular testing are warranted.

Laboratory Testing

Vestibular Laboratory Testing

ELECTRONYSTAGMOGRAPHY: Ocular motor function was normal.

ROTATIONAL TESTING: Not performed

POSTUROGRAPHY: Not performed

Audiometric Testing: Not performed

Imaging: The patient had a normal MRI of the brain.

Other: Right-beating nystagmus during head-fixed body-turned maneuvers was recorded with the body turned to the left. This was seen in both the lying and seated positions.

Question 3: What is the cervico-ocular reflex? What is a possible explanation for this patient's disequilibrium?

Answer 3: The cervico-ocular reflex is an eye movement response to relative movement of the head with respect to the torso, that is, neck movement. The reflex is based upon afferent activity from the *neck* rather than from the *labyrinth*. Relative movement between the head and the torso alters the neural activity relayed to the vestibular nuclei regarding head position. These afferents primarily comprise neck muscle proprioceptive fibers.[3] This innervation may arise from joint afferents in the neck.[3] Also, other nerves may arise from facet joints in the cervical spine. The cervico-ocular reflex is thought to be of minimal importance in normal individuals, because quantitative testing of the reflex has revealed minimal eye movements as a result of relative motion between the head and torso with the head fixed in space.[4–6] However, numerous case reports attest to the dizziness and disequilibrium experienced by patients who have sustained neck injuries, and some patients have demonstrated nystagmus during the head-fixed body-turned maneuver.[7] Also, anesthetizing one side of the neck produces acute disequilibrium and imbalance.[8] This patient appears to have a heightened cervico-ocular reflex when the body is turned to the left, so that clearly visible nystagmus was generated.

Question 4: What is the significance of this patient's episodic neck muscle spasm and its association with symptoms of dizziness?

Answer 4: The cause-and-effect relationship between the patient's neck muscle spasm and his symptoms of dizziness is uncertain. As described above, abnormal afferent activity from the neck could lead to dizziness as a result of the central nervous system receiving aberrant information regarding the position of the head in space. Such aberrant information could be made more unreliable by neck muscle spasm. Conversely, the vestibulocollic and cervicocollic reflexes (see Chap. 1), which are designed to help stabilize the head in space, could be leading to excessive neck muscle activity when the patient is experiencing a vestibular imbalance. Thus, patients with cervical vertigo may experience a "vicious cycle" of excessive neck muscle activity exacerbating their dizziness, which subsequently exacerbates their neck discomfort.

Question 5: What types of injuries can cause cervical vertigo?

Answer 5: Cervical vertigo has been reported in flexion-extension injuries often related to motor vehicle accidents, severe cervical arthritis, herniated cervical disks, and trauma, especially blunt trauma to the top of the head.

DIAGNOSIS/DIFFERENTIAL DIAGNOSIS

This patient was given the diagnosis of *cervical vertigo*.

TREATMENT/MANAGEMENT

Cyclobenzaprine was prescribed as a muscle relaxant to be used on an as-needed basis. A soft cervical collar was also prescribed for the patient, and he was admonished not to use the collar for more than 1 to 2 hours per day so that he did not lose neck muscle strength and so that he continued to stimulate neck proprioception. This patient was treated with physical therapy to improve range of motion of the neck and to reduce neck muscle spasm and discomfort. These treatment interventions afforded him significant relief, but he remained symptomatic, especially if he was required to turn his head repeatedly for several hours, for instance, while driving an automobile for long distances.

SUMMARY

A 49-year-old man presented with the chief complaint of dizziness whose onset was associated with a flexion-extension injury during a motor vehicle accident. Examination revealed nystagmus during head-fixed body-turned maneuvers, suggesting the diagnosis of cervical vertigo. The patient was treated with physical therapy, muscle relaxants, and a soft cervical collar, and gained symptomatic relief.

TEACHING POINTS

1. **Cervical vertigo** is a poorly defined condition that refers to dizziness and disequilibrium thought to be caused by abnormal afferent activity from the neck. The close temporal association of symptoms of dizziness and neck pain following a neck injury should suggest a diagnosis of cervical vertigo. Cervical vertigo can be seen in association with flexion-extension (whiplash) injuries, severe cervical arthritis, herniated cervical disks, and head trauma, especially blunt trauma to the top of the head.
2. **The cervico-ocular reflex,** an eye movement response to neck movement, is thought to be of minimal importance in normal individuals. However, a patient who has sustained a neck injury may have an abnormal or exaggerated cervico-ocular reflex that causes dizziness or disequilibrium when the head is turned.
3. **Neck muscle spasm** and pain are often associated with symptoms of dizziness. The cause-and-effect relationship between these two symptoms is uncertain. In fact, patients with cervical vertigo may experience a "vicious cycle" of excessive neck muscle activity exacerbating their dizziness, which subsequently exacerbates their neck discomfort.
4. **Treatment of cervical vertigo** includes muscle relaxants and physical therapy to improve range of motion of the neck and to reduce neck muscle spasm and discomfort. Use of a cervical collar should be limited to no more than 1 to 2 hours per day.

REFERENCES

1. Ryan, GMS, and Cope, S: Cervical vertigo. Lancet 2:1355–1358, 1955.
2. Jongkees, LBW: Cervical vertigo. Laryngoscope 79:1473–1484, 1969.
3. Neuhuber, WL, and Zenker, W: Central distribution of cervical primary afferents in the rat, with emphasis on proprioceptive projects to vestibular, perihypoglossal, and upper thoracic spinal nuclei. J Comp Neurol 280:231–253, 1989.
4. Huygen, PLM, Verhagen, WIM, and Nicolasen, MGM: Cervico-ocular reflex enhancement in labyrinthine-defective and normal subjects. Exp Brain Res 87:457–464, 1991.
5. Barlow, D, and Freedman, W: Cervico-ocular reflex in the normal adult. Acta Otolaryngol 89:487–496, 1980.
6. Bronstein, A, and Hood, J: The cervico-ocular reflex in normal subjects and patients with absent vestibular function. Brain Res 373:399–408, 1986.
7. Oosterveld, WJ, et al: Electronystagmographic findings following cervical whiplash injuries. Acta Otolaryngol (Stockh) 111:201–205, 1991.
8. De Jong, PTV, Vianney de Jong, JMB, Cohen, B, and Jongkees, BW: Ataxia and nystagmus induced by injection of local anesthetics in the neck. Ann Neurol 1:240–246, 1977.
9. Fitz-Ritson, D: Assessment of cervicogenic vertigo. J Manipulative Physiol Ther 14(3):193–198, 1991.

C8

Labyrinthine
Concussion

HISTORY

A 44-year-old woman who worked as a travel agent complained of dizziness and disequilibrium that were present constantly but fluctuated from day to day. The patient dated her symptoms to head trauma sustained during a motor vehicle accident 10 months before evaluation. The car she was driving was hit on the passenger side, causing the left side of her head to strike the inside of the passenger compartment. The patient had not lost consciousness in the accident. She was particularly symptomatic during rapid head movement and had difficulty ambulating in dimly lit environments. Headaches occurred irregularly. The patient noted that hearing in the right ear was not as good as in the left. Symptoms were not exacerbated by Valsalva maneuvers such as coughing, sneezing, or straining during bowel movements. There was no positional dizziness. There were no neurologic or psychiatric complaints, including anxiety, insomnia, undue fatigue, or personality change. There was no significant past medical history. The family history was noncontributory.

A CT scan of the head obtained by the patient's primary care physician was within the normal limits. The patient had used meclizine with some relief but continued to experience dizziness and disequilibrium.

Question 1: Based on the patient's history, what is the likely diagnosis?

Answer 1: This patient is likely to have suffered from a labyrinthine concussion caused by striking her head during the motor vehicle accident. Other considerations include perilymphatic fistula (Cases C19, C23), brainstem concussion, or cervical vertigo (see Case C7). Other possibilities include conditions that may be unrelated to the motor vehicle accident or exacerbated by it, such as a prior compensated peripheral vestibulopathy or a central nervous system disorder such as demyelinating disease or a mass lesion. These latter two conditions are unlikely, but for uncertain reasons can sometimes come to light following head trauma and so must be considered.

PHYSICAL EXAMINATION

The general and neurologic examinations were normal. Otologic examination revealed normal-appearing tympanic membranes with normal mobility on pneumatic otoscopy. During tuning forks examination using 512- and 1024-Hz forks, Weber's test lateralized to the left and the Rinne tests were positive bilaterally, indicating a possible sensorineural type of hearing loss on the right. Neuro-otologic examination revealed spontaneous left-beating nystagmus with Frenzel glasses and difficulty standing on a compliant foam surface with the eyes closed. Dix-Hallpike maneuvers were negative.

Laboratory Testing

Vestibular Laboratory Testing

ELECTRONYSTAGMOGRAPHY: Ocular motor function was normal. There was no positional nystagmus. A spontaneous left-beating vestibular nystagmus of 6 degrees per second was present. Caloric irrigations revealed a right-reduced vestibular response of 35 percent.

ROTATIONAL TESTING: Rotational testing revealed a mild left-directional preponderance.

POSTUROGRAPHY: Posturography indicated excessive sway only on Condition 6.

Audiometric Testing: Testing revealed a mild to moderate right-sided sensorineural hearing loss that was greatest in the higher frequencies (Fig. C8–1). Hearing in the left ear was normal. Results of electrocochleography, which was performed to evaluate the possibility of post-traumatic endolymphatic hydrops or perilymphatic fistula (see Cases C19, C23), was normal.

Imaging: A CT scan of the brain was normal.

Other: None

Question 2: Based on the patient's history, physical examination, and laboratory studies, what is the most likely diagnosis?

Answer 2: The most likely diagnosis is labyrinthine concussion on the right as a result of head trauma suffered during a motor vehicle accident. This diagnosis is supported by the combination of the asymmetrical sensorineural hearing loss worse in the right ear and right unilateral reduced vestibular response on caloric testing. The fact that the patient described hitting the *left* side of her head against the passenger compartment is somewhat inconsistent with the right-sided audiovestibular loss. However, because the exact mechanism of injury in labyrinthine concussion is not well known, the fact that head trauma occurred is more important than the side of head impact. There is also a possibility that a combination of central and peripheral dysfunction is causing the present symptoms.

Question 3: What is the pathophysiologic basis for labyrinthine concussion?

Answer 3: The mechanism of injury in labyrinthine concussion is poorly understood, and it is likely that several different mechanisms occur. Possible mechanisms of injury to the labyrinth include pressure "shock waves" transmitted directly to the labyrinth by the skull or implosive barotrauma in the form of acoustic energy or barometric pressure waves transmitted via the tympanic membrane and ossicular chain to the labyrinth. Explosive pressure changes can also occur from sudden shifts of the brain or intracranial fluids. Sudden intracranial pressure changes can be transmitted to the

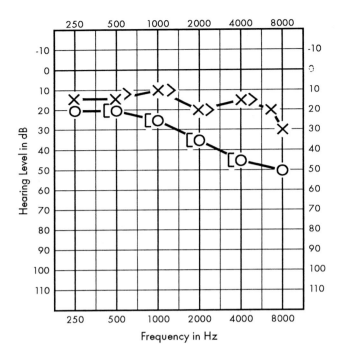

Figure C8-1
Audiogram.

Word Recognition Score			
Right : 90%			
Left : 96%			

			Right	Left
Air	unmasked		O—O	X—X
	masked		△—△	□—□
Bone	unmasked		◄---◄	►---►
	masked		⊏---⊏	⅃---⅃

labyrinth via the cochlear aqueduct, endolymphatic sac, or the cribriform regions of the internal auditory canal that transmit eighth cranial nerve fibers into the labyrinth. Sudden pressure shifts of the labyrinthine fluids can cause hemorrhage or tears of fine labyrinthine membranes, allowing intermixing of perilymph and endolymph and local metabolic disturbances that could result in the formation of endolymphatic hydrops. Sudden pressure shifts can also damage hair cell stereocilia, the organ of Corti, or the various specialized cupular structures; cause collapse or fibrosis of the endolymphatic membranes; or cause the loss of hair cells themselves.[1-3]

Question 4: Why is this patient symptomatic 10 months following the trauma?

Answer 4: As discussed in Case C1, failure to compensate for a peripheral vestibular lesion may be based on several reasons. This patient may be experiencing erroneous or fluctuating peripheral vestibular input as a result of labyrinthine trauma. It is possible that the central vestibular system has more difficulty compensating for erroneous or fluctuating vestibular signals from the peripheral end organ than a complete or fixed peripheral vestibular function deficit. Following any significant head injury, subtle central nervous system dysfunction is also possible that could impair the central compensatory processes. No abnormalities of vision or proprioception are noted, and thus these causes are unlikely to be contributing to the current balance dysfunction. Inadequate sensory input as a result of sedentary behavior also is possible and could have delayed compensation.

Question 5: What are conditions other than failure to compensate for a peripheral vestibular lesion that may underlie persistent dizziness following head trauma?

Answer 5: Conditions that may underlie persistent dizziness following head trauma other than failure to compensate for a peripheral vestibular lesion include benign positional vertigo (discussed in Cases T1, C9, C15), perilymphatic fistula (discussed in Cases C19, C23), and brainstem or cerebral concussion. This patient is unlikely to be suffering from benign positional vertigo considering the absence of a history of positional disequilibrium and dizziness and negative Dix-Hallpike maneuvers. Perilymphatic fistula is more difficult to rule out, but the patient does not report fluctuation of hearing loss, nor are her symptoms exacerbated by Valsalva maneuvers such as those experienced during coughing, sneezing, straining during bowel movements, or by pneumatic otoscopy. Electrocochleography may be positive in either endolymphatic hydrops or perilymphatic fistula, but was negative in this patient. Nevertheless, perilymphatic fistula should remain a possibility because of the inherent difficulty in diagnosing perilymphatic fistula (see Cases C19, C23). The patient is unlikely to have suffered from a brainstem contusion because neurotologic signs are absent. However, it is possible that some degree of the patient's failure to compensate for a peripheral vestibular injury may relate to a mild brainstem concussion. The patient is unlikely to have suffered from a cerebral concussion in that there are no complaints of abnormal memory or personality change. Her headaches, however, suggest the possibility of a mild cerebral concussion, although the headaches could easily be the result of head trauma without cerebral concussion.

DIAGNOSIS/DIFFERENTIAL DIAGNOSIS

The patient was given the diagnosis of *labyrinthine concussion*.

TREATMENT/MANAGEMENT

Because the patient was symptomatic primarily during rapid head movement and while ambulating in dimly lit environments, it was felt that this patient would be likely to benefit from a course of vestibular rehabilitation intended to reduce her symptoms of dizziness and disequilibrium during movement. The patient was also given a vestibular suppressant, meclizine 25 mg, to be used on as-needed basis up to three times per day, only when the patient was particularly symptomatic. The patient was also advised that recovery might be prolonged because of the possibility of a brainstem concussion and that improvement could continue for up to 2 years. The plan was to discontinue meclizine as soon as possible following the hoped-for successful treatment with vestibular rehabilitation.

FOLLOW-UP

The patient's symptoms gradually decreased and her balance improved noticeably following physical therapy. At a 6-month follow-up visit, the patient was using meclizine only a few days each month when her symptoms seemed worse.

SUMMARY

A 44-year-old woman complained of 10 months of dizziness that began following a motor vehicle accident in which she struck the side of her head against the inside of the passenger compartment. The patient's laboratory testing suggested a reduced vestibular response on the right of mild degree as well as mild sensorineural hearing loss. These findings suggested a labyrinthine concussion. The patient's persistent symptoms may have been based on abnormal or fluctuating peripheral vestibular function or sedentary behavior and may have been compounded by a mild brainstem concussion. Treatment consisted of a course of balance therapy and vestibular-suppressant agents to be used for a short time on an as-needed basis.

TEACHING POINTS

1. **The differential diagnosis for post-traumatic dizziness** includes post-traumatic benign positional vertigo, post-traumatic endolymphatic hydrops, labyrinthine concussion, perilymphatic fistula, brainstem concussion, or cervical-related vertigo. Other possibilities include conditions that may be unrelated to the trauma or exacerbated by it, such as a prior compensated peripheral vestibulopathy or a central nervous system disorder such as demyelinating disease or a mass lesion.

2. **A diagnosis of labyrinthine concussion** is suggested by the presence of symptoms or signs of inner ear dysfunction such as asymmetrical sensorineural hearing loss, tinnitus, and a unilateral reduced vestibular response on caloric testing following head trauma.

3. **Prolonged dizziness following head trauma** may relate to failure of central compensation for a trauma-related peripheral vestibular lesion. Poor compensation may be based on aberrant or fluctuating peripheral vestibular input as a result of labyrinthine trauma, subtle central nervous system dysfunction, inadequate sensory input as a result of sedentary behavior, or subclinical damage to the contralateral ear. Following head trauma, other conditions such as benign positional vertigo, perilymphatic fistula, and brainstem or cerebral concussion also may underlie persistent dizziness.

4. **The pathophysiology of labyrinthine concussion** is poorly understood. Possible mechanisms of injury include: (1) implosive barotrauma in the form of acoustic energy or barometric pressure waves transmitted via the surrounding skull bone, the tympanic membrane, or the ossicular chain to the labyrinth; (2) explosive pressure changes from sudden shifts of the brain or intracranial fluids; (3) sudden pressure shifts of labyrinthine fluids that can cause hemorrhage or tears of fine labyrinthine membranes, allowing intermixing of perilymph and endolymph and local metabolic disturbances.

REFERENCES

1. Schuknecht, HF, Neff, WD, and Perlman, HD: An experimental study of auditory damage following blows to the head. Ann Otol Rhinol Laryngol 60:273–289, 1951.
2. Schuknecht, HF: A clinical study of auditory damage following blows to the head. Ann Otol Rhinol Laryngol 59:331–359, 1950.
3. Proctor, B, Guadjian, ES, and Webster, JE: The ear in head trauma. Laryngoscope 66:17–50, 1956.

C A S E

C9

Diagnosis and Treatment of Benign Positional Vertigo

HISTORY

A 45-year-old man who worked as an attorney complained of positional vertigo that had begun 6 weeks before evaluation. Symptoms occurred when he rolled over in bed to the right and when he reached above his head. There were no other neurologic or otologic symptoms. Past history was significant for a 1-day episode of severe vertigo, nausea, and vomiting that had occurred 2 months before evaluation. Family history was noncontributory. An emergency room physician at that time diagnosed "labyrinthitis" and prescribed promethazine, which the patient was still taking on an irregular basis. The patient had several days of nausea and severe imbalance following this acute episode; during this time he was unable to work in his usual occupation as an attorney. Since returning to work, the patient reports a sense of mild disequilibrium and unsteadiness during quick head movements. These symptoms have been gradually improving, and he is almost entirely asymptomatic at rest but still reports positional vertigo.

Question 1: Based on the history, what is the most likely diagnosis?

Answer 1: This patient's history is consistent with an episode of vestibular neuritis (see Cases T5 and C1) 2 months before evaluation. He seems to have largely recovered from the vestibular neuritis but has persistent symptoms related to positional vertigo that probably are a result of benign positional vertigo.

PHYSICAL EXAMINATION

General, neurologic, and otologic examinations were normal. Neuro-otologic examination revealed impaired tandem gait, an inability to stand on a compliant foam pad with the eyes closed, and 90-degree rotation to the right on a stepping test. Dix-Hallpike maneuvers using Frenzel glasses were positive with the right ear down. The nystagmus was upbeating (toward the forehead) and torsional with the upper poles of the eyes beating toward the dependent (right) ear. The nystagmus began several seconds after positioning and was accompanied by a strong sense of vertigo and nausea. The nystagmus lasted for about 15 seconds, after which time the patient's vertigo also stopped.

Question 2: How does the additional information provided by the physical examination influence this patient's diagnosis?

Answer 2: This patient manifests the characteristic symptoms and signs of benign positional nystagmus and vertigo, including the typical nystagmus evoked by Dix-Hallpike maneuvers. Also, the patient's abnormal neuro-otologic examination suggests a lingering vestibular imbalance, probably the result of the vestibular neuritis suffered 2 months earlier.

Laboratory Testing

Vestibular Laboratory Testing

ELECTRONYSTAGMOGRAPHY:	Ocular motor function was normal. There was no static positional nystagmus. Dix-Hallpike maneuvers in the laboratory documented a predominantly upbeating nystagmus with the right ear down. Caloric irrigations revealed a significant (40%) right reduced vestibular response.
ROTATIONAL TESTING:	Rotational testing revealed a mild left directional preponderance.
POSTUROGRAPHY:	Posturography indicated excessive sway on conditions 5 and 6, that is, a vestibular pattern.

Audiometric Testing: Not performed

Imaging: Not performed

Other: None

Taken together, these findings suggested that the patient was suffering from a partial right-sided peripheral vestibular loss, benign positional nystagmus and vertigo affecting the right ear, and an ongoing vestibulo-ocular and vestibulospinal asymmetry.

Question 3: What is the significance of the vestibular laboratory abnormalities?

Answer 3: The right reduced caloric response suggests that the presumed vestibular neuritis, which the patient suffered 2 months earlier, damaged afferent fibers or sensory epithelium of at least the right horizontal semicircular canal. The patient's directional preponderance on rotational testing suggests an ongoing vestibulo-ocular reflex asymmetry, that is, incomplete compensation for a peripheral vestibular deficit. This incomplete recovery may be on the basis of fluctuating peripheral vestibular function on the right, chronic use of vestibular suppressants (see Case C1), or both. The vestibular pattern on platform posturography suggests an ongoing vestibulospinal abnormality, which represents further evidence for incomplete central nervous system compensation. The nystagmus elicited during Dix-Hallpike maneuvers confirms the diagnosis of benign nystagmus and vertigo.

DIAGNOSIS/DIFFERENTIAL DIAGNOSIS

Question 4: Are there any conditions other than benign positional nystagmus and vertigo that should be considered?

Answer 4: Unquestionably, this patient's most likely diagnoses are resolving vestibular neuritis and benign positional vertigo. Other entities that can present with an acute vestibular syndrome followed by benign positional vertigo are labyrinthine concussion (see Cases T7, C8, and C22) and labyrinthine infarction (see Case U4). As discussed in Case T1, few conditions masquerade as benign positional vertigo. Extremely rarely, however, posterior fossa lesions can present with the typical signs and symptoms of benign positional vertigo, although one or more features of the clinical presentation are often atypical, such as the direction of the nystagmus, and suggest a central nervous system abnormality.

Question 5: What features in the clinical presentation of a patient with acute vertigo followed by positional vertigo would lead to a suspicion of a posterior fossa lesion?

Answer 5: Neurologic symptoms such as numbness or weakness of the face or extremities, or visual loss associated with the onset of vertigo should lead to a suspicion of a posterior fossa lesion. Additionally, if the neurologic examination disclosed any central nervous system signs or if the patient's Dix-Hallpike maneuvers were associated with a response atypical of benign positional nystagmus and vertigo, further evaluation, such as MRI of the posterior fossa, would be warranted. Responses during the Dix-Hallpike maneuver that are atypical of benign positional vertigo include nystagmus that (1) is downbeating rather than upbeating in the head hanging position, (2) occurs immediately upon positioning, (3) is not associated with vertigo, or (4) does not fatigue if the patient is repeatedly positioned.

This patient was given a diagnosis of *benign positional vertigo*.

Question 6: What is the pathophysiology of benign positional vertigo?

Answer 6: Benign positional vertigo is thought to result from malfunction of the posterior semicircular canal such that the canal becomes abnormally sensitive to gravity or linear acceleration. Malfunction of the posterior semicircular canal in benign positional vertigo is supported by two observations:

(1) The direction of provoked nystagmus is consistent with the ocular motor connections of the dependent posterior semicircular canal.

(2) Surgical sectioning of the afferent nerve to the posterior semicircular canal abolishes benign positional vertigo.

There are two current theories to explain why the posterior semicircular canal becomes sensitive to gravity: cupulolithiasis and canalithiasis.

Cupulolithiasis refers to the idea that detached otoconia from the utricle or saccule descend to the most inferior portion (when upright) of the labyrinth and become adherent to the cupula of the posterior semicircular canal (Fig. C9–1).[1,2] These adherent particles change the specific gravity of the cupula so that it no longer is isodense with the surrounding endolymph. As a result, the posterior semicircular canal cupula becomes a gravity-sensitive organ. Consequently, the posterior semicircular canal falsely signals continuous rotation for particular head positions, for example, tipping the head backward.

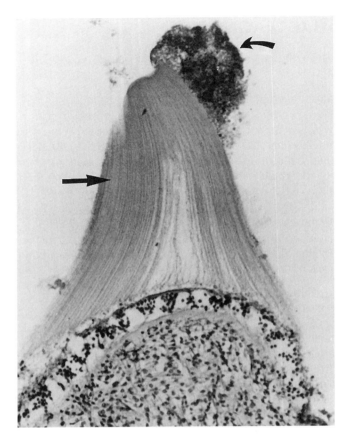

Figure C9-1
Histopathological section of the posterior semicircular canal ampulla demonstrating a large deposit of debris on the cupula. The histological finding has been referred to as cupulolithiasis. Straight arrow = cupula; curved arrow = debris. (With permission of Moriarty, B, et al: The incidence and distribution of cupular deposits in the labyrinth. Laryngoscope 102:56–59, 1992, p 57.[11])

Canalithiasis refers to the idea that debris, possibly degenerating otoconia or other cellular debris, becomes free-floating in the endolymph of the posterior semicircular canal (Fig. C9–2).[3,4] Any head movement that changes the orientation of the posterior semicircular canal with respect to gravity may cause the particles in the endolymph to move within the posterior semicircular canal. Presumably, as the particles move, the endolymph is disturbed in a manner that stimulates the posterior semicircular canal ampulla. Once the particles settle into a dependent position and stop moving, which presumably takes about 10 or 20 seconds, the abnormal stimulation ceases. When the patient returns to the upright position, the particles may again move and again cause an erroneous sensation of motion.

Both the cupulothiasis and the canalithiasis theories have merit, and it is possible that both exist as pathologic conditions. However, the concept of cupulolithiasis cannot explain why the nystagmus provoked by head positioning stops after 15 to 30 seconds. If debris remained attached to the cupula, one would expect nystagmus to continue unabated for a long period of time. It is necessary to hypothesize that another mechanism, for example, central adaptation, is involved in stopping the nystagmus or that the debris is released from the cupula, in which case the debris become free-floating as hypothesized in the concept of canalithiasis. Strong support for the canalithiasis theory includes the recent surgical observations of free-floating particles within the posterior semicircular canals of patients with benign positional

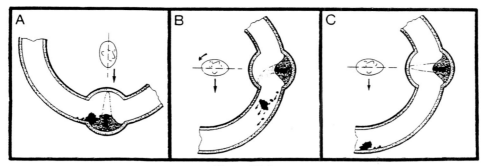

Figure C9-2

Canalithiasis. (*A*) Free-floating debris lies in the nonampullated limb of the posterior semicircular canal (the patient is upright). (*B*) As the patient moves to the supine position, the free-floating debris in the posterior semicircular canal floats to the most gravity-dependent portion of the posterior semicircular canal. This induces turbulence and deflection of the cupula, thereby provoking vertigo typical of benign positional vertigo. (*C*) Once the particles reach the gravity-dependent portion of the semicircular canal, stimulation ceases, no further stimulation of the posterior semicircular canal ampulla occurs, and the vertigo and nystagmus stop. (With permission from Brandt, T, et al: Therapy for benign paroxysmal positional vertigo, revisited. Neurology 44: 796–800, 1994.[12])

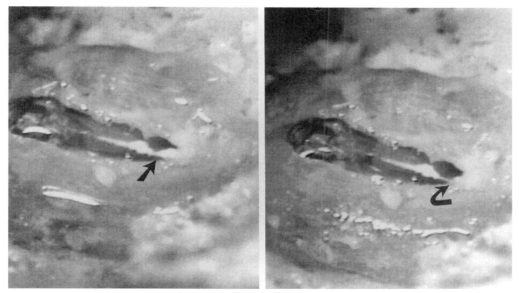

Figure C9-3

Free-floating endolymph particles within the posterior semicircular canal observed during surgery. The posterior semicircular canal had been opened in preparation for a canal plugging procedure. White debris was observed within the endolymph compartment of the posterior semicircular canal. These two photographs are sequential in time and show that the particles shifted during movement of the patient's head; compare shape and position of particles at straight arrow with the curved arrow. (With permission from Parnes, LS, and McClure, JA: Free-floating endolymph particles: A new operative finding during posterior semicircular canal occlusion. Laryngoscope 102:988–992, 1992.[3])

vertigo (Fig. C9–3).[5] Moreover, the latency, duration, and fatigability of the nystagmus that characterizes benign positional vertigo can all be explained by the theory of canalithiasis without invoking other central mechanisms.

Question 7: What conditions often precede the appearance of benign positional vertigo?

Answer 7: Although benign positional vertigo apparently often occurs spontaneously, it has been seen commonly following various peripheral vestibular disorders such as vestibular neuritis (as in this patient), and head trauma, which may be mild.

TREATMENT/MANAGEMENT

Question 8: What are the treatment options for benign positional nystagmus and vertigo? What is the role of medication such as vestibular suppressants? Should this patient continue using promethazine?

Answer 8: Benign positional nystagmus and vertigo is best treated using the particle repositioning maneuver (Fig. C9–4).[4,6] Previously, habituating exercises, such as those

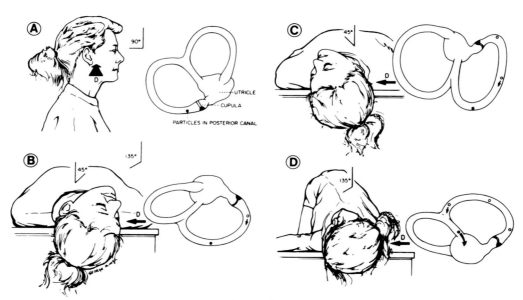

Figure C9-4

The particle-repositioning maneuver. (*A*) The patient is in the sitting position. The position of the vertibular labyrinth is illustrated to the right of the patient. Free-floating endolymph particles lie in the nonampullated end of the posterior semicircular canal. (*B*) The head is turned 45 degrees to the right for treating the right ear and the Dix-Hallpike maneuver is performed. The free-floating endolymph particles shift as a result of the gravity; movement within the posterior semicircular canal is from the open circle to the closed circle. (*C*) Next, the patient's head is turned 90 degrees to the opposite side, keeping the vertex of the head dependent (the head is now 45 degrees to the left). The free-floating endolymph particles continue to shift as a result of gravity. (*D*) The patient moves onto the left side and the head is now facing the floor. The free-floating endolymph particles continue around the semicircular canal toward the vestibule as a result of gravity. Finally, the patient sits upright (without rolling onto their back) to complete the maneuver (not shown). (With permission from Parnes, LS: Treatment of benign paroxysmal positional vertigo. In Myers, EN, et al (eds): Advances in Otolaryngology–Head and Neck Surgery, Vol 8. St. Louis: CV Mosby, 1994, p 330.[13])

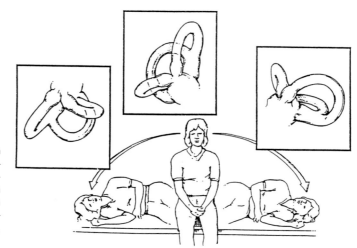

Figure C9-5
Brandt-Daroff exercises for benign positional vertigo. (With permission from Herdman, SJ: Assessment and management of benign paroxysmal positiional vertigo. In Herdman, SJ: Vestibular Rehabilitation. Philadelphia: FA Davis, 1994, p 334.[14])

described by Brandt and Daroff[7] (Fig. C9–5), and other physical maneuvers, such as the "liberatory" maneuver,[8] were most popular. All of these treatments are designed to relocate endolymphatic debris, which is presumed to be near or adherent to the posterior semicircular canal cupula, to the labyrinthine vestibule where the debris no longer affects the semicircular canals and can be naturally reabsorbed. The particle-repositioning maneuver is a "one-time" therapy, whereas the Brandt-Daroff exercises generally require 1 to 2 weeks of twice-daily performance. In the unusual patient who cannot be cured of his or her benign positional nystagmus and vertigo with a physical maneuver or with exercises, surgical treatment consisting of sectioning of the nerve to the posterior semicircular canal (singular neurotomy)[9] or plugging of the posterior semicircular canal[10] is usually successful (see Case C15).

Vestibular-suppressant medication is often helpful at the onset of benign positional nystagmus and vertigo, especially if it follows an acute vestibular loss, as in this patient or if a patient is so apprehensive that he or she refuses to perform the exercise therapy. However, once the acute episode of vestibular imbalance, if present, is over, vestibular-suppressant medication should be avoided, since central vestibular compensation for their peripheral vestibular loss can be delayed. If the patient expects to be exposed to excessive motion, such as prolonged car or air travel, or becomes particularly symptomatic for a brief time, meclizine, diazepam, or promethazine prescribed on an "as-needed" basis (see Case C18) may be beneficial.

A course of vestibular rehabilitation may be useful, even if a patient's positional vertigo is cured by a repositioning maneuver, especially for a patient with evidence on physical examination or laboratory testing of an ongoing vestibular system imbalance such as a directional preponderance or abnormal posturography.

Treatment consisted of a particle-repositioning maneuver, a gradual discontinuation of the patient's vestibular-suppressant medication, and a course of vestibular rehabilitation. The patient had complete relief from his positional symptoms and gradually recovered nearly normal balance. His limitations were noticed only during taxing balance tasks such as waterskiing.

Question 9: What is the natural history of benign positional nystagmus and vertigo? Is this patient likely to recover from this condition?

Answer 9: Benign positional nystagmus and vertigo is usually a self-limited condition. That is, without treatment, most patients recover spontaneously over several weeks or months. The typical patient with benign positional vertigo seeks specialty treatment about 6 weeks after the onset of the vertigo (mean 16 months, range 5 days to many years). It has been shown that without specific intervention, 75 percent of patients have spontaneous resolution of symptoms with a mean duration of about 1 month (range 5 to 42 days) of further symptoms. Thus, for most patients the duration of benign positional vertigo is about 10 weeks. However, in 25 percent of patients, symptoms can continue for years. The natural history of benign positional vertigo speaks to the value of actively treating such patients, especially since the condition can continue for years in a significant minority of patients. Benign positional vertigo also may recur, often between 6 months and 6 years following the initial presentation. The patient should be advised of this possibility. Positional maneuvers are equally effective in treating recurrences.

SUMMARY

A 45-year-old man presented with positional vertigo following acute vestibular neuritis that had occurred 2 months before evaluation. The patient's physical examination was consistent with benign positional vertigo. An ongoing vestibulo-ocular and vestibulo-spinal asymmetry was suggested by both the physical examination and laboratory test results. Treatment consisted of a particle-repositioning maneuver, a gradual discontinuation of the patient's vestibular-suppressant medication, and a course of vestibular rehabilitation. The patient had complete relief from his positional symptoms and gradually recovered nearly normal balance.

TEACHING POINTS

1. **Benign positional vertigo** can be seen following other disorders, such as vestibular neuritis and labyrinthine concussion. Benign positional vertigo may be only one of several manifestations of an ongoing vestibular abnormality. Patients presenting with positional vertigo should be thoroughly evaluated for other evidence of otologic disease. Patients presenting with disequilibrium for any reason should be evaluated for benign positional vertigo with appropriate questioning and physical examination, even if they do not present with a chief complaint of positional vertigo.
2. **Atypical positional vertigo** should suggest a posterior fossa lesion. Atypical features include any neurologic symptoms or signs that cannot be ascribed to a peripheral vestibular localization, any atypical features on the response to Dix-Hallpike maneuvers, and a failure to respond to particle-repositioning maneuvers.
3. **The treatment for benign positional vertigo** is the particle-repositioning maneuver. This is highly successful and provides complete relief in nearly all patients. Some patients with benign positional nystagmus and vertigo do not respond to this maneuver. Vestibular-suppressant medications can be used early in the disorder, but after several days should be used sparingly if at all.

REFERENCES

1. Schuknecht, HF: Positional vertigo: Clinical and experimental observations. Trans Am Acad Ophthalmol Otolaryngol 166:319–332, 1962.
2. Schuknecht, HF: Cupulolithiasis. Arch Otolaryngol 90:113–126, 1969.
3. Parnes, LS, and McClure, JA: Free-floating endolymph particles: A new operative finding during posterior semicircular canal occlusion. Laryngoscope 102:988–992, 1992.
4. Epley, JM: The canalith repositioning procedure: For treatment of benign paroxysmal positional vertigo. Otolaryngol Head Neck Surg 107:399–404, 1992.
5. Hall, SF, Ruby, RRF, and McClure, JA: The mechanics of benign paroxysmal vertigo. J Otolaryngol 8:151–158, 1979.
6. Parnes, LS, and Price-Jones, R: Particle repositioning maneuver for benign paroxysmal positional vertigo. Ann Otol Rhinol Laryngol 102:325–331, 1993.
7. Brandt, T, and Daroff, RB: Physical therapy for benign paroxysmal positional vertigo. Arch Otolaryngol 106:484–485, 1980.
8. Semont, A, Greyss, G, and Vitte, E: Curing the BPPV with a liberatory maneuver 42:290–293, 1988.
9. Gacek, RR: Transection of the posterior ampulary nerve for relief of benign paroxysmal positional vertigo. Ann Otol Rhinol Laryngol 83:596–605, 1974.
10. Parnes, LS, and McClure, JA: Posterior semicircular canal occlusion in the normal hearing ear. Otolaryngol Head Neck Surg 104:52–57, 1991.
11. Moriarty, B, et al: The incidence and distribution of cupular deposits in the labyrinth. Laryngoscope 102:56–59, 1992.
12. Brandt, T, et al: Therapy for benign paroxysmal positional vertigo, revisited. Neurology 44:796–800, 1994.
13. Parnes, LS: Treatment of benign paroxysmal positional vertigo. In Myers, EN, et al (eds): Advances in Otolaryngology–Head and Neck Surgery, Vol 8. St. Louis: CV Mosby, 1994.
14. Herdman, SJ: Assessment and management of benign paroxysmal positional vertigo. In Herdman, SJ: Vestibular Rehabilitation. Philadelphia: FA Davis, 1994.

C A S E

C10

Endolymphatic Hydrops

HISTORY

A 50-year-old female attorney was evaluated 1 week after the onset of acute vertigo. About 1 month before evaluation, the patient noticed a sense of pressure or blocking in her right ear similar to the feeling of water trapped in the ear after swimming. There was also a quiet ringing in her ear, but within a few days the fullness and ringing disappeared. A few weeks later, the full feeling and ringing returned, and she also noticed difficulty hearing on the telephone with the right ear. She went to a neighborhood urgent care center, where a mild ear infection was diagnosed and treated with an oral antibiotic and decongestant. A few days later, she woke up with an aching pressurelike pain in her ear associated with both increased ringing and decreased hearing in the ear. Suddenly she had an episode of acute vertigo that she described as the environment whirling; it was associated with nausea and vomiting that lasted for 3 hours. She was taken to an emergency room and given an intramuscular injection of an antiemetic. The following day, she felt nearly normal, with no vertigo. Her hearing loss, ringing, and fullness in the right ear had almost completely resolved. Some disequilibrium persisted. There was no significant past medical or family history.

Question 1: Based on the patient's history, what is the likely cause of these symptoms?

Answer 1: This patient's history suggests unilateral endolymphatic hydrops (see Cases T3, T9, C14, and C16). The term *endolymphatic hydrops* is used to describe a particular pathologic condition of the inner ear characterized by swelling, or distension, of the endolymphatic compartment of the inner ear (Fig. C10–1 A and B). Clinically, endolymphatic hydrops is associated with recurrent vertigo and other aural symptoms, such as tinnitus, hearing loss, and fullness or a pressure sensation in the ear. Presumably, distension of the delicate membranous labyrinth causes dysfunction of the hair cells involved in hearing and balance.

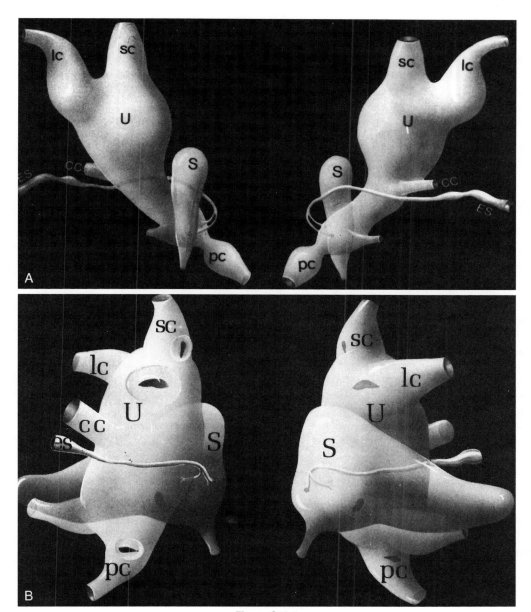

Figure C10-1

(*A*) Three-dimensional reconstruction of the normal membranous labyrinth. Medial and lateral views of the normal membranous labyrinth (right ear). (*B*) Three-dimensional reconstruction of the membranous labyrinth affected by endolymphatic hydrops. Medial and lateral views showing dilation of the membranous labyrinth (utricle and saccule) caused by endolymphatic hydrops (left ear). U = utricle; S = saccule; sc = superior semicircular canal ampulla; hc = horizontal semicircular canal ampulla; pc = posterior semicircular canal ampulla; es = endolymphatic duct and sac; cc = common crus (junction of non-ampullated ends of the superior and posterior semicircular canals). (With permission from Rizvi, SS, and Boston, MA: Investigations into the cause of canal paresis in Meniere's disease. Laryngoscope 96:1258–1271, 1986, p 1260.[8])

Question 2: How does endolymphatic hydrops produce episodic symptoms of hearing loss, tinnitus, aural fullness, and vertigo?

Answer 2: The mechanism underlying episodic hearing loss and vertigo caused by endolymphatic hydrops is not entirely understood. Endolymphatic hydrops characteristically produces transient and fully reversible inner ear dysfunction early in the course of the disorder. Hearing loss, tinnitus, and aural fullness associated with endolymphatic hydrops typically lasts for hours to weeks, whereas the acute vertigo associated with endolymphatic hydrops typically lasts for at least 20 minutes, usually 2 to 4 hours, and can be followed by a day or two of mild disequilibrium. The most popular theory to explain the vertigo associated with endolymphatic hydrops is rupture of membranous labyrinth and subsequent potassium intoxication.[1,2] Normally, thin, delicate membranes, such as Reissner's membrane in the cochlea or the saccular membrane in the vestibule, separate the endolymphatic space from the perilymphatic space. During endolymphatic hydrops, these membranes can rupture, allowing mixing of the high-potassium endolymph with the low-potassium perilymph. The influx of a high concentration of potassium ions into the perilymph can alter the neural discharge rate in the vestibular nerve, thereby causing nystagmus and vertigo. The direction of nystagmus observed during an acute attack of Meniere's disease is variable and complex. In the few cases where eye movements have been observed from the beginning of an attack, the slow component of the nystagmus was initially directed away from the affected labyrinth, thus suggesting abnormal excitatory neural activity in the affected ear. Seconds to minutes later, the direction of nystagmus reversed, thus indicating abnormally reduced neural activity in the affected labyrinth. This biphasic nystagmus response is consistent with the results of animal models of potassium perfusion into the perilymph. A third phase of nystagmus that beats toward the affected side, known as recovery nystagmus, also can occur days to weeks later. Recovery nystagmus is presumably related to a combination of central adaptation and recovery of vestibular function in the affected labyrinth.[3,4]

The resolution of vertigo is probably the result of a combination of restoration of normal potassium levels in the perilymph, normalization of the pressure-volume relationships within the labyrinth following membrane rupture, and central vestibular adaptation. Not uncommonly, hearing loss and aural fullness seem to improve after the vertigo spell (Lermoyez syndrome); however, for unknown reasons aural fullness, tinnitus, and hearing loss generally follow a different, more protracted course than the vertigo.

Following repeated acute episodes, the previously reversible symptoms of Meniere's disease can become permanent and progressive. Hearing loss increases and ceases to return to normal. Tinnitus becomes invariably present and other auditory distortions such as recruitment (sharp or loud sounds are perceived as excessively loud, even painful) and diplacusis (a given tone is heard at a different pitch in the two ears) become permanent. A permanent reduction of vestibular function also occurs. These symptoms and signs are thought to be primarily caused by progressive damage and loss of hair cells within the inner ear and not to direct involvement of the primary afferent neurons of the labyrinth.

PHYSICAL EXAMINATION

General and neurologic examinations were normal. Otoscopic examination was normal. On tuning-fork testing, Weber's test lateralized to the left and the Rinne test was positive bilaterally. Mild diplacusis was noted. Dix-Hallpike maneuvers were negative. Foam and dome testing was normal. On the stepping test, the patient marched 120 degrees to the left.

Question 3: Is this physical examination consistent with a presumptive diagnosis of endolymphatic hydrops? Can the affected side be distinguished from this examination?

Answer 3: In patients with vestibular system dysfunction localized to the inner ear, the neurologic examination should be normal, as was found in this patient. Tuning-fork testing suggests a sensorineural hearing loss in the right ear. The patient's ability to stand on foam with her eyes closed indicates nearly full recovery of postural control. The positive result on the stepping test, however, indicates a residual vestibular system asymmetry. Because endolymphatic hydrops characteristically produces reversible changes in the inner ear, the results of the stepping test depend on when the test was performed in relation to the last episode of vertigo, because vestibular compensation acts to reduce symptoms from any persistent vestibular injury that may occur. Immediately after an abrupt decrease in vestibular function, patients usually march on the stepping test toward the side of the affected ear. However, days to weeks following an acute spell of vertigo, patients often march toward the contralateral ear on the stepping test, suggesting that the combined influence of increasing vestibular function in the diseased ear and vestibular compensation are producing a relative "overcompensation." Thus, the physical examination of this patient supports the preliminary diagnosis of endolymphatic hydrops affecting the right ear. The diminished hearing in the right ear provides the best clue to localization, whereas the abnormal stepping test suggests a recent unilateral vestibular injury.

Question 4: What causes endolymphatic hydrops?

Answer 4: Endolymphatic hydrops represents a common pathologic response to a variety of insults to the inner ear. Etiologic factors include but are not limited to concurrent or preceding viral infection of the inner ear, head trauma, vascular insufficiency, syphilis, autoimmune inner ear disease, abnormal glucose metabolism, hypothyroidism, and inhalant and food allergies.[5] The use of the terms *Meniere's disease* and *endolymphatic hydrops* can be confusing. Many prefer to define Meniere's disease as the idiopathic syndrome of endolymphatic hydrops. When the cause of endolymphatic hydrops is known, it can be clearly defined as syphilitic endolymphatic hydrops or autoimmune-related endolymphatic hydrops, and so on.

In addition to these etiologic factors, other factors known to influence the formation of endolymphatic hydrops include excessive salt intake, stress, and excessive caffeine ingestion.

Question 5: Which laboratory studies should be ordered for this patient and why?

Answer 5: The patient's physical examination increases the likelihood of a peripheral vestibular ailment. Quantitative vestibular testing and audiometric testing help determine the presence of a vestibular abnormality as well as determine the presence of cochlear dysfunction.

Laboratory Testing

Vestibular Laboratory Testing

ELECTRONYSTAGMOGRAPHY: Ocular motor and positional testing were normal. Caloric testing demonstrated a 35 percent reduced vestibular response in the right ear.

ROTATIONAL TESTING: Not performed

POSTUROGRAPHY: Not performed

Audiometric Testing: An audiogram (Fig. C10–2) revealed a unilateral low-frequency sensorineural hearing loss affecting the right ear. Hearing in the left ear was normal. Electrocochleography revealed a summating to action potential ratio of 60 percent in the right ear and 20 percent in the left ear (see Chap. 3).

Imaging: An MRI scan of the brain was normal.

Other: A metabolic blood screen was normal.

Question 6: Why was an MRI performed?

Answer 6: Although the constellation of clinical symptoms is characteristic of Meniere's disease, tumors of the cerebellopontine angle, such as meningioma or

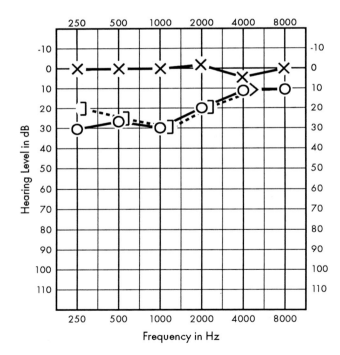

Figure C10-2
Audiogram.

acoustic neuroma, can cause similar symptoms, including fluctuating hearing loss, aural fullness, tinnitus, and dizziness. Thus, it is prudent to always obtain imaging of the central nervous system or a screening brainstem auditory-evoked potential test in cases of suspected Meniere's disease.

DIAGNOSIS/DIFFERENTIAL DIAGNOSIS

This patient was given a diagnosis of *Meniere's disease,* or *endolymphatic hydrops.*

ADDITIONAL HISTORY

Further evaluation of the patient's lifestyle and habits revealed a stressful work environment that included a 10-to-12-hour workday and occasional "all-nighters." In addition, the patient consumed approximately 6 cups of caffeinated coffee per day and 1 liter of caffeinated cola. Other habits that could exacerbate endolymphatic hydrops included a high-salt diet and smoking one pack of cigarettes per day.

TREATMENT/MANAGEMENT

Question 7: What medications have been shown to be efficacious in the treatment of endolymphatic hydrops?

Answer 7: Several controlled clinical trials have demonstrated the efficacy of the combination of a low-salt diet and a diuretic in the treatment of endolymphatic hydrops. The combination of hydrochlorothiazide and triameterene (diazide) is widely accepted as the first choice of diuretic.[6] Oral vasodilators such as nicotinic acid and parenteral treatments such as histamine injections or Papaverine have not been tested in clinical trials of endolymphatic hydrops.[7] However, based on anecdotal experiences, these medications are frequently prescribed for this condition.

Acute attacks of vertigo can be treated with antiemetic and vestibular suppressant medications. Droperidol 1 to 2.5 mg (intravenously, or intramuscularly, or as a sublingual [drop]) can quickly abort severe nausea and vomiting. Promethazine (25 to 50 mg) or compazine (10 mg) (oral or as a rectal suppository) are effective for mild to moderate nausea and vomiting. Meclizine (30 mg) is helpful for mild dizziness but not generally effective for severe nausea or vomiting. Vestibular rehabilitation is not generally helpful in Meniere's disease, because the vertigo usually occurs abruptly and remits spontaneously. Most individuals report normal balance between episodes and thus vestibular rehabilitation offers little advantage.

The initial treatment recommendations included alteration of the patient's lifestyle to include reduction in the use of caffeine, reduced smoking, stress reduction, and a low-salt diet.

FOLLOW-UP

The patient was compliant with treatment recommendations but continued to experience minor episodes of vertigo. Hydrochlorothiazide and triamterene once daily were prescribed, and she became symptom-free aside from one vertiginous episode the following year.

SUMMARY

A 50-year-old female attorney presented with fluctuating aural fullness, hearing loss, and tinnitus followed by an episode of acute prostrating vertigo. The presumptive diagnosis of Meniere's disease was made on the basis of these clinical symptoms. An audiogram, electrocochleography, vestibular laboratory testing, and MRI were performed to further evaluate and confirm the diagnosis. The patient was treated with a diuretic and a salt-restricted diet. This resulted in a significant reduction in the patient's symptoms.

TEACHING POINTS

1. **The typical presentation of Meniere's disease** includes fluctuating aural fullness, tinnitus, hearing loss, and recurrent bouts of vertigo.
2. **Endolymphatic hydrops** (swelling of the endolymphatic space) is the underlying pathophysiologic process of Meniere's disease. Endolymphatic hydrops can be associated with a number of different metabolic, infectious, and immune disorders. Meniere's disease is defined as the idiopathic form of endolymphatic hydrops.
3. **The mechanisms of hearing loss and vertigo** caused by endolymphatic hydrops are uncertain. Possibly, endolymphatic hydrops causes rupture of intralabyrinthine membranes and mixing of endolymph and perilymph with concomitant potassium intoxication.
4. **The medical treatment of endolymphatic hydrops** includes the combination of a diuretic and dietary salt restriction, which can prevent or reduce the recurrence of symptoms.

REFERENCES

1. Schuknecht, HF: Pathology of the Ear. Cambridge, MA: Harvard University Press, 1974.
2. Brown, DH, McClure, JA, and Downar-Zapolski, Z: The membrane rupture theory of Meniere's disease—is it valid? Laryngoscope 98:599–601, 1988.
3. McClure, JA, Copp, JC, and Lycett, P: Recovery nystagmus in Meniere's disease. Laryngoscope 91:1727–1737, 1981.
4. Bance, M, Mai, M, Tomlinson, D, and Rutka, J: The changing direction of nystagmus in acute Meniere's disease: Pathophysiological implications. Laryngoscope 101:197–201, 1991.
5. Paparella, MM: The cause (multifactorial inheritance) and pathogenesis (endolymphatic malabsorption) of Meniere's disease and its symptoms (mechanical and chemical). Acta Otolaryngol (Stockh) 99:445–451, 1985.
6. Jackson, CG, Glasscock, ME, and Davis, WE: Medical management of Meniere's disease. Ann Otol 90:142–147, 1981.
7. Cass, SP: Role of medications in otological vertigo and balance disorders. Semin Hearing 12:257–269, 1991.
8. Rizvi, SS, and Boston, MA: Investigations into the cause of canal paresis in Meniere's disease. Laryngoscope 96:1258–1271, 1986.

C A S E

C11

Cerebellar Degeneration

HISTORY

A 65-year-old man presented with a gradually worsening course of disequilibrium and gait instability. The patient did not complain of vertigo, hearing loss, or tinnitus. His problem had been present for at least 5 years and possibly for as many as 10 years, with gradually increasing difficulty with balance while walking, especially on uneven surfaces while hunting. He did not notice any particular worsening of his balance in dimly lit environments. There was no exacerbation of symptoms with rapid head movements or with position change. The patient had no past medical history of importance and used no medication. His family history was significant; his mother, who died in her early eighties, had suffered from a gradually worsening balance problem and became wheelchair-bound in her mid to late seventies.

Question 1: Based on the patient's history, what are the diagnostic considerations and what further historical information would be helpful?

Answer 1: This patient has a nonspecific balance complaint. There is little in the history to suggest a peripheral vestibular process. Rather, the patient's complaint of abnormal gait suggests a central nervous system, possibly a cerebellar, disorder. Further, the gradual worsening of the patient's problem suggests a degenerative disorder, especially because of the positive family history, but a mass lesion must also be considered. A multisensory disequilibrium should also be considered, although there is nothing in the history that suggests sensory system involvement.

It would be helpful to learn more about the patient's ethanol use and any information regarding toxic exposures. A more detailed family history would also be helpful.

Question 2: How do the effects of acute ethanol intoxication differ from the effects of chronic ethanol abuse on the vestibular system?

Answer 2: Acute ethanol intoxication causes cerebellar dysfunction as evidenced by gaze-evoked nystagmus, incoordination, and gait ataxia. Also, as discussed in Case

151

C13, ethanol causes a direction-changing positional nystagmus, presumably as a result of altering the specific gravity of the semicircular canal cupulae.[1] The central vestibular structures damaged by chronic ethanol use include the cerebellar vermis, flocculo-nodular lobe, and the vestibular nuclei.[2] Although some controversy exists as to the role of malnutrition as opposed to ethanol toxicity directly, it is generally agreed that ethanol, in and of itself, is a neurotoxin.

FURTHER HISTORY

The patient denied significant ethanol consumption. There was no past medical history of pancreatitis, seizures, or cirrhosis of the liver. Family history was significant for his mother and maternal uncle having a late-onset balance disorder (see previous text). The patient's older brother was killed in World War II and his 60-year-old sister had no balance complaints.

PHYSICAL EXAMINATION

The patient's general examination was normal. He had no postural hypotension. Neurologic examination revealed full extraocular movements. However, pursuit tracking was not smooth and a bilateral horizontal gaze-evoked nystagmus was seen. Motor examination was normal. Coordination testing showed very mild abnormalities of rapid alternating movements, finger-to-nose movements, and heel-knee-shin movements. Sensation was normal. The patient's gait was extremely wide-based, and the patient was ataxic and unable to tandem walk. The patient had great difficulty standing with his feet together even with his eyes open, so Romberg's test could not be performed. He had a normal otologic examination.

Question 3: Based on the history and physical examination, what laboratory tests would provide further information regarding this patient's problems?

Answer 3: The patient's history and physical examination suggest a central nervous system abnormality, probably affecting midline cerebellar structures. Diagnostic considerations, as noted, include cerebellar degeneration (unlikely to be on an alcoholic basis) and a posterior fossa mass lesion. Other conditions to be considered, although unlikely, include vasculitis, a paraneoplastic process, or a structural abnormality such as a Chiari malformation. Thus, magnetic resonance imaging (MRI) of the brain with special attention to the posterior fossa is appropriate. Additionally, vestibular laboratory testing to specifically assess cerebellar function should be considered.

Laboratory Testing

Vestibular Laboratory Testing

ELECTRONYSTAGMOGRAPHY:	Ocular motor testing revealed normal velocity saccades with overshoot dysmetria, impaired pursuit, dysrhythmic optokinetic nystagmus, that is, irregular quick component generation and no spontaneous nystagmus.
ROTATIONAL TESTING:	Rotational testing indicated symmetric responses of high-normal response amplitude with an abnormally large phase lead.

Nystagmus dysrhythmia was also noted on rotational testing. Visual-vestibular interaction testing (see Chap. 2) indicated difficulty suppressing vestibular responses while viewing a head-fixed target during sinusoidal rotation. The magnitude of the patient's nystagmus during rotation while viewing earth-fixed stripes was not significantly greater than the magnitude of nystagmus elicited by rotation in darkness. Together, these findings indicated an inability to suppress or augment vestibular responses with vision. The patient's ability to reduce postrotatory nystagmus by changing the orientation of his head with respect to gravity immediately following the cessation of rotation was found to be abnormal. As discussed in Chapter 2, this deficiency suggests an abnormality of semicircular canal–otolith interaction, probably on the basis of abnormalities of the cerebellar uvula and/or nodulus.[3]

POSTUROGRAPHY: Posturography indicated excessive sway in all conditions to a moderate degree in a nonspecific pattern.

Audiometric Testing: Not performed

Imaging: MRI scan of the brain showed midline cerebellar degeneration (Fig. C11–1). There was obvious involvement of the anterior cerebellar vermis and a suggestion of loss of tissue in the caudal midline cerebellum. There were no other abnormalities on MRI scan.

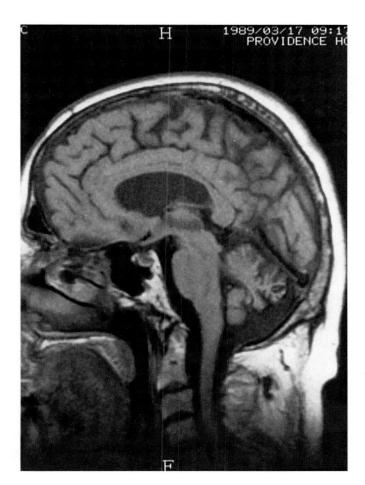

Figure C11-1
Note on this sagittal MRI that the midline cerebellum is atrophied. The cerebellar vermian sulci are larger than normal.

Other: The patient had normal screening blood studies including hematologic, metabolic, rheumatologic, and thyroid studies.

DIAGNOSIS/DIFFERENTIAL DIAGNOSIS

The patient was given the diagnosis of *adult-onset cerebellar degeneration,* probably dominantly inherited.

Question 4: Based on the history, physical examination, and laboratory studies, what is the localization of this patient's abnormality and what is its likely etiology?

Answer 4: The patient's history, physical examination, and laboratory studies all point toward an abnormality of cerebellar function. The MRI scan documents loss of midline cerebellar tissue and quantitative laboratory testing documents ocular-motor and vestibulo-ocular abnormalities consistent with an abnormality of the vestibulocerebellum (flocculonodular lobe), and centers important for the accuracy of saccades. The patient's most likely diagnosis is adult-onset cerebellar degeneration. Because saccades were of normal velocity and there were no corticospinal tract findings on neurologic examination, this patient does not have olivopontocerebellar atrophy. Given the family history, the patient appears to have a dominantly inherited form of parenchymal cerebellar atrophy.

TREATMENT/MANAGEMENT

The patient was treated by discontinuation of vestibular-suppressant medications, a home safety consultation, and referred to a physical therapist for gait training. These measures were associated with a slight improvement in the patient's balance.

Question 5: Under what circumstances is visual-vestibular interaction testing useful? What is the usefulness of measuring tilt suppression of postrotatory nystagmus?

Answer 5: Visual-vestibular interaction testing is useful as an adjunct to quantitative vestibular laboratory testing when information is needed regarding the ability of the patient to modify vestibular reflexes with vision. Visual-vestibular interaction is a particularly sensitive measure when searching for evidence of an abnormality of the vestibulocerebellum.[4] Although most patients with abnormalities of visual-vestibular interaction also have abnormalities of ocular pursuit, several studies have indicated that visual-vestibular interaction provides information over and above that which can be obtained from measuring pursuit.[5] In this patient's case, abnormal visual-vestibular interaction confirms the suspicion of abnormal central vestibular processing and suggests involvement of the cerebellar flocculus in the degeneration syndrome.

The usefulness of tilt suppression of postrotatory nystagmus pertains to its dependence on normal function of the cerebellar uvula and nodulus and their connection with the brainstem vestibular nuclei. Studies have shown that abnormal tilt suppression of postrotatory nystagmus indicates a caudal midline cerebellar lesion.[3,6] Although tilt suppression of postrotatory nystagmus is not considered a routine vestibular test, it can provide additional localizing information. This patient's abnormal tilt suppression of postrotatory nystagmus suggests involvement of the cerebellar uvula and nodulus in the degeneration syndrome.

SUMMARY

A 65-year-old man presented with a gradually worsening course of disequilibrium and gait instability. The patient's complaints did not suggest a peripheral vestibular disorder. Family history was positive for late-onset balance disorder. Examination suggested cerebellar system abnormalities. Brain imaging showed midline cerebellar degeneration. Vestibular laboratory testing indicated abnormal visual-vestibular interaction and abnormal tilt suppression of postrotatory nystagmus. The patient was given the diagnosis of adult-onset cerebellar degeneration, probably dominantly inherited. Symptomatic treatment consisted of vestibular rehabilitation therapy and discontinuation of vestibular-suppressant medication.

TEACHING POINTS

1. **A neurodegenerative disorder** should be suggested by the gradual onset and worsening of imbalance in the absence of vertigo. Other diagnostic considerations for patients with progressively severe symptoms include a posterior fossa mass lesion, vasculitis, a paraneoplastic process, or a structural abnormality such as a Chiari malformation. If a degeneration syndrome is suspected, a family history should be obtained that specifically addresses whether or not other family members have had similar difficulties.
2. **Acute ethanol intoxication** causes both reversible peripheral vestibular and reversible cerebellar dysfunction.
3. **Chronic ethanol abuse** causes cerebellar degeneration, most prominently in the cerebellar vermis, manifested by truncal ataxia and gait instability.
4. **Cerebellar degeneration** may be associated with pontine abnormalities. Thus, patients should be examined carefully for signs of pontine involvement such as slowing of saccadic eye movements and for signs of corticospinal tract involvement. In this way, patients can be categorized as to whether they have an isolated olivocerebellar degeneration or olivopontocerebellar atrophy because pontine involvement causes saccadic slowing and corticospinal tract signs. This categorization may be important because olivopontocerebellar atrophy has a worse prognosis than olivocerebellar degeneration.
5. **Visual-vestibular interaction** testing in the vestibular laboratory provides a quantitative assessment of the ability of a patient to modify vestibular reflexes with vision. Visual-vestibular interaction is a particularly sensitive measure when searching for evidence of an abnormality of the vestibulocerebellum, particularly the flocculus. Although most patients with abnormalities of visual-vestibular interaction also have abnormalities of ocular pursuit, several studies have indicated that visual-vestibular interaction provides information over and above that which can be obtained from measuring pursuit.
6. **Tilt suppression of postrotatory nystagmus** refers to a laboratory measure of the alteration of vestibular responses to a cessation of rotation caused by tilting the head. Although tilt suppression of postrotatory nystagmus is not considered a routine vestibular test, it can provide additional localizing information

about the cerebellar uvula and nodulus and their connection with the brainstem vestibular nuclei.

7. **Vestibular laboratory manifestations of cerebellar dysfunction** may include saccadic dysmetria; impaired pursuit; nystagmus dysrhythmia, that is, irregular quick component generation; abnormal visual-vestibular interaction; and abnormal tilt suppression of postrotatory nystagmus.

REFERENCES

1. Money, K, Johnson, W, and Corlett, R: Role of semicircular canals in positional alcohol nystagmus. Am J Physiol 208:1065–1070, 1965.
2. Victor, M, Adams, RD, and Collins, GH (eds): The Wernicke-Korsakoff Syndrome and Related Neurologic Disorders Due to Alcoholism and Malnutrition, 2d ed. Contemporary Neurology Series. Philadelphia: FA Davis, 1989.
3. Hain, T, Zee, D, and Maria, B: Tilt suppression of vestibulo-ocular reflex in patients with cerebellar lesions. Acta Otolaryngol 105:13–20, 1988.
4. Baloh, RW (ed): The Essentials of Neurotology. Philadelphia: FA Davis, 1984.
5. Chambers, BR, and Gresty, MA: The relationship between disordered pursuit and vestibulo-ocular reflex suppression. J Neurol Neurosurg Psychiatry 46:61–66, 1983.
6. Furman, JM, Wall, C, III, and Pang, D: Vestibular function in periodic alternating nystagmus. Brain 113:1425–1439, 1990.

C A S E

C12

Childhood Vertigo

HISTORY

A 13-year-old boy presented with a chief complaint of 4 months of dizziness occurring once or twice a week. The patient described a spinning sensation associated with a feeling of imbalance and a tendency to fall. He also noted that if he disregarded these symptoms and continued his normal activities, he could become nauseated and on two occasions had actually vomited. The patient had no complaint of hearing loss or tinnitus and did not describe fullness in the ears. His school performance was excellent, but he had experienced some recent difficulty in gym class and performing extracurricular sport.

Question 1: Based on the patient's history, what are the diagnostic considerations?

Answer 1: Causes of episodic vertigo in childhood include benign paroxysmal vertigo of childhood,[1] which is believed to have a migrainous basis,[2] and, infrequently, endolymphatic hydrops (see Cases T3, T9, C10, C14, C16). Less likely disorders include otitis media (see Case C19), perilymphatic fistula (see Case C23), a seizure disorder (see Case U7), and an anxiety disorder (see Case C2). Benign (paroxysmal) *positional* vertigo (see Cases T1, C9, and C15), not to be confused with benign *paroxysmal* vertigo of childhood, is most unusual in children. Rare metabolic abnormalities such as ornithine transcarbamylase deficiency[2] may present with episodic dizziness, as can familial periodic ataxia and vertigo. Structural lesions in the posterior fossa, including mass lesions, and malformations such as a Chiari malformation, would not be expected to produce episodic symptoms. Other unusual abnormalities that rarely present in childhood include familial vestibular areflexia and spinocerebellar degeneration.

Question 2: What further historical information will be helpful in establishing a diagnosis of benign paroxysmal vertigo of childhood?

Answer 2: Associated historical features often include motion sickness; an apparent relationship between vertiginous episodes and certain foods such as aged cheese and chocolate, possibly because of their tyramine or phenylethylamine, that is, vasoactive amines, content;[2] and a positive family history of migraine. Patients may also be bothered by certain visual environments such as flickering candles or open spaces.[3]

ADDITIONAL HISTORY

The patient had a history of car sickness, especially when riding in the back seat. He did not notice a particular association between dizziness episodes and diet. There was a strong family history of migraine on the maternal side; the patient's mother and maternal aunt suffered from throbbing headaches associated with photophobia, phonophobia, and nausea. Also, the patient's mother remembered having car sickness and avoidance of amusement parks during her childhood.

PHYSICAL EXAMINATION

The patient's physical examination was entirely normal, including general, neurologic, otologic, and neurotologic examinations.

Laboratory Testing

Vestibular Laboratory Testing

ELECTRONYSTAGMOGRAPHY:	Ocular motor function and caloric responses were normal. There was no positional nystagmus.
ROTATIONAL TESTING:	Rotational testing revealed a left directional preponderance.
POSTUROGRAPHY:	Not performed

Audiometric Testing: Audiometry testing was scheduled because of the possibility of endolymphatic hydrops or some other associated cochlear abnormality. The results of this testing were normal.

Imaging: Magnetic resonance imaging, which had been ordered by the patient's pediatrician, was normal.

Other: None.

Question 2: Are the vestibular laboratory findings of this patient consistent with a diagnosis of benign paroxysmal vertigo of childhood?

Answer 2: This patient's laboratory studies suggest an ongoing vestibulo-ocular imbalance without evidence for peripheral vestibular involvement. Moreover, there was no evidence of auditory system involvement nor evidence for a structural abnormality of the central nervous system. Taken together, these findings make the diagnosis of benign paroxysmal vertigo of childhood most likely. Although Basser's original description of benign paroxysmal vertigo of childhood[1] suggested that a unilateral caloric reduction was important for this diagnosis, subsequent studies have not suggested this as a diagnostic criterion.[4] A review of vestibular laboratory findings in patients with migraine suggests that a directional preponderance on rotation is a common finding (see Case C4).[5–7]

DIAGNOSIS/DIFFERENTIAL DIAGNOSIS

This patient was diagnosed as having *benign paroxysmal vertigo of childhood*, presumably a manifestation of a migrainous disorder.

TREATMENT/MANAGEMENT

Based on the frequency of attacks, propranolol, 20 mg three times daily, was prescribed. The patient was also advised regarding dietary restriction of foods known to provoke migraine (see Table C12–1).[8] He responded well to this intervention and had a markedly reduced frequency and severity of attacks. Other medications effective in childhood migraine, such as periactin, calcium channel blockers, and anticonvulsants, could also have been tried.[2]

SUMMARY

A 13-year-old boy presented with episodic vertigo associated with nausea but no vomiting. The patient had a history of car sickness and a family history of migraine. Magnetic resonance imaging and audiometry were normal. Vestibular laboratory testing

TABLE C12–1
Foods That May Provoke Migraine

Alcohol
Foods containing tyramine
  Aged cheeses
  Chianti wine
  Pickled herring
  Dried smoked fish
  Sour cream
  Yogurt
  Yeast extracts
  Chicken liver
Chocolate
Citrus fruit
Dairy products
Onions
Nuts
Beans
Caffeine (excess, withdrawal)
Avocado
Banana
Food additives
  Nitrates (e.g., in hot dogs, luncheon meats)
  Monosodium glutamate
  Aspartame artificial sweetener (NutraSweet, Equal)

Source: Adapted from American Council for Headache, Constantine, LM, and Scott, S: Migraine: The Complete Guide. New York: Dell Publishing, 1994, p 66.[8]

showed a vestibulo-ocular asymmetry on rotational testing, although caloric testing was normal. The patient was given a diagnosis of benign paroxysmal vertigo of childhood. Treatment consisted of dietary restriction of migraine-provoking foods and a prescription for a beta blocker. The patient responded well to this intervention and had markedly reduced frequency and severity of attacks.

TEACHING POINTS

1. **Causes of episodic vertigo in childhood** include benign paroxysmal vertigo of childhood, endolymphatic hydrops, otitis media, perilymphatic fistula, seizure disorder, and anxiety disorder. Several metabolic, anatomic, and degenerative disorders may also present with episodic dizziness. These include ornithine transcarbamylase deficiency, cranial-cervical junction malformations such as Chiari malformation, familial periodic ataxia and vertigo, familial vestibular areflexia, olivopontocerebellar atrophy, familial recurrent ataxia, and familial benign paroxysmal vertigo. Mass lesions in the posterior fossa do not generally cause episodic vertigo.

2. **Benign paroxysmal vertigo of childhood,** a common cause of vertigo in childhood, is probably a childhood manifestation of migraine. The diagnosis of benign paroxysmal vertigo of childhood is established by the presence of episodic vertigo in a child without auditory or neurologic symptoms in conjunction with associated historical features such as motion sickness sensitivity, an apparent relationship between vertiginous episodes and certain foods such as aged cheese and chocolate, and a positive family history of migraine.

3. **Vestibular test results in benign paroxysmal vertigo of childhood** usually include evidence of an ongoing vestibulo-ocular imbalance without evidence for peripheral vestibular involvement. Unilateral caloric reduction is sometimes found but is not important for this diagnosis. Directional preponderance on rotational testing is a common finding.

4. **Treatment of benign paroxysmal vertigo of childhood** depends in part on the frequency and severity of symptoms. Identification and avoidance of dietary triggers is recommended (Table C12–1). Potentially beneficial medications that may be tried in more severe cases include propranolol, periactin, amitriptyline, and depakote.

REFERENCES

1. Basser, L: Benign paroxysmal vertigo of childhood. Brain 87:141–152, 1964.
2. Hockaday, JM (ed): Migraine in Childhood. London: Butterworths, 1988.
3. Davidoff, RA: Migraine: Manifestations, Pathogenesis, and Management. Philadelphia: FA Davis, 1995.
4. Lanzi, G, et al: Benign paroxysmal vertigo of childhood: A long follow-up. Cephalalgia 14:458–460, 1994.
5. Cass, SP, et al: Migraine-related vestibulopathy. Ann Otol Rhinol Laryngol (in press).
6. Kayan, A, and Hood, J: Neuro-otological manifestations of migraine. Brain 107:1123–1142, 1984.
7. Toglia, J, Thomas, K, and Kuritzky, A: Common migraine and vestibular function electronystagmographic study and pathogenesis. Ann Otol 90:267–271, 1981.
8. American Council for Headache, Constantine, LM, and Scott, S: Migraine: The Complete Guide. New York: Dell Publishing, 1994.

C13

Solvent Exposure

HISTORY

A 30-year-old welder presented with a chief complaint of dizziness after a mishap at work 3 months before evaluation. The patient was welding inside a large tank that previously had been used for storing industrial solvents. He was not wearing any breathing protection. He remembers vaporizing some "goo." Then he felt giddy, and was observed by fellow workers giggling and rolling in the snow outside the storage tank. The patient was taken to a local emergency room, where no abnormalities were found. He experienced persistent dizziness and disequilibrium characterized by a sense of lightheadedness and worsened by head movement. The patient's symptoms were also worsened by standing for prolonged periods and by walking on uneven surfaces. He also complained of intolerance to exposure to any solvents or household cleaning agents. The patient had no complaint of hearing loss, tinnitus, or fullness or stuffiness of the ears. There was no positional sensitivity. He had no prior history of dizziness or any other significant prior medical history. Family history was noncontributory. The patient had undergone an extensive evaluation before presentation because of the legal implications of the accident. These revealed normal brain imaging, normal blood studies, and normal audiometric testing.

Question 1: Based on the patient's history, what is the likely diagnosis?

Answer 1: This patient is likely to have suffered from industrial chemical or solvent exposure.[1] The chance occurrence of any unrelated illness or exacerbation of a pre-existing condition is unlikely. He also seems to have acquired an intolerance to solvents.[2]

PHYSICAL EXAMINATION

The general and otologic examinations were normal. Neurologic examination showed that the patient had full extraocular movements with saccadic pursuit. There was bilateral horizontal gaze-evoked nystagmus. With Frenzel glasses, there was direction-changing positional nystagmus with left-beating nystagmus in the head-left and left-lateral positions and right-beating nystagmus in the head-right and right-lateral positions. Romberg's test was normal. Stepping in place revealed wide-based and ataxic stepping but not rotational deviation. The patient had a wide-based gait and unsteady tandem gait and could not stand on a foam pad with his eyes closed. The remainder of the neurologic examination was normal. There was no paroxysmal positional nystagmus on Dix-Hallpike maneuvers.

Laboratory Testing

Vestibular Laboratory Testing

ELECTRONYSTAGMOGRAPHY:	Ocular motor and positional testing confirmed the abnormalities seen during physical examination that included saccadic pursuit, bilateral horizontal gaze-evoked nystagmus, and a direction-changing positional nystagmus. Additionally, the patient could suppress his positional nystagmus with vision. There was a 35 percent left reduced vestibular response on caloric testing.
ROTATIONAL TESTING:	Rotational testing revealed a mild right directional preponderance.
POSTUROGRAPHY:	Posturography indicated excessive sway on all conditions in a nonspecific pattern.

Audiometric Testing: Not performed

Imaging: Not performed

Other: None

Question 2: Based on the patient's history, physical examination, and laboratory studies, what structures are likely to be involved in this patient's problem?

Answer 2: Some of this patient's abnormalities, such as gaze-evoked nystagmus and saccadic pursuit, suggest brainstem and cerebellar involvement, whereas peripheral vestibular involvement (on the left) is suggested by caloric testing. His posturography is nonlocalizing and thus does not support or rule out a peripheral vestibular disorder. The patient's directional preponderance on rotational testing suggests an ongoing vestibulo-ocular asymmetry either on the basis of poor compensation for his peripheral vestibular disorder (see Cases C1 and C16) or on the basis of a central vestibular abnormality.

Question 3: What is the pathophysiology of direction-changing positional nystagmus and what is its localizing value?

Answer 3: Direction-changing positional nystagmus was at one time thought to be indicative of a central nervous system disorder, but more recent studies have suggested that direction-changing positional nystagmus can be caused by either a peripheral or a central vestibular disorder.[3] A well-recognized peripheral vestibular cause for direction-changing positional nystagmus is acute ethanol intoxication. However, direction-changing positional nystagmus that is not acute and not a result of ethanol cannot be localized. Direction-changing positional nystagmus of peripheral vestibular origin, either alcoholic or otherwise, is probably based on an inequality between the specific gravity of the cupula of the horizontal semicircular canal and the specific gravity of the surrounding endolymph.[4] Such an inequality of specific gravity could result from either a heavy cupula, a light cupula, or from debris adherent to the cupula.

Well-documented cases of direction-changing positional nystagmus resulting from central nervous system lesions have been described,[5] but the underlying pathophysiology for this association is unknown. Thus, this patient's direction-changing positional nystagmus may be based upon either a central or a peripheral vestibular involvement.

Question 4: What are some of the industrial solvents known to cause vestibular system impairment and what is the pathophysiologic basis for this impairment?

Answer 4: Very little is known about industrial solvent exposure, including exactly which chemicals are responsible and the underlying pathophysiology. However, xylene, styrene, trichlorethylene, and methylchloroform are industrial agents thought to be toxic to the vestibular system.[6] The most consistent vestibular abnormalities following exposure to these agents in animals are a static, that is, a nonparoxysmal, positional nystagmus[6] and impaired visual-vestibular interaction.[7-9] Other reported abnormalities include an increased vestibulo-ocular response.[10]

The pathophysiology of the vestibular dysfunction seen in industrial solvent exposure probably relates to central vestibular pathways, including the cerebellum. The direction-changing positional nystagmus seen with solvent exposure is not thought to be caused by a cupula-endolymph specific gravity mismatch (see above), because the positional nystagmus can be blocked by the GABA agonist baclofen.[6]

Chronic exposure to volatile hydrocarbons can cause chronic toxic encephalopathy, which can be associated with abnormal visual-vestibular interaction and abnormal smooth pursuit.[11]

DIAGNOSIS/DIFFERENTIAL DIAGNOSIS

This patient was given the diagnosis of *industrial solvent toxicity* causing a combination of peripheral and central vestibular disorders.

TREATMENT/MANAGEMENT

This patient was treated with a course of balance rehabilitation therapy. He was advised to avoid exposure to all industrial solvents, including paint fumes and household cleaning products. The patient was also advised to avoid situations that required balance for safety. His symptoms improved somewhat, but he was unable to return to work as a welder.

SUMMARY

A 30-year-old male welder was accidentally exposed to a vaporized mixture of industrial solvents and became acutely dizzy. He gradually recovered but was left with a chronic imbalance. The patient was found to have objective evidence of a vestibular system disorder, including direction-changing positional nystagmus, which is a non-localizing abnormality. Other abnormalities, such as a unilateral caloric reduction and abnormal ocular motor testing, suggested impairment of both peripheral and central vestibular structures, respectively. The patient was treated with a course of balance rehabilitation therapy and gained some decrease in symptoms, but he could not return to work.

TEACHING POINTS

1. **Industrial solvents** can cause vestibular system impairment. Xylene, styrene, trichlorethylene, and methylchloroform are industrial agents thought to be toxic to the vestibular system. The most consistent vestibular abnormality following exposure to these agents is a static positional nystagmus.
2. **The pathophysiology of industrial solvent–induced vestibular dysfunction** is unknown but probably involves central vestibular pathways including the cerebellum.
3. **Treatment for industrial solvent–induced vestibular dysfunction is nonspecific.** Affected individuals should be advised to avoid subsequent exposure to all industrial solvents, including paint fumes and household cleaning products, and to avoid situations that require balance for safety. Vestibular rehabilitation may help promote improved balance and adaptation to vestibular deficits.

REFERENCES

1. Hodgson, MJ, et al: Encephalopathy and vestibulopathy following short-term hydrocarbon exposure. J Occup Med 31:51–54, 1989.
2. Gyntelberg, F, et al: Acquired intolerance to organic solvents and results of vestibular testing. Am J Ind Med 9:363–370, 1986.
3. Brandt, T: Background, technique, interpretation, and usefulness of positional and positioning testing. In Jacobson, GP, Newman, CW, and Kartush, JM (eds): Handbook of Balance Function Testing. St Louis: Mosby Year Book, 1993.
4. Money, K, Johnson, W, and Corlett, R: Role of semicircular canals in positional alcohol nystagmus. Am J Physiol 208:1065–1070, 1965.
5. Lin, J, Elidan, J, Baloh, RW, and Honruba, V: Direction-changing positional nystagmus: Incidence and meaning. Am J Otolaryngol 7:306–310, 1986.
6. Odkvist, LM, et al: Vestibular and oculomotor disturbances caused by industrial solvents. J Otolaryngol 9:53–59, 1980.
7. Niklasson, M, Tham, R, Larsby, B, and Eriksson, B: Effects of toluene, styrene, trichloroethylene, and trichloromethane on the vestibulo- and opto-oculo motor system in rats. Neurotoxicol Teratol 15:327–334, 1993.
8. Hyden, D, et al: Impairment of visuo-vestibular interaction in humans. ORL J Otorhinolaryngol Relat Spec 45:262–269, 1983.
9. Odkvist, LM, et al: Vestibulo-oculomotor disturbances in humans exposed to styrene. Acta Otolaryngol 94:487–493, 1982.
10. Biscaldi, GP, et al: Acute toluene poisoning. Electroneurophysiological and vestibular investigations. Toxicol Eur Res 3:271–273, 1981.
11. Odkvist, LM, Moller, C, and Thuomas, K-A: Otoneurologic disturbances caused by solvent pollution. Otolaryngol Head Neck Surg 106:687, 1992.

C14

Surgical Treatment of Meniere's Disease

HISTORY

A 36-year-old woman who worked as a cashier in a large grocery store presented with a complaint of recurrent bouts of vertigo that had occurred every 7 to 14 days for 6 months before evaluation. The spells consisted of severe rotatory vertigo, nausea, and often retching or vomiting that usually lasted for a few hours. For 1 or 2 days after the acute vertigo, she felt somewhat unsteady and dizzy when moving her head. Subsequently, her symptoms resolved within several days. The episodes of vertigo occurred irregularly and without an obvious precipitant. She reported being quite embarrassed on a number of occasions when incapacitating vertigo occurred suddenly at work. One year before evaluation, the patient had suffered a few spells of vertigo and was evaluated by her primary care physician, who thought that the vertigo might possibly be caused by Meniere's disease. The primary care physician prescribed meclizine and a diuretic, with a low-salt diet. The patient had faithfully used the diuretic and restricted salt intake and was symptom free for about 6 months. She felt quite frustrated by the return of episodic vertigo.

In addition to the episodes of vertigo, the patient reported the recent onset of some hearing disturbances in her right ear. She described her hearing as sometimes muffled or clogged with intermittent tinnitus, and fullness in her right ear before the vertigo. On the day of evaluation, the patient noticed that loud noises sounded abnormally sharp and almost painful.

PHYSICAL EXAMINATION

General examination was normal. The neurologic examination was normal except that the patient had increased sway on Romberg's test. Gait was normal. On tests of sensory interaction and balance, the patient was able to maintain her balance while standing on foam with her eyes open or closed. The stepping test revealed a 100-degree deviation to the right. The Dix-Hallpike maneuver was negative. Otoscopy was normal. Pressure

165

changes induced in the external auditory canal by pneumatic otoscopy produced no dizziness or nystagmus.

DIAGNOSIS/DIFFERENTIAL DIAGNOSIS

Question 1: What is this patient's most likely diagnosis?

Answer 1: This patient is likely to have Meniere's disease (see Cases T3, T9, C10, and C16). The symptoms of recurrent vertigo, hearing loss, tinnitus, and aural fullness are characteristic of Meniere's disease. However, Meniere's disease is a clinical diagnosis. No test is absolutely diagnostic for this disease, and the presence of endolymphatic hydrops can be proved with certainty only by postmortem histologic examination of the temporal bones. It is important that the term Meniere's disease not be used to describe all forms of dizziness, but be restricted to patients who manifest the full symptom complex described above. Patients manifesting only part of the syndrome, such as Meniere-like vertigo without hearing loss, tinnitus, and aural fullness without vertigo, can be described as possibly having Meniere's disease. In these individuals, the true diagnosis often becomes evident over time.

This patient was given the diagnosis of *Meniere's disease.*

TREATMENT/MANAGEMENT

Question 2: What are the options for treating this patient?

Answer 2: It is essential that treatable causes of endolymphatic hydrops, such as metabolic and endocrine disorders, infectious diseases, and central nervous system abnormalities, be considered and ruled out. A number of factors such as stress, smoking, excessive salt intake, and the use of alcohol and caffeine are known to be capable of exacerbating Meniere's disease, and the patient should be encouraged to adjust his or her lifestyle accordingly. The use of a diuretic and dietary salt restriction is an effective treatment of Meniere's disease.[1] Other medications that have been used include vasodilators, vestibular suppressants, and calcium channel blockers. It is estimated that about 20 percent of individuals with Meniere's disease will eventually fail medical therapy.[1] Individuals such as this patient, who have failed medical therapy, are faced with using symptomatic relief for each episode or considering surgical intervention, which is discussed extensively in the following text.

Question 3: What surgical procedures are available to treat vertigo caused by Meniere's disease?

Answer 3: The surgical alternatives for treating vertigo caused by Meniere's disease include endolymphatic sac surgery, labyrinthectomy, and vestibular nerve section. It is essential that the patient understand that none of these procedures benefit the hearing loss, tinnitus, or aural fullness associated with Meniere's disease. In fact, any otologic surgical procedure, including endolymphatic sac surgery or vestibular nerve section, may cause further hearing loss. Labyrinthectomy always produces complete deafness.

Endolymphatic sac surgery presumably reduces vertigo by affecting the underlying pathologic process of endolymphatic hydrops, that is, by reducing endolymphatic pressure.[2] The endolymphatic sac is illustrated in Figure C14–1. Endolymphatic sac surgery is a safe and uncomplicated procedure. It is usually performed as outpatient surgery and requires only 3 to 5 days of postsurgical convalescence. Unfortunately, the success rate for control of vertigo ranges between 50 to 70 percent. Many surgeons recognize that this low success rate approximates what would be expected from a placebo procedure, and thus do not routinely recommend sac surgery.[3] Interestingly, despite the relatively low success rate of endolymphatic sac surgery, patients often choose to undergo sac surgery because of the prospect of improving their vertigo without undergoing a more involved surgical procedure.

The goal of both labyrinthectomy and vestibular nerve section is to permanently ablate all vestibular function in the ear affected by Meniere's disease. The dysfunctional ear can then no longer produce vertigo because the vestibular apparatus has been destroyed (labyrinthectomy) or disconnected from the brain (vestibular nerve section). Labyrinthectomy is a highly successful procedure (90 to 95 percent

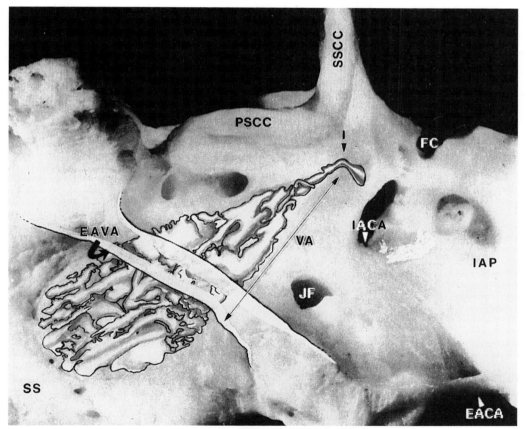

Figure C14-1

Three-dimensional computer-aided reconstruction of the vestibular aqueduct and endolymphatic sac anatomically positioned within a microdissected left human temporal bone. VA = vestibular aqueduct; EAVA = external aperture of the vestibular aqueduct; FC = facial canal; EACA = external aperture of the cochlear aqueduct; IACA = internal aperture of the cochlear aqueduct; IAP = internal auditory canal; JF = jugular foramen; PSCC = posterior semicircular canal; SS = sigmoid sinus; SSCC = superior semicircular canal. (With permission from Wackym, PA, et al: Re-evaluation of the role of the human endolymphatic sac in Meniere's disease. Otolaryngol Head Neck Surg 102:732–744, 1990.[10])

vertigo control) and has a relatively low risk, but always results in permanent loss of hearing in the treated ear.[4] Surgical labyrinthectomy is illustrated in Figure C14–2. The advantages of labyrinthectomy include brief operating time, technical ease, and the ability to visualize clearly and remove all vestibular neuroepithelium, which ensures the reliable control of vertigo. Vestibular nerve section is also highly successful (85 to 90 percent vertigo control) and has the advantage that hearing is usually preserved in the operated ear.[5,6] Vestibular nerve section is illustrated in Figure C14–3. The disadvantage of vestibular nerve section is that it is a more complicated procedure, and although the incidence of complications is low, the potential complications can be severe.

Another form of treatment called *chemical labyrinthectomy* is currently under active investigation.[7] In chemical labyrinthectomy, an ototoxic medication that is preferentially toxic to vestibular as compared to auditory hair cells, such as

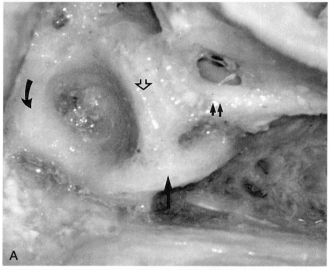

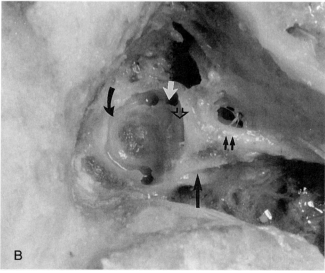

Figure C14-2
(*A*) Gross anatomical view of the semicircular canals from a micro-dissected right human temporal bone. (*B*) Surgical labyrinthectomy performed by opening each of the canals and the vestibule with direct visualization and removal of the neuroepithelium. Curved arrow = superior semicircular canal; open arrow = horizontal semicircular canal; straight arrow = posterior semicircular canal; double arrows = facial nerve; white arrow = vestibule.

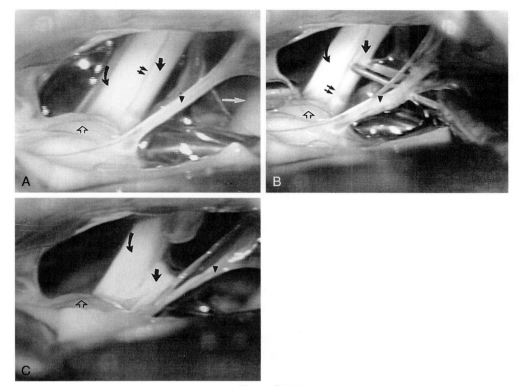

Figure C14-3
(*A*) Surgical view of the vestibular and cochlear nerves through a small craniotomy posterior to the left mastoid. (*B*) Selective vestibular nerve section is performed using micro-scissors. Note the small blood vessel running on the posterior surface of the vestibular-cochlear nerve complex, which helps to define the plane between the vestibular and cochlear nerve bundles. (*C*) Completed vestibular nerve section. Open arrow = cerebellar flocculus; curved arrow = cochlear division of eight cranial nerve; double black arrows = blood vessel demarcating border of between cochlear and vestibular divisions of the eighth cranial nerve; white arrow = fifth cranial nerve; arrowhead = strand of anarchnoid tissue.

gentamicin, is injected into the middle ear space (Fig. C14–4). Once in the middle ear, the medication reaches the inner ear through the round window membrane and exerts a toxic effect on the vestibular hair cells, resulting in ablation of vestibular function in the ear. Chemical labyrinthectomy is performed in the office setting using topical anesthesia. Preliminary results suggest that control of vertigo using chemical

Figure C14-4
Schematic view of the injection of gentamicin into the middle ear space for chemical labyrinthectomy. (With permission from Monsell, EM, et al: Chemical labyrinthectomy: Methods and results. In Brackmann, DE (ed): Otologic Surgery. Philadelphia: WB Saunders, 1994, p 517.[11])

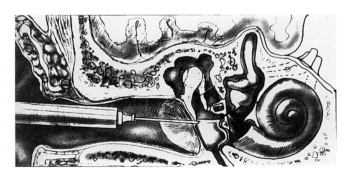

labyrinthectomy is similar to that achieved using vestibular nerve section. Severe
hearing loss induced by chemical labyrinthectomy may occur in 10 to 20 percent of
patients as compared to about 5 percent of patients following vestibular nerve
section. It is unclear, however, if the long-term hearing results differ among patients
undergoing vestibular neurectomy, chemical labyrinthectomy, and the natural
progression of hearing loss that characterizes Meniere's disease.

Patients with profound loss of hearing are ideal candidates for surgical or
chemical labyrinthectomy. Patients with normal or nearly normal hearing are ideal
candidates for vestibular nerve section. The patient and surgeon need to discuss the
pros and cons of labyrinthectomy and vestibular nerve section. Our general view is
that younger patients (under age 65) with any measurable hearing should first
consider vestibular nerve section. This view recognizes that (1) hearing in Meniere's
disease typically fluctuates over time and could improve spontaneously after surgery;
(2) individuals with many years of life expectancy have a chance of unexpectedly
losing hearing in their contralateral ear. If this should happen, any hearing that is
preserved may be of critical importance; and (3) speech reception threshold and word
recognition levels do not fully describe all the beneficial aspects of hearing. "Useful"
hearing is difficult to define and must be individualized. Older patients (over age 65)
with moderate to severe hearing loss that has stopped fluctuating and who do not
receive any benefit from using a hearing aid are generally better candidates for
labyrinthectomy.

In the setting of bilateral Meniere's disease (see Case T9) or in the setting of
unilateral Meniere's disease complicated by a contralateral hearing loss of any cause,
treatment decisions regarding surgical treatment can be complex.

Question 4: What are the characteristics of patients with Meniere's disease for
whom surgery is an appropriate treatment option?

Answer 4: As a general rule, the following three criteria should be met before
considering surgery for vertigo. First, the vertigo should be caused by unilateral
peripheral vestibular dysfunction and the offending ear must be localized with
certainty. Meniere's disease is one of the most common forms of unilateral peripheral
vestibular dysfunction, and the affected side is usually unambiguously identified by
the presence of unilateral hearing loss, tinnitus, and aural fullness. Second, the vertigo
should be disabling to the patient. There are no hard-and-fast rules to determine
disability, and each patient's situation and desires must be considered individually.
Third, there should be no signs or symptoms of central vestibular system dysfunction
that could impair vestibular compensation (see Chap. 1 and Case C1).[8,9] Central
nervous system dysfunction can be detected by the neurologic portion of the physical
examination and confirmed by vestibular function testing. Aging also adversely affects
vestibular compensation, and therefore the patient's age, both chronologic and
physiologic, must be considered before recommending surgery.

Question 5: At what stage in a patient's clinical course should surgery be considered
for Meniere's disease?

Answer 5: Surgical candidates should have failed at least a 6-month trial of medical
therapy (diuretic and dietary salt restriction) and the vertigo should be disabling to the
patient. Vertigo caused by Meniere's disease is usually incapacitating, producing
violent spinning vertigo, loss of postural control, nausea, and often vomiting. These

episodes usually last a few hours, and most patients need to rest or sleep afterward. When these episodes are frequent, employment, family life, and personal well-being are threatened and surgical intervention is appropriate. As noted above, the Meniere's disease should not be bilateral and there should be no evidence of central nervous system dysfunction. Younger individuals with financial and family responsibilities are more likely to feel disabled by the recurrent vertigo and often seek a surgical remedy earlier in their disease than nonworking or retired individuals, who can usually tolerate this condition without much disruption of their lifestyle. Thus, because Meniere's disease is not a life-threatening disorder, surgical intervention should be emphasized only when vertigo is causing a significant and unacceptable change in a patient's lifestyle.

Question 6: What laboratory testing is indicated before surgery for Meniere's disease?

Answer 6: Vestibular function testing is indicated to search for evidence of coexisting central nervous system dysfunction. Central nervous system dysfunction is a contraindication to surgery because of its potential adverse effect on postsurgical vestibular compensation, which is required for a successful clinical outcome. Also, it is helpful to know whether the contralateral ear has normal caloric function. Moreover, the degree of caloric weakness in the affected ear can be used to estimate the severity of the postsurgical acute vestibular syndrome. If the ear to be operated on has absent responses preoperatively, the patient's immediate postoperative vestibular imbalance may be mild because the patient probably already has compensated for a unilateral vestibular deficit.

An audiogram is indicated to (1) confirm the involved ear and to be sure it fits into a Meniere-type pattern, and (2) to document the amount and usefulness of the remaining hearing to the patient because, as noted above, this information is an important factor in deciding which surgical procedure to consider. Brainstem auditory-evoked potentials or brain imaging is also indicated in all patients before surgical intervention to assess the central nervous system.

Laboratory Testing

Vestibular Laboratory Testing

ELECTRONYSTAGMOGRAPHY:	Ocular motor function including saccades, pursuit, and optokinetic nystagmus was normal. A low-amplitude left-beating spontaneous vestibular nystagmus was noted. There was no positional nystagmus. Caloric irrigation revealed a significant right reduced vestibular response.
ROTATIONAL TESTING:	Rotational testing revealed normal gain and phase with a mild left directional preponderance.
POSTUROGRAPHY:	Posturography was normal.

Audiometric Testing: The audiogram showed normal hearing in the left ear and a mild low-frequency sensorineural hearing loss in the right ear. Word recognition scores were 100 percent in each ear.

Imaging: An MR scan of the brain with and without gadolinium enhancement was normal.

Other: None

TREATMENT/MANAGEMENT

The patient elected to undergo right selective vestibular nerve section. The surgical procedure was performed without complication and required approximately 3 hours. After surgery, the patient remained in the hospital for 4 days. On the first postoperative day, the patient was very nauseated and vomited when she rolled over in bed. She stayed in bed the entire day and required intravenous hydration and intramuscular antiemetics. Interestingly, she stated that an acute Meniere attack was worse than the way she felt after surgery. Third-degree left-beating vestibular nystagmus, that is, a horizontal-torsional left-beating vestibular nystagmus that was present in all fields of gaze but worst on leftward gaze was noted. On the second postoperative day, she was able to get out of bed, ambulate with assistance, and drink fluids without vomiting. Her gait was wide-based and slow. She consistently veered to the right and restricted head movement. Examination of her extraocular movements revealed the presence of second-degree vestibular nystagmus, that is, a nystagmus that was like the third-degree nystagmus seen the previous day except that now the nystagmus was present only with the gaze straight ahead and to the left. There was no nystagmus on rightward gaze. Consultation with a physical therapist was obtained and the patient was instructed regarding the use of head, eye, and body exercises to promote vestibular compensation (see Chapt. 4). The patient was discharged home on the fourth postoperative day. On the day of discharge, a first-degree vestibular nystagmus was noted, that is, a nystagmus that was present only on gaze to the left but absent on rightward or straight-ahead gaze. The patient was able to return to work about 1 month later.

SUMMARY

A 36-year-old woman presented with a 1-year history of recurrent vertigo. She was diagnosed as having unilateral Meniere's disease. Medical therapy was unsuccessful. She was treated with surgery consisting of a selective vestibular nerve section. Her hearing was unchanged. Vertiginous episodes ceased. The patient underwent vestibular rehabilitation with a physical therapist and returned to work 1 month following surgery.

TEACHING POINTS

1. **Meniere's disease** is characterized by recurrent vertigo, hearing loss, tinnitus, and aural fullness. Meniere's disease is a clinical diagnosis, and no test is absolutely diagnostic for it. Meniere's disease may be considered the idiopathic form of endolymphatic hydrops. It is essential that known treatable causes of endolymphatic hydrops such as metabolic, endocrine, and infectious diseases be considered and ruled out. Several factors such as stress; excessive salt intake; and use of tobacco, alcohol, and caffeine can exacerbate Meniere's disease.
2. **Medical treatment of Meniere's disease** includes the use of a diuretic and dietary salt restriction. However, about 20 percent of individuals with Meniere's disease will eventually fail medical therapy.
3. **Surgical treatment for Meniere's disease** includes endolymphatic sac surgery, labyrinthectomy, and vestibular nerve section. It is essential that the patient

understand that none of these procedures benefit the hearing loss, tinnitus, or aural fullness associated with Meniere's disease. Surgical candidates should have failed at least a 6-month trial of medical therapy (diuretic and dietary salt restriction) and the vertigo should be disabling to the patient.

4. **Chemical labyrinthectomy**, an alternative to surgery, is a new nonsurgical procedure. Chemical labyrinthectomy is able to produce ablation of vestibular function without surgery or general anesthesia. This procedure consists of instillation of an ototoxic agent, typically an aminoglycoside antibiotic, into the middle ear. Chemical labyrinthectomy is especially applicable to elderly or infirm patients with disabling vertigo.

5. **Vestibular function testing in Meniere's disease** may uncover coexisting central nervous system dysfunction. Central nervous system dysfunction is a contraindication to surgery because of its potential adverse effect on postsurgical vestibular compensation, which is required for a successful clinical outcome.

REFERENCES

1. Jackson, CG, Glasscock, ME, and Davis, WE: Medical management of Meniere's disease. Ann Otol 90:142–147, 1981.
2. Monsell, EM, and Wiet, RJ: Endolymphatic sac surgery: Methods of study and results. Am J Otol 9:396–402, 1988.
3. Silverstein, H, Smouha, E, and Jones, R: Natural history vs. surgery for Meniere's disease. Otolaryngol Head Neck Surg 100:6–16, 1989.
4. Kemink, JL, et al: Transmatoid labyrinthectomy: Reliable surgical management of vertigo. Otolaryngol Head Neck Surg 101:5–10, 1989.
5. Silverstein, H, and Norell, H: Retrolabyrinthine vestibular neurectomy. Otolaryngol Head Neck Surg 90:778–782, 1982.
6. Monsell, EM, et al: Surgical treatment of vertigo with retrolabyrinthine vestibular neurectomy. Laryngoscope 98:835–839, 1988.
7. Monsell, EM, Cass, SP, and Rybak, LP: Chemical labyrinthectomy: Methods and results. In Brackmann, DE (ed): Otologic Surgery. Philadelphia: WB Saunders, 1994.
8. Monsell, EM, Brackmann, DE, and Linthicum, FH: Why do vestibular destructive procedures sometimes fail? Otolaryngol Head Neck Surg 99:472–479, 1988.
9. Konrad, HR: Intractable vertigo—When not to operate. Otolaryngol Head Neck Surg 95:482–484, 1986.
10. Wackym, PA, et al: Re-evaluation of the role of the human endolymphatic sac in Meniere's disease. Otolaryngol Head Neck Surg 102:732–744, 1990.
11. Monsell, EM, et al: Chemical labyrinthectomy: Methods and results. In Brackmann, DE (ed): Otologic Surgery. Philadelphia: WB Saunders, 1994.

C15

Surgical Management of Benign Positional Vertigo

HISTORY

A 70-year-old retired woman complained of bouts of vertigo that occurred daily for 8 months before evaluation. The patient reported that vertigo could be provoked by lying down in bed, rolling over in bed, or getting out of bed. She expressed a fear of falling and was unable to leave her home because of fear of her vertigo. The patient reported that similar vertiginous episodes had recurred intermittently for the previous 20 years.

Recently, the patient was treated using particle-repositioning maneuvers (see Cases T1 and C9). Although the maneuvers were repeated at six different office visits, she continued to suffer from positional vertigo. After the particle-repositioning maneuvers failed, the patient underwent a 3-month course of vestibular rehabilitation therapy that focused on Brandt-Daroff exercises. After physical therapy, the positional vertigo continued unabated.

Question 1: This patient reported a 20-year history of symptoms consistent with benign positional vertigo. Is it unusual for benign positional vertigo to persist for this long?

Answer 1: A history of recurrent periods of positional vertigo spanning 20 years is not unusual. Studies that reflect the natural history of benign positional vertigo show that up to 25 percent of patients with benign positional vertigo report symptoms that have persisted for greater than 1 year, and many report vertigo lasting 5 to 20 years.[1] Most patients have symptoms intermittently, but some have positional vertigo that is always present. These individuals have learned never to sleep on the affected side, bend over, or pitch their head backward. Interestingly, by sleeping with the head turned away from the affected side, these individuals have probably inadvertently prolonged their benign positional vertigo, because the presumed free-floating endolymph particles that cause benign positional vertigo never have a chance to escape the posterior semicircular canal. Typically, periods of benign positional vertigo can last 6 to 8 weeks and then spontaneously disappear. Recurrent episodes of benign positional vertigo may occur multiple times each year.

Question 2: This patient presented with what appears to be "typical" benign positional vertigo. However, the positional vertigo was unresponsive to treatment using particle repositioning maneuvers and physical therapy that included Brandt-Daroff exercises. Is it unusual for benign positional vertigo to be unresponsive to these treatments?

Answer 2: Benign positional vertigo that is unresponsive to particle-repositioning maneuvers or to Brandt-Daroff exercises is unusual but does occasionally occur. More commonly, benign positional vertigo disappears either spontaneously or after treatment, but recurs later. It is estimated that approximately 30 percent of individuals with one episode of benign positional vertigo will have a recurrence within 1 year.[1]

Question 3: What other conditions should be considered in patients with benign positional vertigo that is unresponsive to treatment?

Answer 3: Even if a patient's description is quite typical of benign positional vertigo, it is important to rule out: (1) a central nervous system cause of apparent benign positional vertigo,[2–4] (2) bilateral benign positional vertigo, (3) horizontal semicircular canal benign positional vertigo (see below), and (4) an associated chronic peripheral vestibular disorder other than benign positional vertigo that is contributing to the patient's symptoms.

Rarely, patients with symptoms and signs identical to those characteristic of benign positional nystagmus and vertigo have been diagnosed as having a brainstem neoplasm or brainstem infarction.[3,4]

Bilateral benign positional vertigo occurs infrequently in patients with benign positional vertigo and can be ruled out by performing the Dix-Hallpike maneuver with the head turned both to the right and to the left. If benign positional vertigo is present bilaterally, sequential particle-repositioning maneuvers can be performed. Horizontal semicircular canal benign positional vertigo (HCBPV), presumably caused by debris in the horizontal rather than the posterior semicircular canal,[5] can be detected by placing the individual into the supine position and then turning the head rapidly to the head right or right lateral position and then quickly to the head left or left lateral position (see Case U17). HCBPV produces horizontal right-beating nystagmus with the head turned to the right and left-beating with the head turned to the left. HCBPV can be seen in patients who have undergone a particle-repositioning maneuver for typical, that is, posterior semicircular canal, benign positional vertigo. Presumably, these patients have debris that moved from the posterior to the horizontal semicircular canal. HCBPV can be treated using a modified particle-repositioning maneuver (see Case U17).[6]

A peripheral vestibulopathy associated with benign positional vertigo is not unusual,[5] especially if benign positional vertigo follows an acute labyrinthine disorder. Presumably, an acute vestibulopathy, whether viral, traumatic, or other, can produce degeneration within the inner ear that results in the formation of free-floating endolymphatic debris that causes benign positional vertigo (see Case C9). Thus, in a patient with symptoms persisting despite treatment for benign positional vertigo, the symptoms may actually be based on the prior peripheral labyrinthine injury. The patient may not have fully compensated from a peripheral disorder, or the peripheral disorder may be fluctuating and thereby producing intermittent symptoms. Such symptoms should be easily distinguished from those of typical benign positional vertigo.

Although benign positional vertigo is usually caused by free-floating endolymph particles, it has been postulated that occasionally a *fixed* cupular density may occur. In this situation, particle repositioning or exercises may not cause dispersion of the cupular density. This situation is called *cupulolithiasis* rather than *canalithiasis*. The direction of typical positional nystagmus and its fatigability, when present, are difficult to explain physiologically using the cupulolithiasis theory. As a result, even the existence of cupulolithiasis is now controversial.

PHYSICAL EXAMINATION

The patient's general, neurologic, and otologic examinations were normal. On performance of the Dix-Hallpike maneuver with the head turned to the right, a torsional-upbeat nystagmus typical of benign positional vertigo was provoked. The patient experienced vertigo. The nystagmus and vertigo began approximately 5 seconds following positioning and lasted approximately 30 seconds. A particle-repositioning maneuver was performed (see Case C9), but upon repeat Dix-Hallpike testing, nystagmus and vertigo, although decreased in intensity, remained present. The Dix-Hallpike maneuver with the head turned to the left was negative for vertigo or nystagmus. Testing for horizontal canal benign positional vertigo (see Case U17) by rapidly positioning the patient into the head left or head right position from the supine position was negative.

Laboratory Testing

Vestibular Laboratory Testing

ELECTRONYSTAGMOGRAPHY:	Ocular motor and static positional testing were normal. However, Dix-Hallpike maneuvers produced vertigo and upbeating nystagmus typical of benign positional vertigo in the head-hanging right position.
ROTATIONAL TESTING:	Not performed
POSTUROGRAPHY:	Not performed

Audiometric Testing: Not performed

Imaging: An MRI scan of the brain was performed and was normal.

Other: None

Question 4: Based on the additional information from physical examination and laboratory testing, what are the diagnostic considerations?

Answer 4: This patient appears to have typical benign positional vertigo that is refractory to conventional treatments. Examination and laboratory testing have ruled out bilateral benign positional vertigo, HCBPV, and a posterior fossa lesion. An associated vestibulopathy is also unlikely.

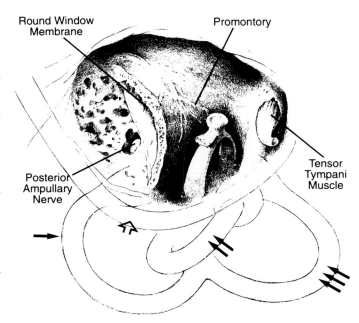

Round Window
Membrane

Promontory

Posterior
Ampullary
Nerve

Tensor
Tympani
Muscle

Figure C15-1
Schematic anatomical drawing showing the location of the singular nerve (posterior ampullary nerve) near the round window membrane. Singular neurectomy is performed by lifting the eardrum and exposing the singular nerve in the middle ear, usually under local anesthesia. The promontory represents the region of the basal turn of the cochlea and vestibule. Single arrow = posterior semicircular canal; double arrow = horizontal semicircular canal; triple arrow = superior semicircular canal; open arrow = facial nerve. (With permission from Epley, JM: Singular neurectomy: Hypotympanotomy approach. Otolaryngol Head Neck Surg 88:304–309, 1980.[10])

Question 5: What surgical procedures are available for treatment of patients with benign positional vertigo that has been unresponsive to treatment with physical maneuvers?

Answer 5: Three types of surgical procedures have been performed for patients with benign positional vertigo refractory to other nonsurgical treatments. These include: (1) singular neurectomy[7] (Fig. C15–1), (2) posterior semicircular canal "plugging" (occlusion)[8] (Fig. C15–2), and (3) vestibular nerve section.[9] Because the singular nerve is composed of only eighth-nerve afferent fibers that innervate the ampulla of the posterior semicircular canal, singular neurectomy, a procedure in which the singular

Figure C15-2
Semicircular canal plugging for benign positional vertigo. (*A*) Posterior semicircular canal is exposed within the mastoid cavity and a small oval island of bone is drilled free. (*B*) The island of bone is removed with a pick, revealing the perilymphatic and endolymphatic compartments within the bony semicircular canal. (*C*) Bone wax or bone paté is then inserted into the opening in the semicircular canal. (*D*) Plugging of the bony canal results in compression and occlusion of the endolymphatic compartment, which physiologically inactivates the posterior semicircular canal. (With permission from Hirsch BE, et al: Translabyrinthine approach to skull base tumors with hearing preservation. Am J Otol 14(6):533–543, 1993.[11])

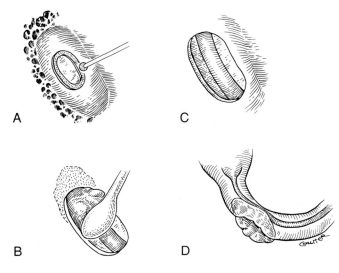

A

C

B

D

nerve is selectively sectioned, removes all afferent activity arising from the posterior semicircular canal. Posterior semicircular canal "plugging" refers to a procedure in which the bony posterior semicircular canal is opened surgically and then occluded with bone wax or a "paté" of bone dust and fibrin glue. This procedure inactivates the posterior semicircular canal ampulla. Vestibular nerve section refers to the sectioning of the entire vestibular nerve (see also Case C14).

Question 6: How do these three alternative surgical procedures address the underlying pathophysiology of benign positional vertigo?

Answer 6: Singular neurectomy (see Figure C15–1) takes advantage of the fact that the posterior semicircular canal ampulla is abnormally stimulated in patients with benign positional vertigo. Thus, by sectioning the afferent nerve to the posterior canal ampulla, erroneous signals that result from abnormal stimulation of the posterior semicircular canal that occur with certain head movements are not transmitted to the central nervous system and thus vertigo and nystagmus are prevented.

Occlusion (plugging) of the posterior semicircular canal (see Fig. C15–2) prevents the flow of endolymph in the posterior semicircular canal. By preventing endolymph flow, the posterior semicircular canal is effectively inactivated. Thus, free-floating particles either become locked in place and cannot provoke vertigo with head movement, or are no longer able to cause deflection of the posterior semicircular canal cupula because they are physically separated from the ampulla. Vestibular nerve section does not specifically address the pathophysiology of benign positional vertigo and is generally not indicated for patients with benign positional vertigo because this procedure results in denervation of the entire vestibular portion of the inner ear. However, vestibular nerve section may be indicated in selected patients with concomitant labyrinthine dysfunction in addition to benign positional vertigo.

Question 7: How often is a surgical remedy required for benign positional vertigo?

Answer 7: We estimate that fewer than 1 in 100 cases of benign positional vertigo require surgical intervention. Both the natural history of benign positional vertigo and the success of particle-repositioning maneuvers and vestibular exercises ensure that most patients with benign positional vertigo can be cured without surgery.

DIAGNOSIS/DIFFERENTIAL DIAGNOSIS

This patient has *benign positional vertigo* recalcitrant to medical management. Causes other than a unilateral posterior semicircular canal lesion, including a central nervous system disease, bilateral benign positional vertigo, horizontal canal benign positional vertigo, and an associated labyrinthine injury, were ruled out.

TREATMENT/MANAGEMENT

This patient was successfully treated with surgical occlusion (plugging) of the posterior semicircular canal. In the immediate postoperative period, the patient had mild disequilibrium that was treated with additional physical therapy. Three months after treatment, the patient was asymptomatic.

SUMMARY

A 70-year-old retired woman with a complaint of positional vertigo was diagnosed as having benign positional vertigo. The patient's condition was unresponsive to physical therapy, including particle-repositioning maneuvers and Brandt-Daroff exercises. Central nervous system causes for apparent benign positional vertigo, associated labyrinthine dysfunction, bilateral benign positional vertigo, and horizontal canal benign positional vertigo were all ruled out. A semicircular canal occlusion (plugging) procedure was performed. The patient was cured of her benign positional vertigo.

TEACHING POINTS

1. **Benign positional vertigo may be long-standing;** 25 percent of patients with benign positional vertigo report symptoms that have persisted for longer than 1 year, and many report vertigo lasting 5 to 20 years. Most patients have intermittent symptoms, but some have positional vertigo that is always present. Typically, periods of benign positional vertigo can last 6 to 8 weeks and then spontaneously disappear.
2. **Benign positional vertigo may remit and then recur.** It is estimated that approximately 30 percent of individuals with one episode of benign positional vertigo will have a recurrence within 1 year. Recurrent episodes of benign positional vertigo may occur multiple times each year.
3. **Benign positional vertigo that is recalcitrant to treatment** may be caused by: (1) a central nervous system abnormality that manifests itself as apparent benign positional vertigo, (2) bilateral benign positional vertigo, (3) horizontal semicircular canal benign positional vertigo, and (4) an associated chronic peripheral vestibular disorder other than benign positional vertigo that is contributing to the patient's symptoms.
4. **Surgical procedures for patients with benign positional vertigo** that is refractory to nonsurgical treatments include: (1) singular (posterior semicircular canal nerve) neurectomy, (2) posterior semicircular canal plugging (occlusion), and (3) vestibular nerve section.

REFERENCES

1. LeLiever, WC: Comparative repositioning maneuvers for benign paroxysmal positional vertigo. Proceedings from the COSM Meeting, Palm Beach, Florida, May 7–13, 1994.
2. Drachman, DA, Diamond, ER, and Hart, CW: Posturally-evoked vomiting: Association with posterior fossa lesions. Ann Otol 86:97–101, 1977.
3. Watson, P, Barber, HO, Deck, J, and Terbrugge, K: Positional vertigo and nystagmus of central origin. Journal Canadien des Sciences Neurologiques 8:133, 1981.
4. Watson, CP, and Terbrugge, K: Positional nystagmus of the benign paroxysmal type with posterior fossa medullobastoma. Arch Neurol 39:601–602, 1982.
5. Baloh, RW, Honrubia, V, and Jacobson, K: Benign positional vertigo: Clinical and oculographic features in 240 cases. Neurology 37:371–378, 1987.

6. Baloh, RW, Jacobson, K, and Honrubia, V: Horizontal semicircular canal variant of benign positional vertigo. Neurology 43:2542–2549, 1993.

7. Gacek, RR: Singular neurectomy update II: Review of 102 cases. Laryngoscope 101:855–862, 1991.

8. Parnes, LS, and McClure, JA: Posterior semicircular canal occlusion for intractable benign paroxysmal positional vertigo. Ann Otol Rhinol Laryngol 99:330–334, 1990.

9. Cass, SP, Kartush, JM, and Graham, MD: Patterns of vestibular function following vestibular nerve section. Laryngoscope 102:388–394, 1992.

10. Epley, JM: Singular neurectomy: Hypotympanotomy approach. Otolaryngol Head Neck Surg 88:304–309, 1980.

11. Hirsch, BE, et al: Translabyrinthine approach to skull base tumors with hearing preservation. Am J Otol 14(6):533–543, 1993.

C16

Impaired Central Compensation Following Acute Vestibular Injury / Combined Central and Peripheral Vestibular Dysfunction

HISTORY

A 66-year-old woman presented with a complaint of constant disequilibrium that became noticeable following a left-sided vestibular nerve section for episodic vertigo 1 year before evaluation (see Case C14). The patient previously had attacks of acute vertigo that occurred in discrete episodes. Her symptoms during those acute attacks were characterized by severe rotatory vertigo associated with nausea and vomiting. The attacks were preceded by fullness in her left ear. The attacks lasted for several hours. In association with the acute vertigo were a fluctuating unilateral left-sided hearing loss, aural fullness, and tinnitus. Between episodes, the patient did not have positional dizziness and was asymptomatic when sitting or lying still. The increasing frequency of these vertigo attacks had led the patient to have surgery.

In addition to the previous acute attacks of vertigo, the patient also reported 5 years of chronic disequilibrium and unsteadiness. These chronic symptoms were associated with a persistently unsteady gait and blurring of her vision when she moved her head quickly. Despite resolution of her acute attacks of vertigo following surgery, these chronic symptoms continued.

The patient's past medical history was significant for severe peripheral vascular disease. Also, she had suffered two "ministrokes" approximately 10 years earlier that had completely resolved. Family history was noncontributory.

Question 1: Based on the patient's history what is the most likely diagnosis?

Answer 1: The combination of episodic acute vertigo associated with unilateral fluctuating sensorineural hearing loss, aural fullness, and tinnitus is suggestive of unilateral Meniere's disease (see Cases T3 and C10). However, this patient's presentation is somewhat unusual because, in addition to the acute episodes of vertigo, she has chronic disequilibrium. Typically, patients with Meniere's disease are asymptomatic between their episodes of vertigo. Moreover, after surgery, the patient's disequilibrium persisted despite resolution of her episodic vertigo. Although this could indicate poor compensation, to account for her prior intercurrent and now chronic symptoms, the past medical history of possible cerebrovascular disease raises the additional possibility of a problem involving the central nervous system.

PHYSICAL EXAMINATION

General examination was normal. Neurologic examination revealed a bilateral gaze-evoked nystagmus, poor ocular pursuit, and saccadic overshoot dysmetria. There were no changes in strength or sensation and no incoordination. The patient's gait was wide-based and mildly ataxic. Romberg's test was negative. The patient could not stand on a compliant surface with her eyes open or closed. There was no nystagmus seen with Frenzel glasses. Dix-Hallpike maneuvers were negative.

Otoscopic examination was normal. Weber's test lateralized to the right and the Rinne test was positive bilaterally. On the stepping test, the patient's stepping was wide-based and slightly ataxic and she rotated approximately 90 degrees to the left.

Question 2: How does this patient's physical examination influence the diagnostic considerations?

Answer 2: The patient's examination suggests that there is an ongoing central nervous system abnormality affecting the ocular motor system. Specifically, the presence of a bilateral gaze-evoked nystagmus, saccadic pursuit, and saccadic dysmetria suggest dysfunction of the brainstem and cerebellum. Also, the patient falls on foam and, her gait and her stepping test indicate a postural control abnormality and a vestibulospinal asymmetry. The combination of these findings suggests the presence of central nervous system dysfunction and an uncompensated peripheral vestibular lesion (see Case C1).

Laboratory Testing

Vestibular Laboratory Testing:

ELECTRONYSTAGMOGRAPHY: Ocular motor function was abnormal. Specifically, there was saccadic overshoot dysmetria both to the right and left, impaired pursuit in both directions, and bilateral gaze-evoked nystagmus. As expected, caloric testing revealed an absent caloric response on the left including an absent ice water response. The caloric response on the right was normal.

ROTATIONAL TESTING: Rotational testing revealed responses of normal amplitude but with an increased phase lead at low frequency suggesting a diminished time constant (see Chapt. 2). In addition, there was a right directional preponderance.

POSTUROGRAPHY: Posturography indicated excessive sway on conditions 5 and 6, that is, a surface-dependent pattern.

Audiometric Testing: Audiometric testing revealed normal hearing in the right ear and a low-frequency sensorineural hearing loss in the left ear with an abnormal word recognition score of 65 percent.

Imaging: The patient had undergone MRI scanning previously that revealed multiple small infarctions in the deep cerebral white matter and in the cerebellar hemispheres.

Other: None.

Question 3: How does the laboratory testing influence the diagnostic considerations?

Answer 3: Laboratory testing indicates that the patient has both a unilateral peripheral vestibular loss, presumably as a result of the previous surgery for Meniere's disease, and poor compensation for this unilateral peripheral vestibular loss as evidenced by a directional preponderance on rotational testing and impaired postural control. In addition, the abnormalities of ocular motor function suggest an underlying central nervous system dysfunction that may be the cause of the patient's impaired compensation following surgery and chronic disequilibrium. The patient's MRI scan further suggests that her central nervous system abnormalities may be based on cerebrovascular disease.

Question 4: How important is vestibular compensation for successful recovery following ablative vestibular system surgery?

Answer 4: Vestibular compensation is critically important for the success of vestibular ablative surgery such as vestibular nerve section or labyrinthectomy, two procedures that are commonly performed for disabling Meniere's disease (see Case C14). These surgical procedures are ablative in that the vestibular function in the affected ear is either disconnected from the brain (vestibular nerve section) or destroyed (labyrinthectomy). After ablative vestibular surgery, the central nervous system must compensate for the unilateral loss of vestibular function. Although the exact mechanisms of central vestibular compensation are unknown, it is known that restoration of both static and dynamic vestibular function occurs in such a way that a single intact labyrinth can provide sufficient vestibular function for successful recovery[1] (see Chap. 1). Without vestibular compensation, a patient would not be expected to recover balance following vestibular surgery, and thus therapeutic vestibular injury for vertigo would have devastating effects on the patient both symptomatically and functionally.

Question 5: What are the symptoms and signs of incomplete vestibular compensation? What are the signs and symptoms of central nervous system dysfunction that imply that a patient will have difficulty with vestibular compensation?

Answer 5: Incomplete vestibular compensation is manifested by symptoms and signs of vestibular imbalance such as dizziness and disequilibrium and other signs such as blurred vision and gait ataxia. Abnormal ocular motor function such as saccadic dysmetria, saccadic slowing, abnormal smooth pursuit, and gaze-evoked nystagmus can suggest central nervous system dysfunction of the type that corresponds with an impaired ability to compensate for peripheral vestibular injury. Also, vestibular compensation can be adversely influenced by certain medications (see Case C1) and by sedentary behavior.

Question 6: How is laboratory testing used to distinguish between incomplete vestibular compensation and abnormalities of the central nervous system that imply an impaired ability to compensate?

Answer 6: Incomplete vestibular compensation is generally associated with asymmetries in either static or dynamic vestibular dysfunction.[2] Static vestibular asymmetry includes the presence of a spontaneous vestibular or positional nystagmus. Dynamic vestibular asymmetry includes a directional preponderance on rotational testing and a vestibular pattern on dynamic posturography testing. Abnormalities of ocular motor function and structural abnormalities of the posterior fossa on brain imaging are poor prognostic indicators for the process of vestibular compensation and suggest an impaired ability to compensate rather than incomplete compensation.[3–5]

DIAGNOSIS/DIFFERENTIAL DIAGNOSIS

This patient's history, physical examination, and laboratory studies suggest chronic disequilibrium and *poor compensation* following a vestibular nerve section for *Meniere's disease*. Both the disequilibrium and poor compensation are likely to be a result of pre-existing central nervous system dysfunction as evidenced by the presence of gaze-evoked nystagmus, saccadic pursuit, and saccadic dysmetria. Magnetic resonance imaging suggests that the basis for the central nervous system dysfunction may be cerebrovascular disease.

TREATMENT/MANAGEMENT

This patient was treated with a course of vestibular rehabilitation to enhance compensation for her peripheral vestibular deficit. Vestibular-suppressant agents were discontinued. The patient was advised to institute measures to reduce the likelihood of a fall at home. Her balance function improved modestly, but she continued to complain of dizziness.

SUMMARY

A 66-year-old woman presented with a history of Meniere's disease that was treated by vestibular nerve section. Episodic vertigo stopped. However, the patient developed symptoms of constant disequilibrium and unsteadiness that continued unabated and remained disabling. Physical examination suggested the presence of both incomplete vestibular compensation and central nervous system dysfunction. This clinical impression was confirmed by laboratory testing. Thus, the patient was felt to have incomplete vestibular compensation as a result of pre-existing central nervous system dysfunction.

An MRI scan suggested cerebrovascular disease. The patient was advised to discontinue vestibular-suppressant medications and was enrolled in a course of vestibular rehabilitation.

TEACHING POINTS

1. **The success of vestibular ablative surgery** such as vestibular nerve section or labyrinthectomy depends on vestibular compensation. Without vestibular compensation, therapeutic vestibular injury for vertigo has devastating effects on the patient both symptomatically and functionally. Thus, an assessment of central vestibular function to rule out central nervous system disorders before performing ablative vestibular system surgery is essential.

2. **Poor vestibular compensation following an ablative surgical procedure** may be the result of a number of different causes, including use of vestibular-suppressant medication, an incomplete surgical procedure, unrecognized disease of the contralateral ear, sedentary lifestyle, and coexistent central nervous system dysfunction.

3. **Incomplete vestibular compensation** is manifested by symptoms and signs of vestibular imbalance such as dizziness, disequilibrium, blurred vision, and gait ataxia.

4. **Abnormal ocular motor function** such as saccadic dysmetria, abnormal smooth pursuit, and gaze-evoked nystagmus suggest central nervous system dysfunction of the type associated with an impaired ability to compensate for peripheral vestibular injury.

5. **Laboratory testing can be used to assess vestibular compensation.** Poor vestibular compensation is manifested by both static and dynamic vestibular asymmetries. Static vestibular asymmetry includes the presence of a spontaneous vestibular or positional nystagmus. Dynamic vestibular asymmetry includes a directional preponderance on rotational testing and a vestibular pattern on dynamic posturography testing.

6. **Treatment of poor vestibular compensation** includes aggressive vestibular rehabilitation to enhance compensation, gradual discontinuation of vestibular suppressant agents, and measures to help reduce the likelihood of a fall at home.

REFERENCES

1. Smith, PF, and Curthoys, IS: Mechanisms of recovery following unilateral labyrinthectomy: A review. Brain Res Rev 14:155–180, 1989.
2. Cass, SP, Kartush, JM, and Graham, MD: Patterns of vestibular function following vestibular nerve section. Laryngoscope 102:388–394, 1992.
3. Konrad, HR: Intractable vertigo—When not to operate. Otolaryngol Head Neck Surg 95:482–484, 1986.
4. Monsell, EM, Brackmann, DE, and Linthicum, FH: Why do vestibular destructive procedures sometimes fail? Otolaryngol Head Neck Surg 99:472, 1988.
5. Hamid, MA, et al: ENG-MRI correlates in cerebellar oculomotor dysfunction. Otolaryngol Head Neck Surg 99:302–308, 1988.

C17

Aging and the Vestibular System

HISTORY

An 80-year-old woman presented with a complaint of disequilibrium when walking. The patient noted occasional lightheadedness but had no complaint of vertigo or of hearing loss or tinnitus. She did not complain of positional sensitivity when lying supine. Symptoms had been present for several years but had been especially noticeable in the last 6 months. The patient dated the onset of her problem to cataract surgery in the right eye that resulted in a marked improvement in her vision. The patient's family indicated that her balance had been gradually worsening for several years. Her primary care physician ordered a CT scan of the head, which revealed a small (0.5 cm) meningioma in the cerebellopontine angle without evidence of mass effect. An MRI scan confirmed this finding and revealed diffuse increased signal intensity in the deep white matter. The patient was using meclizine, 25 mg twice daily without obvious benefit.

Question 1: Based on this patient's history, what are the diagnostic considerations and what further information would be helpful in the evaluation of this patient?

Answer 1: This patient's history suggests a nonspecific abnormality of the balance system. With the information available, it is difficult to localize the problem to the vestibular system specifically. Further information regarding past medical history, medication use, any remote history of a vestibular disorder, family history, and habits such as smoking and alcohol consumption, would all be helpful. Additionally, a physical examination is likely to provide helpful information.

ADDITIONAL HISTORY

The patient had had essential hypertension for the past 20 years and was being treated with a diuretic. There was no remote history of dizziness or disequilibrium. She had smoked one pack of cigarettes per day for 40 years and had used ethanol socially.

The patient has no family history of balance disorder.

PHYSICAL EXAMINATION

The patient's general examination was normal. Neurologic examination revealed no specific abnormalities of cranial nerves aside from difficulty pursuing a slowly moving target. Examination of the motor and sensory systems was normal. Coordination was normal. However, the patient had a slightly widened base to her gait and was unable to tandem walk without assistance. She was quite unsteady on a compliant foam surface with eyes open or closed but did not fall. Otologic examination was normal.

Question 2: Based on the history and physical examination, what is this patient's likely diagnosis? What laboratory testing might assist in the diagnosis?

Answer 2: This patient has no obvious cause for disequilibrium, although several factors might be contributing, including age, probable atherosclerotic disease considering the risk factors of hypertension and tobacco use, recent cataract surgery that changed her vision, and a diminished level of activity.

Further information from laboratory testing may be helpful. Vestibular laboratory testing would provide information regarding the presence of a vestibular system abnormality. Brain imaging has already been performed. The patient was found to have evidence of small-vessel disease on MRI. The role of the patient's small cerebellopontine angle mass is uncertain but it is probably asymptomatic. If not already performed by the patient's primary care physician, the patient's metabolic, hematologic, and thyroid status should be assessed.

Laboratory Testing

Vestibular Laboratory Testing

ELECTRONYSTAGMOGRAPHY:	Ocular motor testing revealed a difficulty performing smooth pursuit. There was a direction-changing positional nystagmus of 5° per second, which was considered borderline abnormal. Caloric irrigations revealed symmetric responses somewhat larger than average amounting to about 50° per second peak slow component velocity for each irrigation.
ROTATIONAL TESTING:	Rotational testing revealed responses of normal magnitude and symmetry with an increased phase lead. Trapezoidal rotations revealed a time constant of about 9 seconds, which is somewhat short.
POSTUROGRAPHY:	Posturography testing indicated excessive sway in all conditions in a nonspecific pattern. Also, the patient had an inability to adapt to repeated platform rotations.

Audiometric Testing: Not performed

Imaging: Not performed

Other: None

These findings suggest a nonspecific central vestibular, possibly a cerebellar, abnormality because of the abnormally large caloric responses and abnormal timing of rotational responses.

DIAGNOSIS/DIFFERENTIAL DIAGNOSIS

Question 3: Based on the information available, what is this patient's likely diagnosis?

Answer 3: The patient's disequilibrium cannot be ascribed to a single causative factor. Patients like the one under discussion have been given a diagnosis of "presbyastasis" and "disequilibrium of the elderly".[1,2]

   Presumably, such patients have disequilibrium on the basis of abnormal sensory input or inputs, abnormal sensory processing by the central nervous system, abnormal control mechanisms for balance, and an aged musculoskeletal system with its concomitant decreased range of motion and diminished strength.

Question 4: What is the influence of age on vestibular function?

Answer 4: Although balance function is known to be adversely affected by aging, manifested by an increase in the incidence of falls in the elderly,[3] the cause of this decline is not known. Many structures in the *peripheral* vestibular system are known to be affected by increased age. Specifically, vestibular hair cell degeneration,[4] saccular otoconia degeneration,[5] changes in vestibular hair cell synaptic membranes,[6] a decline of vestibular ganglion cells,[7] and a decline in the number of vestibular fibers[8] are all associated with increased age. Aging also influences *central* vestibular function. There are modest changes in vestibulo-ocular dynamics;[9–11] a reduction in the ability to combine visual and vestibular signals, that is, impaired visual-vestibular interaction (see Case C11); and a preserved ability to modify (adapt) vestibular reflexes in response to altered visual input.[10] Also, postural sway increases with advanced age, particularly under circumstances that require vestibular sensation such as standing on a compliant surface with a distorted visual surround.[12]

   This patient was given a diagnosis of *disequilibrium of aging*.

TREATMENT/MANAGEMENT

This patient was enrolled in a balance rehabilitation therapy program that emphasized gait training. Vestibular suppressant medications were discontinued. The patient's disequilibrium improved slightly.

SUMMARY

An 80-year-old woman presented with gradually worsening balance during walking without specific complaints of vertigo. The patient had a past medical history of hypertension. Physical examination did not suggest a specific localization for her disequilibrium. Laboratory studies suggested cerebrovascular disease and nonspecific vestibular system impairment. A diagnosis of *disequilibrium of aging* was given. Treatment consisted of discontinuation of vestibular-suppressant medications and balance therapy.

TEACHING POINTS

1. **Aging affects the vestibular system.** In the vestibular periphery, otoconia, hair cells, and ganglion cells and fibers degenerate with increased age. Centrally, there is a decline in vestibular processing that includes a reduction in the ability to combine visual and vestibular signals and a decline in the ability to modify (adapt) vestibular reflexes.

2. **Disequilibrium of the elderly,** also known as *presbyastasis* and *presbylibrium*, is used to describe elderly patients who present with imbalance and disequilibrium that cannot be ascribed to a particular disease state or to a single causative factor. Presumably, such patients have disequilibrium on the basis of abnormal sensory input, abnormal sensory processing by the central nervous system, abnormal control mechanisms for balance, and an aged musculoskeletal system with a concomitant decreased range of motion and diminished strength.

3. **Vestibular rehabilitation may benefit** patients with disequilibrium of the elderly despite physical limitations and the decline of sensory function and sensorimotor processing. Also, such individuals should be counseled regarding prevention of falls, including use of a cane if necessary and use of appropriate home safety devices such as rails in the bathroom.

REFERENCES

1. Jenkins, HA, et al: Dysequilibrium of aging. Otolaryngol Head Neck Surg 100:272–282, 1989.
2. Belal, A, and Glorig, A: Disequilibrium of ageing (presbyastasis). J Laryngol Otol 100:1037–1041, 1986.
3. Tinetti, ME, Speechley, M, and Ginter, SF: Risk factors for falls among elderly persons living in the community. N Engl J Med 319:1701–1707, 1988.
4. Rosenhall, U, and Rubin, W: Degenerative changes in the human vestibular sensory epithelia. Acta Otolaryngol 79:67–80, 1975.
5. Ross, MD, et al: Observations on normal and degenerating human otoconia. Ann Otol 85:310–326, 1976.
6. Engstrom, H, et al: Structural changes in the vestibular epithelia in elderly monkeys and humans. Adv Otorhinolaryngol 22:93–110, 1977.
7. Richter, E: Quantitative study of human Scarpa's ganglion and vestibular sensory epithelia. Acta Otolaryngol 90:199–208, 1980.
8. Bergstrom, B: Morphology of the vestibular nerve. II. The number of myelinated vestibular nerve fibers in man at various ages. Acta Otolaryngol 76:173–179, 1973.
9. Baloh, RW, Jacobson, KM, and Socotch, TM: The effect of aging on visual-vestibuloocular responses. Exp Brain Res 95:509–516, 1993.
10. Paige, GD: Senescence of human visual-vestibular interactions. J Vestibular Res 2:133–151, 1992.
11. Peterka, R, Black, F, and Schoenhoff, M: Age-related changes in human vestibulo-ocular reflexes: Sinusoidal rotation and caloric tests. J Vestibular Res 1:49–59, 1990.
12. Peterka, R, and Black, F: Age-related changes in human posture control: Sensory organization tests. J Vestibular Res 1:73–85, 1990.

C A S E
C18

Treatment of "Nonspecific Vestibulopathy"

HISTORY

A 30-year-old female data processor presented with a chief complaint of dizziness and disequilibrium. The patient's complaints were of approximately 1 year's duration, worse in the last several months, especially premenstrually. There was a constant sense of dizziness and disequilibrium with periodic exacerbations lasting for several days. There was no positional dizziness. When the patient was symptomatic, she noticed that rapid head movements were bothersome and that looking at her computer screen at work caused her discomfort, including mild nausea and "eye strain." She had no neurologic complaints. The patient walked regularly for exercise and noticed that when symptomatic, she would veer slightly both to the right and to the left. There was no history of headache and no family history of migraine headache. The patient had no complaint of hearing loss or tinnitus and no complaint of fullness, pain, or stuffiness in the ears. She was evaluated extensively by her primary care physician with no diagnosis reached. An MRI scan revealed that the cerebellar tonsils were 2 mm below the foramen magnum without evidence of compression of brainstem or caudal midline cerebellar structures. The patient noted some increase in symptoms in shopping malls and grocery stores but was able to carry on her homemaking activities. She had not experienced panic attacks. The patient used meclizine on an as-needed basis. This provided some relief, but she was still symptomatic.

Question 1: Based on the history, what is this patient's probable diagnosis?

Answer 1: This patient has a symptom complex that is nonspecific but does suggest some impairment of the balance system. Although she has a Chiari malformation by imaging criteria, it is unlikely to be "symptomatic" considering her history and the lack of compression of posterior fossa structures.[1] However, physical examination will be

190

helpful in establishing whether a Chiari malformation could be causing some or all of the patient's symptoms (see Case C3). The fact that the patient benefitted from meclizine also suggests that she may have a vestibular system abnormality, a mild anxiety condition, or both. From the information available, there are many conditions that are *unlikely*, including endolymphatic hydrops, benign positional vertigo, migraine, and multiple sclerosis.

PHYSICAL EXAMINATION

The patient's general, neurologic, otologic, and neuro-otologic examinations were normal, with the exception of some difficulty standing on a complaint foam surface with eyes closed. Also, the patient's gait had a slightly widened base.

Laboratory Testing

Vestibular Laboratory Testing

ELECTRONYSTAGMOGRAPHY:	Ocular motor function, positional testing, and caloric responses were normal.
ROTATIONAL TESTING:	A mild right directional preponderance was seen on rotational testing.
POSTUROGRAPHY:	Posturography indicated minimally excessive sway on conditions 5 and 6.

Audiometric Testing: Not performed

Imaging: Not performed

Other: As noted, the patient had normal blood studies including metabolic, hematologic, rheumatologic, and thyroid tests.

DIAGNOSIS/DIFFERENTIAL DIAGNOSIS

Question 2: Based on all of the information available, what diagnosis can be given to this patient?

Answer 2: This patient does not have a well-defined disease process. As noted previously, this patient's evaluation does not suggest a "symptomatic" Chiari malformation (see Case C3). The patient could be given the diagnosis of "vestibulopathy" of unknown origin. This is a diagnosis of exclusion, so it must be remembered that other conditions that are difficult to rule out, such as migraine, are possibilities. Follow-up care may allow a specific diagnosis.

This patient was given the diagnosis of *nonspecific vestibulopathy*.

TREATMENT/MANAGEMENT

Question 3: What are the treatment options for a patient with nonspecific vestibulopathy?

Answer 3: In patients in whom a specific diagnosis cannot be uncovered but in whom vestibular system involvement is highly suspected, treatment may consist of one or more of the modalities listed in Table C18–1. The choice of medication will depend on the physician's judgment as to the importance and predominance of symptoms of nausea, dizziness, anxiety, depression, or a functional impairment of balance.[3] This judgment will also influence the decision to enroll the patient in a course of vestibular rehabilitation (see Chap. 4).

Medications commonly used to decrease *dizziness* and nausea are listed in Table C18–2. Note that the medications in Table C18–2 have multiple effects. Specifically, medications used to decrease nausea may also reduce dizziness, whereas drugs used to decrease dizziness often have antinausea properties. The primary action of these medications and their major side effects are listed in Table C18–2.

Some patients respond favorably to antianxiety or antidepressant medications, even when their complaints of dizziness are quite prominent. We have also found that adding a sympathomimetic agent such as pseudoephedrine to agents that cause lethargy, such as promethazine hydrochloride, can be a useful combination. In our experience, droperidol should be reserved for patients with acute vestibular symptoms, such as those experienced during the very early stages of vestibular neuritis or during a severe episode of endolymphatic hydrops. We have found little use for transdermal scopolamine in patients with vestibulopathy. In addition to the minimal relief provided to the patient, there is frequently a complaint of anticholinergic side effects including blurred vision, which may actually worsen the symptoms of dizziness.

The patient was given oral diazepam, 2 mg twice daily. She was also encouraged to increase her physical activity. She had some relief of symptoms but continued to experience mild dizziness and disequilibrium.

SUMMARY

A 30-year-old woman presented with nonspecific dizziness and disequilibrium of a constant nature with periodic exacerbations. The patient's evaluation did not reveal a specific diagnosis but suggested a vestibular system abnormality that could not definitely be localized to the central or peripheral vestibular system. Treatment was therefore symptomatic. The patient was given oral diazepam, 2 mg twice daily. She was also encouraged to increase her physical activity. She had some relief of symptoms but continued to experience mild dizziness and disequilibrium.

TABLE C18–1
Treatment Modalities for Nonspecific Vestibulopathy

Antinausea agents
Vestibular agents
Antianxiety agents
Antidepressants
Physical therapy

TABLE C18–2

Medications Commonly Used to Reduce Dizziness, Vertigo, and Associated Nausea

Generic Name	Trade Name	Class	Dosage	Primary Symptom Treated	Side Effects
Prochlorperazine	Compazine	Phenothiazine	10 mg orally or IM every 6 hours or 25 mg rectally every 12 hours	Nausea	Extrapyramidal reactions, drowsiness, anticholinergic effects
Promethazine with pseudoephedrine	Phenergan	Phenothiazine	25 mg orally or rectally every 6 hours (promethazine) 60 mg orally every 6 hours (pseudoephedrine)	Nausea	Extrapyramidal reactions, drowsiness Restlessness
Meclizine	Antivert, Bonine	Piperazine (H_1-blocking agent)	25 mg orally every 4 to 6 hours	Dizziness	Drowsiness
Dimenhydrinate	Dramamine	Ethanolamine (H_1-blocking agent)	50 mg orally every 4 to 6 hours	Dizziness	Drowsiness
Scopolamine	Transderm Scop	Amine antimuscarinic	0.5-mg adhesive skin patches every 3 days	Dizziness	Dry mouth, blurred vision, drowsiness, disorientation
Cyclizine	Marezine	Piperazine (H_1-blocking agent)	50 mg orally or IM every 4 to 6 hours	Dizziness	Drowsiness
Diazepam	Valium	Benzodiazepine	2–10 mg orally, IM, or IV every 4 to 6 hours	Dizziness	Lethargy
Droperidol	Inapsine	Butyrophenone	2.5 or 5 mg IM	Nausea	Extrapyramidal reaction, drowsiness, respiratory depression
Trimethobenzamine	Tigan	Substituted ethanolamine	250 mg orally every 6 to 8 hours or 200 mg rectally or IM every 6 to 8 hours	Nausea	Extrapyramidal (unusual)
Diphenhydramine	Benadryl	Ethanolamine (H_1-blocking agent)	25–50 mg orally, IM, or IV every 6 hours	Nausea	Drowsiness
Hydroxyzine	Vistaril, Atarax	Piperazine derivative	25–100 mg orally every 8 hours	Nausea	Drowsiness

TEACHING POINTS

1. **Vestibulopathy of unknown origin** or *nonspecific vestibulopathy* are terms used to describe a complex of nonspecific symptoms that are suggestive of some impairment of the balance system but do not fit any well-known vestibular syndromes.

2. **Nonspecific vestibulopathy is a diagnosis of exclusion.** Conditions that should be considered and ruled out include endolymphatic hydrops, benign positional vertigo, migraine, anxiety and panic disorders, and potential central nervous system abnormalities such as multiple sclerosis, Chiari malformation, or neoplasm. Follow-up care is important because a specific diagnosis may become evident over time.

3. **Treatment of nonspecific vestibulopathy** includes medications and a course of balance rehabilitation therapy. The choice of treatment depends on the physician's judgment as to the importance and predominance of symptoms of nausea, dizziness, anxiety, depression, or a functional impairment of balance. Medications commonly used to decrease dizziness, vertigo, and nausea are listed in Table C18–2.

REFERENCES

1. Weber, PC, and Cass, SP: Neurotologic manifestation of Chiari 1 malformation. Otolaryngol Head Neck Surg 109:853–860, 1993.
2. Cass, SP: Role of medications in otological vertigo and balance disorders. Semin Hearing 12:257–269, 1991.

C A S E
C19

Chronic Middle Ear Disease

HISTORY

A 45-year-old insurance agent presented with 1 week of disequilibrium that had started after a day of vertigo, nausea, and vomiting 3 days after the onset of malodorous discharge and pain in his left ear. Since resolution of the acute spell of vertigo, the patient had disequilibrium that fluctuated in intensity. He noted occasional staggering, but otherwise was only mildly unsteady. The patient did not complain of any positional symptoms but felt mildly lightheaded and dizzy even at rest. In addition, he reported that recently he could provoke brief vertigo by putting his finger in his left ear to relieve itching. He also occasionally noticed momentary vertigo when he heard a loud sound. The patient reported a lifelong history of recurrent ear infections and had undergone mastoid surgery on the left at age 10 years. Medicated ear drops were prescribed for him by his primary care physician before evaluation.

Question 1: Based on the patient's history, what is the most likely diagnosis?

Answer 1: The history of chronic ear infections and the occurrence of malodorous discharge immediately preceding the onset of vertigo suggest that the patient's vertigo may be related to infection involving the middle ear and mastoid. Considering his long history of middle ear problems, the patient may simply be experiencing an acute exacerbation of chronic otitis media, or there may be an ongoing chronic middle ear infection related to recurrent cholesteatoma (see later text). Alternatively, the patient's complaints may have no relationship whatever to past and present middle or outer ear problems. If so, the differential diagnosis is broad.

Question 2: What is a cholesteatoma of the ear?

Answer 2: A cholesteatoma of the ear is a skin cyst that behaves like a localized tumor (see Fig. C19–1). It causes destruction of bone and predisposes to repeated acute middle ear infections. Cholesteatoma of the ear is usually found in the presence of chronic middle ear infection (chronic otitis media).

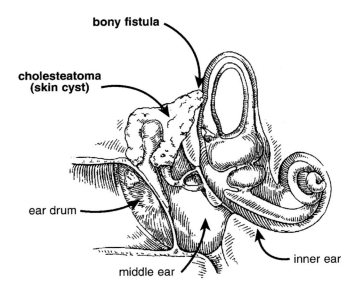

bony fistula

cholesteatoma (skin cyst)

ear drum

middle ear

inner ear

Figure C19-1
Schematic drawing of the ear drum, cholesteatoma within the middle ear space, and inner ear. Cholesteatoma is shown causing erosion of the lateral semicircular canal, resulting in a bony fistula. (Modified with permission from Glasscock, ME, et al: Handbook of Vertigo. New York: Raven Press, 1990.[6])

Question 3: How do chronic otitis media and cholesteatoma cause vertigo?

Answer 3: An acute exacerbation of chronic otitis media can cause vertigo and dizziness as a result of bacterial toxins contained in the middle ear inflammatory exudate reaching the vestibular labyrinth, usually by transmission through the round window membrane. This process is referred to as *serous labyrinthitis* and also may be associated with sensorineural hearing loss, primarily affecting the high frequencies. Cholesteatoma of the ear may cause dizziness by creating a perilymphatic fistula as a result of erosion of the bony vestibular labyrinth (see Fig. C19–1). The combination of an erosive perilymphatic fistula and otitis media can cause both serous labyrinthitis and bacterial labyrinthitis.[1–4]

Question 4: How can an acute exacerbation of chronic otitis media be distinguished from a cholesteatoma of the ear?

Answer 4: Chronic otitis media and cholesteatoma of the ear cannot be distinguished on the basis of the history. Diagnosis of a cholesteatoma of the ear can be made by debridement of the external ear followed by an otologic examination using an operative microscope by a physician skilled in the management of otologic disease. If a cholesteatoma is found, CT imaging is indicated to aid in evaluating the bony labyrinth for erosion and fistula formation. Imaging studies are not indicated before cleaning and examining the ear.

PHYSICAL EXAMINATION

The patient's general and neurologic examinations were normal, including a negative Romberg's test and normal gait. He was able to stand on compliant foam with his eyes open but not with his eyes closed, indicating an ongoing vestibular system abnormality. On the stepping test, the patient rotated 120 degrees to the left. Compression of the tragus produced both nystagmus and sensation of vertigo. Otologic examination revealed a malodorous yellow discharge draining from the left ear, a tympanic membrane perforation, and thickened polypoid mucosa in the middle ear space. With the operative microscope, the ear was cleaned using suction and debrided to reveal minimal bony erosion of the posterior semicircular canal wall and a large cholesteatoma pocket with a moist cholesteatoma matrix overlying the area of the lateral semicircular canal. On tuning fork examination, the Weber's test lateralized to the right and the Rinne test was positive on the right but not detected on the left.

Question 5: What do the results of the physical examination suggest about the cause of this patient's vertigo?

Answer 5: The presence of a large cholesteatoma with active inflammation overlying the lateral semicircular canal suggests that the patient's vertigo may be caused by the presence of fistulization of either the posterior or the lateral semicircular canal. The positive Hennebert's symptoms and signs, that is, vertigo and nystagmus induced by pressure changes in the external auditory canal using pneumatic otoscopy or tragal pressure, are highly suggestive of bony labyrinthine fistula. The tuning forks or tragal pressure suggest a profound sensorineural hearing loss in the left ear.

Question 6: What is the value of vestibular laboratory testing at this point in the evaluation of this patient?

Answer 6: The presence of a cholesteatoma and positive Hennebert's sign strongly suggest that a bony fistula in the left ear is the source of the patient's vestibular symptoms. The presence of profound sensorineural hearing loss in the left ear further suggests that the fistula has produced both auditory and vestibular damage. Although caloric testing can provide information regarding responsiveness of the vestibular labyrinth, vestibular laboratory testing is not indicated because of the presence of the severe acute infection. Also, vestibular testing in the setting of an acute middle ear infection is very uncomfortable and does not provide further significant information needed for diagnosis at this time.

Question 7: What is the value of obtaining a CT scan at this point in the patient's evaluation? What is the value of MRI?

Answer 7: A high-resolution CT scan of the temporal bone can define the bony architecture of the vestibular labyrinth and mastoid and can confirm the presence of a bony labyrinthine fistula. In addition, other potential life-threatening conditions such as a sigmoid sinus thrombosis or a dural abscess may be detected. A CT scan is indicated rather than MRI because of the ability of CT to image the bony anatomy of the labyrinth; MRI of the temporal bone could reveal widespread inflammation but could not provide the anatomic detail necessary to confirm the diagnosis of a bony labyrinthine fistula.

Laboratory Testing

Vestibular Laboratory Testing: Vestibular laboratory function testing was deferred because of the presence of acute infection and discharge.

ELECTRONYSTAGMOGRAPHY:	Not performed
ROTATIONAL TESTING:	Not performed
POSTUROGRAPHY:	Not performed

Audiometric Testing: An audiogram was performed and showed normal hearing in the right ear but the presence of a profound sensorineural hearing loss in the left ear.

Imaging: A CT scan confirmed the presence of a bony fistula of the horizontal semicircular canal.

Other: None

DIAGNOSIS/DIFFERENTIAL DIAGNOSIS

The patient was given the diagnosis of *chronic otitis media with cholesteatoma formation and a fistula of the horizontal semicircular canal.*

TREATMENT/MANAGEMENT

Following debridement of the ear, the patient was placed on an oral antibiotic and a medicated otic drop. He was asked to return in 1 week for further debridement and examination.

The patient returned in 1 week with significant improvement in his symptoms. The drainage had greatly diminished, and the dizziness had improved but had not resolved completely. Otologic examination revealed significant improvement in the amount of discharge and inflammation present in the middle ear and mastoid space, which was visible because of previous surgery at age 10. The patient's medications were changed from medicated otic drops to daily boric acid irrigation of the ear. He was counseled as to the need for future revision mastoid surgery, which was performed.

Question 8: What constitutes surgery for cholesteatoma? When is surgery indicated for a patient who presents with vertigo and is found to have otitis media and a cholesteatoma? Should this patient be advised to undergo repeat mastoid surgery?

Answer 8: Surgery for cholesteatoma consists of opening the mastoid cavity and excising cholesteatoma or widely exteriorizing the cholesteatoma skin cyst.[5] If a bony fistula of a semicircular canal is found, the skin covering the fistula is usually not dissected off the fistula because this can cause further deterioration of hearing and vestibular symptoms. However, by preventing further progression and inflammation associated with the cholesteatoma, further acute vertiginous symptoms are usually eliminated. Unfortunately, in this case there is no treatment for the hearing loss, which is permanent.

Surgery is indicated for a patient with a cholesteatoma that is not "self-cleaning," that is, that produces repeated acute infections, or that is associated with complications such as vertigo, hearing loss, facial nerve paralysis, or central nervous system complications such as meningitis, dural venous sinus thrombosis, or a dural abscess. In this patient's case, there is a large cholesteatoma that has produced a bony labyrinthine fistula with concomitant hearing loss and vertigo. If this cholesteatoma is treated only medically, it is likely that the patient would undergo additional repeated acute attacks of vertigo, suffer persistent imbalance, and be at risk for central nervous system complications of bacterial infection.

Question 9: What is the proper treatment of patients with chronic otitis media that is not associated with cholesteatoma?

Answer 9: Acute exacerbations of chronic otitis media are primarily treated with frequent debridement, local antibiotics, and otic cleansing solutions. Occasionally, tympanoplasty and mastoid surgery are required, but only after the failure of local care.

SUMMARY

A 45-year-old man with a previous history of chronic ear disease and mastoid surgery at age 10 years presented with disequilibrium following the onset of acute vertigo after 3 days of a malodorous discharge from his left ear. The patient's ear was debrided, revealing the presence of a cholesteatoma. He had a positive Hennebert's sign and a profound loss of hearing in the left ear, suggesting the presence of a bony labyrinthine fistula. A fistula of the horizontal semicircular canal was confirmed by CT imaging. Treatment consisted of repeated debridement and local otic cleansing solutions followed by a revision mastoidectomy.

TEACHING POINTS

1. **Acute otitis media** or an acute exacerbation of chronic otitis media can cause vertigo and dizziness as a result of bacterial toxins contained in the middle ear inflammatory exudate reaching the vestibular labyrinth, usually by transmission through the round window membrane. This process is referred to as serous labyrinthitis and may also be associated with sensorineural hearing loss, primarily affecting the high frequencies.
2. **A cholesteatoma of the ear** is a skin cyst that behaves like a localized tumor. It causes destruction of bone and predisposes to repeated acute middle ear infections. Cholesteatoma of the ear is often found in the presence of chronic middle ear infection and can cause dizziness by creating a perilymphatic fistula as a result of erosion of the bony vestibular labyrinth. The combination of an erosive perilymphatic fistula and otitis media can cause both a serous labyrinthitis and bacterial labyrinthitis.
3. **A bony labyrinthine fistula** should be considered in a patient with a history of chronic otitis media who presents with Hennebert's symptoms and signs, vertigo and nystagmus induced by pressure changes in the external auditory canal. A high-resolution CT scan of the temporal bone can define the bony architecture of the vestibular labyrinth and mastoid and should be used to confirm the presence of a bony labyrinthine fistula. An MRI of the temporal bone can reveal widespread inflammation but cannot provide the anatomic detail necessary to confirm the diagnosis of a bony labyrinthine fistula.
4. **Treatment of vertigo caused by acute otitis media** in an otherwise normal ear includes drainage and both topical and oral antibiotics.
5. **Treatment of vertigo associated with an acute exacerbation of chronic otitis media** or cholesteatoma requires repeated debridement of the ear, a combination of an oral and topical antibiotic, and CT imaging of the ear. Surgery is indicated for a patient with a cholesteatoma that is not "self-cleaning," that is, that produces repeated acute infections, or that is associated with complications such as vertigo, hearing loss, facial nerve paralysis, or central nervous system complications such as meningitis, dural venous sinus thrombosis, or a dural abscess.

REFERENCES

1. Paparella, M, and Sugiura, S: The pathology of suppurative labyrinthitis. Ann Otol Rhinol Laryngol 76:554–586, 1967.
2. Walby, PA, Barrerra, A, and Schuknecht, HF: Cochlear pathology in chronic suppurative otitis media. Ann Otol Rhinol Laryngol 103 (Suppl):3–19, 1983.
3. Meyerhoff, WL, Kim, CS, and Paparella, MM: Pathology of chronic otitis media. Ann Otol 87:749–760, 1978.
4. Paparella, MM, et al: Sensorineural hearing loss in otitis media. Ann Otol Rhinol Laryngol 93:623–629, 1984.
5. Sheehy, JL, Brackmann, DE, and Graham, MD: Cholesteatoma surgery: Residual and recurrent disease. Ann Otol Rhinol Laryngol 86:1–12, 1977.
6. Glasscock, ME, et al: Handbook of Vertigo. New York: Raven Press, 1990.

C20

Otosclerosis

HISTORY

A 47-year-old woman employed as a social worker reported having experienced dizziness for 6 months. The dizziness had been quite variable, consisting of one major episode of vertigo 3 months earlier associated with nausea and vomiting that lasted for hours and several minor episodes of vertigo lasting for seconds. Between episodes, the patient noticed daily dizziness symptoms that were worsened by rapid head movements. She also noted some unsteadiness and veering of her gait to the left, especially in darkness.

The patient also complained of a bilateral hearing loss, first noticed at age 25, which has been slowly progressive in both ears. There was no fluctuation of hearing and no aural fullness. A bilateral low-pitch roaring sound was present, worse in the right ear than the left ear. There was no past medical history of otitis media, noise exposure, or trauma. The family history was positive for hearing loss in her mother and two maternal aunts.

PHYSICAL EXAMINATION

General and neurologic examinations were normal except that the patient's casual walking was slow. Tandem walking was performed with slight difficulty. Romberg's test was negative. Otoscopy was normal. Tuning fork examination using a 512-Hz fork revealed that Weber's test lateralized to the right and the Rinne test was negative (bone conduction was greater than air conduction) bilaterally.

Question 1: What is the most likely cause of this patient's hearing loss?

Answer 1: The Rinne tuning fork examination suggests the presence of a bilateral conductive hearing loss. The result on Weber's test suggests either that the conductive hearing loss is slightly greater on the right than the left or that a combined conductive and sensorineural hearing loss is present on the left. The finding of a conductive hearing loss with no previous history of otitis media or trauma and normal otoscopy suggests a diagnosis of otosclerosis. The positive family history of hearing loss reinforces this diagnosis.

Question 2: What is otosclerosis?

Answer 2: Otosclerosis is a disorder of the bony labyrinth and ossicles caused by a progressive stiffening and fixation of the stapes footplate by the formation of abnormal otosclerotic bone that most commonly causes a conductive hearing loss. The conductive hearing loss typically begins in the second or third decade of life.

Question 3: What pathologic changes are seen in the inner ear in otosclerosis?

Answer 3: Otosclerotic bone occurs when the original endochondral bone of the bony labyrinth is destroyed and replaced by highly cellular fibrous tissue. This fibrous tissue contains abundant lysosomes containing hydrolytic enzymes that are thought to be involved in the bony resorption. After destruction of the endochondral bone, bony remodeling and production of immature otosclerotic bone occurs. Repetition of the remodeling process results in areas of otosclerotic bone that often contain both inactive and active regions of bony remodeling. About 85 percent of otosclerotic foci are located in the oval window region area. This process of bony remodeling often results in fixation of the stapes footplate and progressive conductive hearing loss. Interestingly, as normal bone is replaced by otosclerotic bone, the original anatomic configuration of the bony labyrinth is usually preserved. Actual invasion of the labyrinthine spaces is rare and occurs only in the most active lesions.

Question 4: Is otosclerosis a common disorder?

Answer 4: Clinically diagnosed otosclerosis has an estimated incidence of 0.5 to 2 percent in a Caucasian population. The incidence of subclinical otosclerosis, that is, otosclerosis found in the temporal bones of individuals without symptoms during life, ranges between 8 to 12 percent. In African Americans, otosclerosis is found in only 1 percent of temporal bones and has a clinical incidence of only 0.1 percent. The disease is rare to nonexistent in Asians and Native Americans. There is a female-to-male ratio of clinical otosclerosis of about 2:1.[1] Otosclerosis commonly has a hereditary basis, although the exact mode of inheritance is unknown. Recently, evidence has been presented suggesting that viral infection may be a predisposing factor in the development of otosclerosis.[2]

Laboratory Testing

Vestibular Laboratory Testing

ELECTRONYSTAGMOGRAPHY:	Ocular motor function was normal. A low-amplitude left-beating spontaneous vestibular nystagmus was noted. There was no positional nystagmus. Caloric testing revealed a significant right reduced vestibular response.
ROTATIONAL TESTING:	Rotational testing revealed responses of normal amplitude and timing with a significant left directional preponderance.
POSTUROGRAPHY:	Posturography was normal.

Audiometric Testing: An audiogram was performed and showed a bilateral mixed conductive and sensorineural hearing loss (Fig. C20–1). The sensorineural component of the hearing loss was mild, ranging from 20 decibels (dB) in the low frequencies to 30 dB in the higher

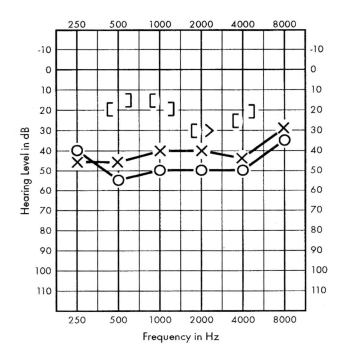

Figure C20-1
Audiogram.

Word Recognition Score			
Right : 100%			
Left : 100%			

			Right	Left
Air	unmasked		O——O	✕——✕
	masked		△——△	☐——☐
Bone	unmasked		◄---◄	►---►
	masked		Ɛ---[	]---]

frequencies. The conductive component of the hearing loss produced a 40- to 50-dB hearing loss primarily affecting the lower frequencies in each ear. The conductive hearing loss was slightly greater in the right ear.

Imaging: Not performed

Other: None

Question 5: This patient reported tinnitus and the audiogram showed some sensorineural hearing loss. Are these symptoms and findings commonly associated with otosclerosis, a disorder that primarily affects conduction of sound through the middle ear?

Answer 5: Although conductive hearing loss is the most common manifestation of otosclerosis, tinnitus is also very common and may be related to either fixation of the stapes or damage to the sensorineural elements of the cochlea. Sensorineural hearing loss is also frequently associated with otosclerosis. If sensorineural hearing loss is present, it is most commonly seen in combination with stapes fixation, which presumably causes a mixed conductive and sensorineural hearing loss. Occasionally, patients present with pure cochlear otosclerosis, that is, sensorineural hearing loss without a conductive component. Establishing that a sensorineural hearing loss is the result of otosclerosis is difficult. In advanced cases of cochlear otosclerosis, it is possible to detect the presence of abnormal otosclerotic bone surrounding the inner ear on high-resolution CT imaging of the temporal bone.

Question 6: Is dizziness commonly associated with otosclerosis? Are vestibular abnormalities common?

Answer 6: Vestibular symptoms are more common in individuals with otosclerosis than in the general population. The reported prevalence of dizziness in individuals with otosclerosis ranges from 7 to 40 percent.[3–5] Unilateral or bilateral reduced caloric function has been observed in up to 60 percent of otosclerosis patients complaining of vertigo.[5] It has also been suggested that the incidence of vestibular symptoms correlates with the presence of an associated sensorineural hearing loss.[5,6]

Question 7: What is the cause of dizziness associated with otosclerosis?

Answer 7: Dizziness in patients with otosclerosis may be caused by either the co-occurrence of a disorder other than otosclerosis, such as Meniere's disease, or by the pathologic process of otosclerosis itself, which can produce vestibular symptoms as a result of the *otosclerotic inner ear syndrome* discussed below. Surprisingly, the otosclerotic inner ear syndrome appears to occur less frequently than combined otosclerosis and Meniere's disease.[4]

The combination of Meniere's disease and otosclerosis has been reported by a number of authors[7,8] and has also been confirmed by temporal bone histopathology.[9] The clinical diagnosis of combined Meniere's disease and otosclerosis is based on the findings of a low-frequency sensorineural hearing loss, fluctuation of hearing, aural fullness, and vertigo, that is, a symptom complex typical of endolymphatic hydrops.[4,7,8]

The pathophysiology underlying the otosclerotic inner ear syndrome is uncertain. One proposed mechanism of vestibular injury caused by otosclerosis involves the encroachment of the cribriform area of the vestibule by otosclerotic bone[10] (Fig. C20–2). The cribriform area is pierced by vestibular nerve fibers from the internal auditory canal that innervate the vestibular end organs within the inner ear. Otosclerotic bone encroachment causes vestibular nerve degeneration, which has been observed in temporal bone specimens. Histopathologic studies have also demonstrated reduced cell counts in Scarpa's ganglion without evidence of otosclerotic encroachment of the cribriform areas, so other pathologic mechanisms are probably involved.[11] The otosclerotic inner ear syndrome seems to be more prevalent in individuals with cochlear otosclerosis and thus may share a common pathophysiology. The most popular theory of cochlear otosclerosis hypothesizes the release of toxic proteolytic enzymes into the inner ear by active areas of otosclerosis.[12,13] This pathologic mechanism may also affect the vestibular side of the inner ear and result in symptoms of the otosclerotic inner ear syndrome.

Question 8: Are there any characteristic symptoms or signs of the otosclerotic inner ear syndrome?

Answer 8: No, historically the diagnosis of otosclerotic inner ear syndrome was created to describe vertigo in a patient with otosclerosis whose audiovestibular symptoms do not suggest Meniere's disease or any other known vestibular syndrome. Symptoms of otosclerotic inner ear syndrome can include episodic vertigo

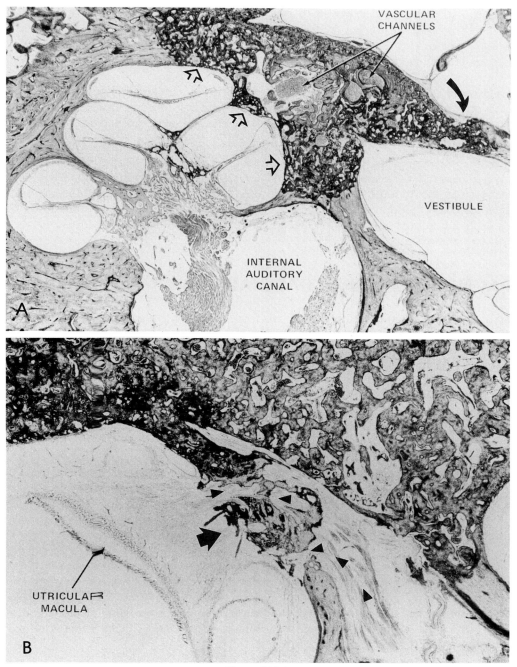

Figure C20-2

Histopathology of otosclerosis. (*A*) Low-power view of temporal bone showing a focus of otosclerotic bone bordering the cochlea and vestibule, and infiltrating the stapes footplate. Note the presence of abnormal vascular channels within the otosclerotic bone. Open arrowheads = portion of cochlea bordered by otosclerosis; curved arrow = stapes footplate. (Reprinted by permission of the publisher from Schuknecht, HF: Pathology of the Ear. Cambridge, MA: Harvard University Press. Copyright 1974 by the President and Fellows of Harvard College.[15]) (*B*) High-power view of temporal bone showing otosclerotic encroachment of the lamina cribosa (the region that transmits the vestibular nerve from the internal auditory canal to the labyrinth). Thick arrow = lamina cribosa; arrowheads = vestibular nerve fibers. (Compliments of Dr. Isamu Sando, Department of Otolaryngology, University of Pittsburgh School of Medicine.)

lasting 20 minutes to 6 hours, vague feelings of floating or lightheadedness, and nonspecific imbalance or disequilibrium.

Question 9: Why is it important to distinguish between vestibular system dysfunction solely on the basis of otosclerotic inner ear syndrome versus vestibular system dysfunction on the basis of combined Meniere's disease and otosclerosis?

Answer 9: Surgical treatment of the conductive hearing loss associated with otosclerosis is highly successful.[14] Although there is no contraindication to surgery for otosclerosis in an ear with the otosclerotic inner ear syndrome, surgery, for whatever reason, in an ear affected by Meniere's disease is associated with an increased incidence of profound hearing loss. In fact, there are multiple reports of reduced vestibular symptoms following otosclerosis surgery in patients with the otosclerotic inner ear syndrome.

DIAGNOSIS/DIFFERENTIAL DIAGNOSIS

The patient was given the diagnosis of *otosclerosis and otosclerotic inner ear syndrome*.

TREATMENT/MANAGEMENT

The patient elected to undergo surgical correction of the conductive hearing loss in the right ear. A stapedectomy was performed under local anesthesia and resulted in substantial improvement in hearing and reduction of tinnitus. The vestibular symptoms remained unchanged. The patient requested surgical correction of hearing in her left ear, but this was deferred for at least 6 months.

The presence of a sensorineural component of the hearing loss is suggestive of mild cochlear otosclerosis. Sodium fluoride supplementation has been proposed as a treatment of cochlear otosclerosis. Sodium fluoride is thought to reduce the amount of proteolytic enzymes released into the inner ear by an active focus of otosclerosis, and for this reason reduce the progression of sensorineural hearing loss. However, the lack of controlled clinical trials, potential complications (gastritis, skeletal fluorosis), and the cost of large doses of sodium fluoride has limited its widespread use.

The vestibular symptoms in this patient consisted of both episodic vertigo and daily dizziness and unsteadiness associated with quick movements. A course of vestibular rehabilitation was recommended to improve the chronic movement-induced disequilibrium and a vestibular suppressant (promethazine [25 mg PO bid]) was provided on an as-needed basis for the episodic spells.

SUMMARY

A 47-year-old woman presented with 6 months of dizziness. A long-standing bilateral hearing loss was also a problem. The family history was significant for hearing loss. The patient's hearing loss was found to be primarily conductive, and a diagnosis of otosclerosis was reached. Additionally, she had a sensorineural hearing loss and vestibular laboratory abnormalities that suggested the otosclerotic inner ear syndrome. The patient underwent surgery for otosclerosis, which improved her hearing. A course of vestibular rehabilitation was also ordered.

TEACHING POINTS

1. **Otosclerosis** is a disorder of the bony labyrinth and ossicles that most commonly causes a progressive stiffening and fixation of the stapes footplate by the formation of abnormal otosclerotic bone.
2. **Otosclerosis is a common disorder** with a subclinical incidence of about 10 percent and a clinical incidence of up to 2 percent of the population. The incidence of otosclerosis varies by ethnic background and is greatest in Caucasians, uncommon in African Americans, and rare in Asians and Native Americans. There is a female-to-male ratio of clinical otosclerosis of about 2:1.
3. **Otosclerosis causes a conductive hearing loss.** The finding of a conductive hearing loss with no previous history of otitis media or trauma and normal otoscopy suggests a diagnosis of otosclerosis. The presence of a conductive hearing loss can be inferred clinically through the use of the Rinne and Weber's tuning fork tests.
4. **Tinnitus and sensorineural hearing loss** may be associated with otosclerosis. Cochlear otosclerosis (that is, sensorineural hearing loss without a conductive component) can also occur but is difficult to diagnose. In suspected cases of cochlear otosclerosis, CT imaging of the temporal bones can confirm the diagnosis.
5. **Vestibular symptoms** are more common in individuals with otosclerosis than in the general population. The reported prevalence of dizziness in individuals with otosclerosis ranges from 7 to 40 percent. Dizziness in patients with otosclerosis may be caused by either the co-occurrence of a disorder other than otosclerosis, such as Meniere's disease, or by the pathologic process of otosclerosis itself, which can produce vestibular symptoms as a result of the *otosclerotic inner ear syndrome*.
6. **The otosclerotic inner ear syndrome** is used for patients with vertigo and otosclerosis whose audiovestibular symptoms do not suggest Meniere's disease or any other known vestibular syndrome. Symptoms of the otosclerotic inner ear syndrome can include episodic vertigo, vague feelings of floating or lightheadedness, and nonspecific imbalance or disequilibrium.
7. **Stapedectomy,** the surgical treatment for the conductive hearing loss associated with otosclerosis, is highly successful. However, it is important to distinguish the otosclerotic inner ear syndrome from combined Meniere's disease and otosclerosis because surgery in an ear affected by Meniere's disease is associated with an increased incidence of profound hearing loss, whereas there is no contraindication to surgery in patients with the otosclerotic inner ear syndrome alone.
8. **Treatment for the otosclerotic inner ear syndrome is nonspecific.** Occasionally, patients report improvement of their vestibular symptoms following stapedectomy. Treatment may include vestibular-suppressant medications as needed and vestibular rehabilitation therapy. Sodium fluoride supplementation has been advocated as a treatment for progressive sensorineural hearing loss associated with cochlear otosclerosis. The efficacy of sodium fluoride in the otosclerotic inner ear syndrome has not been established.

REFERENCES

1. Mackenzie, M, and Wolfenden, N: Otosclerosis. J Laryngol Otol 69:437–456, 1955.
2. McKenna, MJ, and Mills, BG: Immunohistochemical evidence of measles virus antigens in active otosclerosis. Otolaryngol Head Neck Surg 102:415–421, 1989.
3. Paparella, MM, and Chasen, WD: Otosclerosis and vertigo. J Laryngol Otol 80:511–517, 1966.
4. McCabe, BF: Otosclerosis and vertigo. Transactions of Pacific Coast Oto-Ophthalmological Society Annual Meeting 47:37–42, 1966.
5. Cody, DT, and Baker, HL: Otosclerosis: Vestibular symptoms and sensorineural hearing loss. Ann Otol 87:778–796, 1978.
6. Morales-Garcia, C: Cochleo-vestibular involvement in otosclerosis. Acta Otolaryngol 73:484–492, 1972.
7. Paparella, MM, Mancini, F, and Liston, SL: Otosclerosis and Meniere's syndrome: Diagnosis and treatment. Laryngoscope 94:1414–1417, 1984.
8. Shea, JJ, Ge, X, and Orchik, DJ: Endolymphatic hydrops associated with otosclerosis. Am J Otol 15:348–357, 1994.
9. Black, FO, Sando, I, Hildyard, VH, and Hemenway, WG: Bilateral multiple otosclerotic foci and endolymphatic hydrops. Ann Otol Rhinol Laryngol 78:1062–1073, 1969.
10. Sando, I, et al.: Vestibular pathology in otosclerosis temporal bone histopathological report. Laryngoscope 84:593–605, 1974.
11. Richter, E, and Schuknecht, HF: Loss of vestibular neurons in clinical otosclerosis. Arch Otorhinolaryngol 234:1–9, 1982.
12. Lawrence, M: Possible influence of cochlear otosclerosis on inner ear fluids. Ann Otol Rhinol Laryngol 75:553–558, 1966.
13. Causse, JR, et al: The enzymatic mechanism of the otospongiotic disease and NaF action on the enzymatic balance. Am J Otol 3:297, 1982.
14. Hillel, AD: History of stapedectomy. Am J Otolaryngol 4:131–140, 1983.
15. Schuknecht, HF: Pathology of the Ear. Cambridge, MA: Harvard University Press, 1974.

Multisensory Disequilibrium

HISTORY

A 55-year-old man who owned a clothing store presented with the chief complaint of disequilibrium. The patient dated the onset of his problem to a vertiginous episode experienced 6 months before evaluation. Since that time, he noted difficulty with ambulation, especially in dimly lit environments, and great difficulty while trying to shower. He had no complaint of vertigo since recovery from the single vertiginous episode 6 months before evaluation, and no complaints of hearing loss or tinnitus. The patient did not report positional sensitivity.

The patient's past history was significant for insulin-dependent diabetes mellitus for 10 years. There was no family history of a balance problem.

Question 1: Based on the history provided, what are the diagnostic considerations and what further historical information would be helpful in reaching a diagnosis?

Answer 1: This patient's history is consistent with a balance system abnormality. A diagnostic consideration is residual dysfunction from his vertiginous episode 6 months previously. The patient's lack of vertigo and difficulty with ambulation suggests that he may not have compensated for a peripheral vestibular loss (see Case C1). His diabetes mellitus may have caused a visual loss or proprioceptive loss or both. Along with vestibular dysfunction, the patient may be suffering from a combination of sensory deficits. Further important historical information includes any history of retinopathy, any symptoms suggestive of a peripheral neuropathy, and more details regarding the vertiginous episode 6 months before presentation.

ADDITIONAL HISTORY

The patient's vertiginous episode 6 months previously was associated with the acute onset of vertigo, nausea, and vomiting. He had severe gait ataxia and was bedridden for nearly a day. The patient did not require hospitalization or IV hydration despite his insulin-dependent diabetes mellitus, but was nauseated with poor appetite for 3 days, after which he noticed disequilibrium when walking. His gait instability improved somewhat, but by 2 weeks after the acute vertiginous episode, his symptoms became constant. He was evaluated by his primary care physician and was told that he had "labyrinthitis" and was given meclizine. The patient obtained additional symptomatic relief from dizziness from the meclizine for the first month after the vertiginous episode. Because the meclizine caused him to feel lethargic, he discontinued this medication with no worsening of his dizziness or imbalance.

The patient had required laser treatments in both eyes in the past for diabetic retinopathy, but had not required such treatment in the last year. He also related numbness and tingling in both feet that was more or less constant but especially noticeable when he was cold. Also, the patient occasionally had a sense of burning in the feet that was annoying when he was trying to fall asleep.

PHYSICAL EXAMINATION

The patient had a normal general examination without postural hypotension. Funduscopic examination revealed evidence of diabetic nonproliferative retinopathy. On neurologic examination, extraocular movements were full without nystagmus, and no nystagmus was seen with Frenzel glasses. Motor system examination and coordination were normal. Decreased vibratory sensation below the knee bilaterally was noted. The patient made several errors during assessment of joint position in both feet. Ankle jerks were absent. His gait was wide-based, and he was very cautious when walking. He did not veer to the right or to the left, nor was there a reeling quality. Romberg's test was negative. However, the patient could not stand on a compliant foam surface with his eyes open or closed. The stepping test was wide-based and ataxic but without significant deviation. Otologic examination was normal.

Laboratory Testing
Because of the history of a recent vertiginous episode and the high likelihood of a vestibular involvement, vestibular laboratory testing was undertaken.

Vestibular Laboratory Testing

ELECTRONYSTAGMOGRAPHY:	There was no spontaneous or positional nystagmus. Caloric testing revealed absent responses during alternate bithermal testing on the left with reduced responses (6° per second peak velocity for both warm and cold irrigations) on the right. Ice water irrigation of the left ear revealed that responses were present but markedly reduced. Ice water irrigation of the right ear was not performed.
ROTATIONAL TESTING:	Rotational testing revealed symmetric responses of reduced magnitude with an increased phase lead at low frequency (0.02 and 0.05 Hz) and a short time constant of 9 seconds. Responses were symmetric.
POSTUROGRAPHY:	Posturography indicated excessive sway on conditions 4, 5, and 6, that is, a surface dependence pattern (see Chap. 2).

Audiometric Testing: Not performed

Imaging: Not performed

Other: None

Question 2: How does the information from physical examination alter the diagnostic considerations in this case?

Answer 2: The physical examination suggests that the patient has diabetic retinopathy and a peripheral neuropathy, probably the result of diabetes. On examination, the patient had no evidence of an ongoing vestibular asymmetry with no spontaneous nystagmus and no veering of gait. Thus, although impaired sensation other than vestibular function predisposes to impaired compensation, the patient's physical examination does not suggest poor compensation. Rather, he may be suffering from the combined effects of loss of several sensory modalities that are important for balance.

DIAGNOSIS/DIFFERENTIAL DIAGNOSIS

Question 3: Based on the history, physical examination, and laboratory tests, what is this patient's likely diagnosis?

Answer 3: This patient is likely to be suffering from *multisensory disequilibrium* caused by diabetes mellitus. He has a history consistent with an acute vestibular syndrome, possibly from diabetic vascular disease, with involvement of either the vestibular labyrinth or the vestibular nerve. The patient's vestibular dysfunction is coupled with evidence of both visual and proprioceptive impairment, considering the history of diabetic retinopathy and a history of tingling and burning paresthesias. Also, decreased sensation in the feet and absent ankle jerks support the idea of a peripheral neuropathy.

Question 4: What is multisensory disequilibrium? In what clinical settings is multisensory disequilibrium often seen?

Answer 4: Multisensory disequilibrium describes a condition wherein a patient is suffering from dysfunction in all three of the sensory systems most important for balance, including vestibular, visual, and somatic and proprioceptive sensation. Such patients typically complain of unstable gait worsened by environments that further impair or distort their sensory input, such as dimly lit environments, slanted surfaces, soft or compliant surfaces, or moving surfaces such as walkways or escalators.[1] Like patients with vestibular system abnormalities, those with multisensory disequilibrium may find it helpful to lightly touch a wall or furniture while standing or walking indoors or lightly touch a companion while walking outdoors. Such patients also may find benefit when carrying a walking stick that can provide supplemental proprioceptive information regarding spatial orientation through the upper extremities.

Multisensory disequilibrium is most commonly seen in patients with diabetes mellitus because the disease can cause vestibulopathy, retinopathy, and peripheral neuropathy. In addition to diabetes, multisensory disequilibrium can be seen in any combination of disorders that impair all three sensory modalities that are important for balance.

This patient was given a diagnosis of *multisensory disequilibrium* based on diabetes mellitus.

TREATMENT/MANAGEMENT

Question 5: What is the treatment for patients with multisensory disequilibrium?

Answer 5: The treatment of patients with multisensory disequilibrium is aimed at increasing the amount of sensory input available and training such patients how to best use their remaining sensory inputs to control balance. Vestibular-suppressant medications should be discontinued. Refractive errors should be corrected. If patients have cataracts, they should be evaluated by an ophthalmologist for possible surgery. A cane should be prescribed for patients with multisensory disequilibrium to add to their somatosensory input. Medication use should be scrutinized for the presence of any agents known to impair central nervous system function, and these also should be discontinued if possible. Ergonomic factors should be optimized, including proper footwear, night lights in the home, removal of throw rugs, and installation of handrails. Also, these patients should be referred for vestibular rehabilitation, including gait training (see Chap. 4).

   This patient was advised not to use meclizine or any other vestibular-suppressant medication. A cane was prescribed for him and he was referred for a course of vestibular rehabilitation. With these measures, his disequilibrium improved somewhat.

SUMMARY

A 55-year-old man with a history of diabetes mellitus presented with a complaint of disequilibrium that had been persistent for 6 months after a vertiginous episode. The examination suggested evidence of diabetic retinopathy and peripheral neuropathy. Laboratory testing confirmed the presence of a bilateral peripheral vestibular loss coupled with a vestibular asymmetry. The patient was given the diagnosis of multisensory disequilibrium. Treatment consisted of discontinuation of vestibular-suppressant medication, the use of a cane, enrollment in a course of balance therapy, and counseling regarding the benefit of using proper footwear, night lights in the home, removal of throw rugs, and the installation of handrails.

TEACHING POINTS

1. **The three sensory systems most important for balance** include vestibular, visual, and somatic-proprioceptive sensation.
2. **Multisensory disequilibrium refers to combined dysfunction** of vestibular, visual, and somatic-proprioceptive sensation. Patients with multisensory disequilibrium typically complain of unstable gait worsened by environments that further impair or distort their sensory input, such as dimly lit environments, slanted surfaces, soft or compliant surfaces, or moving surfaces such as walkways or escalators.
3. **Diabetes mellitus is a common cause of multisensory disequilibrium** because the disease can cause vestibulopathy, retinopathy, and peripheral neuropathy. In addition to diabetes, multisensory disequilibrium can be seen in any combination of disorders that impair all three sensory modalities important for balance, such as a combination of peripheral vestibulopathy and poor vision from

cataracts and peripheral neuropathy resulting from a chronic lumbar spine disorder.

4. **Supplemental proprioceptive information** regarding spatial orientation via the upper extremities may benefit patients with multisensory disequilibrium. Patients often find it helpful to lightly touch a wall or furniture while standing or walking indoors, or to touch a companion while walking outdoors. Such patients also may gain benefit from carrying a walking stick.

5. **The treatment of multisensory disequilibrium** is aimed at increasing the amount of sensory input available and training patients how to best use their remaining sensory inputs to control balance. Vestibular-suppressant medications should be discontinued. Refractive errors should be corrected. If patients have cataracts, they should be evaluated by an ophthalmologist for possible surgery. Patients with multisensory disequilibrium should use a cane to add to their somatosensory input. Medication use should be scrutinized for the presence of any agents known to impair central nervous system function and these should be discontinued if possible. Ergonomic factors should be optimized, including proper footwear, night lights in the home, removal of throw rugs, and installation of handrails. Also, these patients should be referred for vestibular rehabilitation, including gait training.

REFERENCE

1. Brandt, T, and Daroff, R: The multisensory physiological and pathological vertigo syndromes. Ann Neurol 7:195–203, 1980.

C A S E
C22

Nystagmus Types

HISTORY

A 49-year-old man presented with a chief complaint of dizziness for 5 years. The patient had daily symptoms that were characterized by a sense of lightheadedness, difficulty focusing his vision, a sense of movement just after turning his head, and poor balance while walking. He stated that his symptoms had been particularly noticeable since a head injury sustained 1 year ago while working as a corrections officer. The patient had no complaints of vertigo, positional sensitivity, hearing loss, or tinnitus. His past history was significant for 10 years of high blood pressure, for which he was under the care of a physician. The family history was noncontributory.

Question 1: Based on the patient's history, what are the diagnostic considerations? What further historical information should be obtained?

Answer 1: This patient's complaints suggest a vestibular system abnormality. There are features that suggest both peripheral and central nervous system involvement. The patient's long course of symptoms suggests either a chronic stable condition or a slowly progressive abnormality. The role of the head trauma sustained 1 year earlier is uncertain. Additional history regarding the patient's head trauma would be useful, as well as information about any prior evaluations for dizziness because his problem is so long-standing.

ADDITIONAL HISTORY

The patient related that the head trauma suffered 1 year before evaluation was minor. Evidently he was pushed to the ground and struck his head against a wall, but did not lose consciousness and was able to stand and to return to work immediately. He did note, however, a worsened problem with balance following that episode. He was evaluated by his primary care physician, who was uncertain as to the cause of the patient's disequilibrium but noted unusual eye movements. His physician ordered a CT scan of the head, which was normal, and prescribed meclizine, which was of no benefit to the patient.

PHYSICAL EXAMINATION

The general examination was normal. The patient had full extraocular movements but was noted to have a primary position nystagmus that did not have a clearly defined fast and slow component. The nystagmus appeared irregular with both quick and slow components to the right and to the left. With Frenzel glasses, the nystagmus did not change. On horizontal gaze deviation, the patient had a typical gaze-evoked nystagmus, which was also seen on upward gaze but not on downward gaze. In fact, on downgaze, the nystagmus diminished somewhat. The patient was unable to follow a target smoothly. The remainder of the cranial nerve examination was normal. The patient's motor, sensory, and coordination examinations were normal. Romberg's test was negative. The gait was slightly wide-based and slow. Otologic examination was normal. The patient could stand on a foam pad without falling even with his eyes closed.

Question 2: Based on the history and physical examination, what is this patient's likely diagnosis and what further information would be helpful?

Answer 2: This patient's examination revealed unusual eye movements. It would be helpful to know how long he has had these eye movements. Moreover, since this may represent *congenital nystagmus*, it would be helpful to assess the influence of convergence. An oculographic recording of the patient's nystagmus to assess the influence of eye closure on the nystagmus also might help to determine its origin. A vestibular laboratory evaluation might help uncover the basis for the patient's complaints of dizziness.

ADDITIONAL HISTORY AND ADDITIONAL PHYSICAL EXAMINATION INFORMATION

The patient was unaware of his nystagmus, but said that as a child he was evaluated by an ophthalmologist for "jumpy eyes." With convergence, his nystagmus decreased in amplitude.

Laboratory Testing

Vestibular Laboratory Testing:

ELECTRONYSTAGMOGRAPHY:	Ocular motor testing revealed nystagmus in the primary position during visual fixation that had an unusual pattern. The nystagmus decreased markedly with eye closure but was still present with the eyes open in darkness. With horizontal gaze deviation, the patient developed gaze-evoked nystagmus. He was unable to track a slowly moving target smoothly. Optokinetic nystagmus was severely impaired. During positional testing, the nystagmus persisted without change. Caloric testing revealed bilaterally reduced responses with about 5° per second peak velocity of nystagmus during each irrigation of a binaural bithermal caloric testing sequence.
ROTATIONAL TESTING:	Rotational testing revealed reduced responses with extremely abnormal dynamics, that is, a large phase lead and a short time constant of only about 5 seconds.

POSTUROGRAPHY: Not performed
Audiometric Testing: Not performed
Imaging: Not performed
Other: None

DIAGNOSIS/DIFFERENTIAL DIAGNOSIS

Question 3: What is this patient's diagnosis, and what is the significance of the laboratory testing? What role did the patient's head trauma have in the generation of his symptoms?

Answer 3: The patient's laboratory studies are consistent with congenital nystagmus. The characteristics of congenital nystagmus are listed in Table C22–1. This patient had many of the typical features, although there was no null region; that is, there was no direction of gaze wherein the nystagmus was minimal. Also, he did not have perverted, that is, wrong-direction, optokinetic nystagmus. His vestibular studies suggested bilateral vestibular loss. However, the vestibulo-ocular studies also demonstrated abnormal vestibulo-ocular reflex dynamics. Because congenital nystagmus is usually associated with abnormalities of the vestibulo-ocular reflex even in the absence of dizziness,[1–3] it is impossible to say whether or not the reduced vestibulo-ocular reflex was a feature of the patient's congenital nystagmus, a sign of vestibular abnormality, or in any way related to head trauma. Thus, it is impossible to say whether or not the patient suffered from a labyrinthine or brainstem concussion related to the head trauma suffered 1 year before evaluation. The history alone, however, suggests some exacerbation of the patient's underlying disability from the head trauma, but his abnormal eye movements complicate interpretation of both the physical examination and laboratory abnormalities. Possibly, the patient did suffer a peripheral vestibular injury and his ability to compensate was impaired by a central nervous system abnormality, one of whose manifestations was congenital nystagmus.

Question 4: What is pendular nystagmus? What are its subtypes?

Answer 4: Jerk nystagmus, by definition, has a clearly defined fast and slow component; pendular nystagmus, by definition, is a to-and-fro movement of the eyes *without* a clearly defined quick movement direction. By convention, the direction of

TABLE C22–1
Characteristics of Congenital Nystagmus

Present since infancy
Irregular waveforms
Conjugate
Horizontal almost always
Accentuated by fixation, attention, anxiety
Decreased by convergence, active eyelid closure
Often a null region
No complaint of oscillopsia
Occasionally inverted optokinetic nystagmus

jerk nystagmus is named for the direction of the quick movement, because this is what is most apparent clinically. There are numerous varieties of jerk nystagmus. Defining features include direction, influence of gaze, conjugacy, effect of visual fixation, and waveform.

Pendular nystagmus may be congenital or acquired. *Congenital* pendular nystagmus is known simply as congenital nystagmus, whereas *acquired* pendular nystagmus, which is very unusual, is called just that. Pendular nystagmus is more or less sinusoidal, but it can have an unusual pattern such as that of this patient, whose pendular nystagmus had a pseudoperiodic waveform.

The underlying pathophysiology of pendular nystagmus, congenital or acquired, is unknown. Patients with congenital (pendular) nystagmus have abnormalities of gaze-holding mechanisms that manifest as gaze-evoked nystagmus (see Case C3) and abnormalities of ocular tracking. Patients with congenital nystagmus also have abnormal vestibulo-ocular reflex dynamics.[1,2,3]

Acquired pendular nystagmus has been seen in patients with multiple sclerosis and in those with brainstem infarctions. Although congenital nystagmus is almost always horizontal, acquired pendular nystagmus often has nonhorizontal components and may even be elliptical, presumably as a result of a simultaneous horizontal and vertical pendular oscillation.[4] Although congenital nystagmus is often associated with excellent visual acuity, presumably because the pattern of eye movement allows brief periods of visual fixation, acquired pendular nystagmus is typically associated with oscillopsia and poor vision. Acquired pendular nystagmus is typically unaffected by visual fixation.

A variant of acquired pendular nystagmus is a purely vertical oscillation of the eyes that can be seen in association with palatal myoclonus as a result of interruption of the so-called Mollaret's triangle, which includes the fiber pathways linking the inferior olive, the dentate nucleus, and the red nucleus.[5] Pendular nystagmus should not be confused with saccadic oscillations, which are discussed elsewhere (see Case U2).

This patient was given the diagnoses of *congenital nystagmus* and *labyrinthine concussion*.

TREATMENT/MANAGEMENT

There is no specific treatment for congenital nystagmus. Several medications have been tried with limited success, as have optical remedies,[4,6,7] also with limited success. Based on the possibility that this patient had a vestibular system imbalance that could not be adequately assessed because of the patient's congenital nystagmus, a course of vestibular rehabilitation was instituted. This intervention had little effect on the patient's condition or complaints. A vestibular-suppressant medication was prescribed. This, too, was not beneficial. The patient continued working but planned to take early retirement.

SUMMARY

A 49-year-old man complained of long-standing disequilibrium that worsened following minor head trauma. Examination revealed pendular nystagmus that was diminished by convergence. Laboratory testing documented a marked reduction of the nystagmus with eye closure. The diagnosis of *congenital nystagmus* was made. Vestibular laboratory testing also suggested abnormal vestibulo-ocular reflex dynamics and reduced magnitude of responses. The vestibular laboratory abnormalities may have been the result of congenital nystagmus rather than on the basis of peripheral vestibular dysfunction. The patient's worsening of balance following minor head trauma may have been a result of labyrinthine concussion, but this could neither be confirmed nor ruled out. Treatment with both balance therapy and vestibular-suppressant medication was unsuccessful.

TEACHING POINTS

1. **Pendular nystagmus,** a to-and-fro movement of the eyes without a clearly defined quick movement direction, differs from jerk nystagmus, which has a clearly defined fast and slow component. Pendular nystagmus may be congenital or acquired. Congenital pendular nystagmus is known simply as congenital nystagmus, whereas acquired pendular nystagmus, which is very unusual, is called just that. Pendular nystagmus is more or less sinusoidal, but it can have an unusual pattern.
2. **Congenital nystagmus differs from acquired pendular nystagmus.** Congenital pendular nystagmus is almost always horizontal. Acquired pendular nystagmus often has both horizontal and nonhorizontal components. Also, although congenital nystagmus is often associated with excellent visual acuity, presumably because the pattern of eye movement allows brief periods of visual fixation, acquired pendular nystagmus is typically associated with oscillopsia and poor vision. The characteristics of congenital nystagmus are listed in Table C22–1.
3. **The pathophysiology of pendular nystagmus**, whether congenital or acquired, is unknown. Abnormalities associated with congenital (pendular) nystagmus include poor gaze holding, poor ocular tracking, and a diminished vestibulo-ocular reflex.

REFERENCES

1. Carl, JR, et al: Head shaking and vestibulo-ocular reflex in congenital nystagmus. Invest Ophthalmol Vis Sci 26:1043–1050, 1985.
2. Demer, JL, and Zee, DS: Vestibulo-ocular and optokinetic deficits in albinos with congenital nystagmus. Invest Ophthalmol Vis Sci 25:739–745, 1984.
3. Gresty, MA, et al: Assessment of vestibulo-ocular reflexes in congenital nystagmus. Ann Neurol 17:129–136, 1985.
4. Leigh, JR, and Zee, DS (eds): The Neurology of Eye Movements, ed 2. Philadelphia: FA Davis, 1991.
5. Nakada, T, and Kwee, I: Oculopalatal myoclonus. Brain 109:431–441, 1986.
6. Yee, C, Baloh, R, and Honrubia, V: Effect of Baclofen on congenital nystagmus. In Lennerstrand, G, Zee, D, and Keller, E (eds): Functional Basis of Ocular Motility Disorders. Oxford: Pergamon Press, 1982, pp 151–158.
7. Traccis, S, et al: Successful treatment of acquired pendular elliptical nystagmus in multiple sclerosis with isoniazid and base-out prisms. Neurology 40:492–494, 1990.

C23

Perilymphatic Fistula

HISTORY

A 42-year-old woman who was a social worker presented with a chief complaint of dizziness. The major symptom was a sense of lightheadedness that worsened with rapid head movements. Dizziness was present daily and was exacerbated by bending, coughing, and sneezing, and occasionally by bowel movements. The patient also complained of some difficulty with hearing and tinnitus in the left ear. She dated the onset of her symptoms to head trauma sustained 14 months earlier during a family dispute. The patient was reluctant to provide details of this event. She had no significant past medical history other than the head trauma and was not using any medications prior to her dizziness. The family history was noncontributory. The patient's evaluation by her primary care physician included a normal CT scan. Meclizine was prescribed and provided some benefit, but the patient continued to be symptomatic.

Question 1: Based on the patient's history, what are the diagnostic considerations in this case?

Answer 1: Although this patient does not report the episodic vertigo typical of an acute peripheral vestibular disorder, her complaint of dizziness worsened by head movements is suggestive of a peripheral vestibular disorder. Her associated unilateral auditory symptoms suggest involvement of the inner ear as well. Because her symptoms followed head trauma, diagnostic considerations include labyrinthine concussion, post-traumatic endolymphatic hydrops, and perilymphatic fistula. The symptoms worsened with Valsalva maneuvers, which is particularly suggestive of perilymphatic fistula.

PHYSICAL EXAMINATION

General examination was normal. The patient had full extraocular movements but was noted to have an exophoria, that is, a latent ocular lateral misalignment when fusion was broken. There was no nystagmus. She had decreased pinprick sensation on the left side of her face that did not follow a dermatomal pattern, but according to the patient corresponded to the region injured in the trauma 14 months prior to evaluation. She had normal strength and extremity sensation and normal coordination. Her gait was normal except for slight difficulty with tandem walking. Romberg's test was negative. The patient had great difficulty standing on a compliant foam surface with her eyes open and could not stand on foam at all with her eyes closed.

On otologic examination, the left ear drum had a normal appearance, but within the middle ear space the incus appeared to be dislocated. The long process of the incus had moved laterally and anteriorly from its normal position. On pneumatic otoscopy, the ear drum was freely mobile, and with repeated pressure changes the patient began to feel dizzy and nauseous. No nystagmus was observed during pneumatic otoscopy. The right ear appeared normal. On tuning fork examination, the Rinne test was negative on the left and positive on the right. Weber's test lateralized to the left.

Question 2: Based on the history and physical examination, what is this patient's likely diagnosis and what further laboratory testing is indicated?

Answer 2: This patient has a post-traumatic peripheral vestibulopathy that may be caused by labyrinthine concussion or perilymphatic fistula and traumatic ossicular chain disruption. The tuning fork examination and otoscopy suggest the presence of a conductive hearing loss on the left, probably the results of dislocation of the incus. The association of ongoing dizziness and traumatic dislocation of the incus raises the possibility of additional ossicular dislocation involving the stapes and possible perilymphatic fistula involving the oval window. Appropriate laboratory testing includes audiometry and vestibular laboratory studies to document the character and extent of injury and to serve as a baseline should the patient require surgery for repair of the ossicular chain or perilymphatic fistula.

Laboratory Testing

Vestibular Laboratory Testing

ELECTRONYSTAGMOGRAPHY:	Ocular motor function was normal. There was no spontaneous or positional nystagmus. Caloric testing revealed a borderline normal left reduced vestibular response of 21 percent.
ROTATIONAL TESTING:	Rotational testing revealed a left directional preponderance.
POSTUROGRAPHY:	Posturography indicated excessive sway on conditions 4, 5, and 6, that is, a surface dependence pattern.

Audiometric Testing: An audiogram revealed normal hearing in the right ear. The left ear had a mixed conductive and sensorineural hearing loss with good word recognition scores (see Fig. C23–1).

Imaging: Not performed

Other: None

DIAGNOSIS/DIFFERENTIAL DIAGNOSIS

Question 3: Based on the additional information from laboratory testing, what is the patient's likely diagnosis and what course of management should be taken?

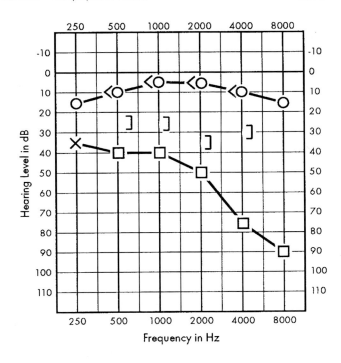

Figure C23-1
Audiogram.

Word Recognition Score		
Right :	100%	
Left :	100%	

			Right	Left
Air	unmasked		o——o	x——x
	masked		△——△	□——□
Bone	unmasked		<---<	>--->
	masked		[---[	]---]

Answer 3: The presence of a conductive hearing loss on audiologic testing supports the impression of a traumatic ossicular chain disruption. The sensorineural portion of the hearing loss raises the possibility that more than an ossicular dislocation occurred. The sensorineural hearing loss could have been caused by labyrinthine concussion or perilymphatic fistula. The results of vestibular testing support the presence of ongoing vestibular system dysfunction and the unilateral caloric weakness supports a peripheral vestibulopathy as the cause. The vestibular symptoms and signs could be the result of either a perilymphatic fistula or labyrinthine concussion.

Surgical exploration of the middle ear is indicated to restore hearing by reconstructing the ossicular chain and to rule out a perilymphatic fistula as a cause of the continuing vestibular symptoms.

Question 4: What is a perilymphatic fistula?

Answer 4: A perilymphatic fistula is an abnormal connection between the middle and inner ear spaces, specifically between the air-filled middle ear and the perilymphatic space of the inner ear. A perilymphatic fistula can occur through the bony labyrinth (so-called bony fistula); through the oval window (so-called oval window fistula); or through the round window (so-called round window fistula) (Fig. C23–2). Bony fistulas were once common as a result of erosion of the horizontal semicircular canal caused by cholesteatoma (see Case C19) or syphilis. Oval window fistulas can be produced

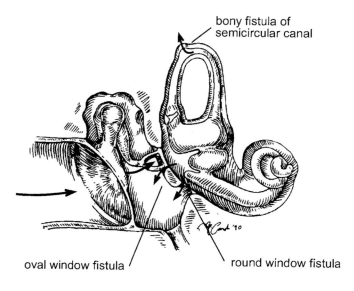

bony fistula of
semicircular canal

oval window fistula

round window fistula

Figure C23-2
Schematic drawing of the middle and inner ears showing common sites of perilymphatic fistulas. Curved arrows highlight the movement of perilymph through the round window membrane, the oval window, and a semicircular canal fistula. (Modified with permission from Glasscock, ME, et al: Handbook of Vertigo. New York: Raven Press, 1990.[10])

iatrogenically, as a result of stapedectomy for otosclerosis, and can be caused by blunt trauma, barotrauma, or heavy lifting, which presumably transmits excessive pressure to the footplate of the stapes. Both oval window and round window fistulas are not uncommonly observed in association with anatomic malformations of the inner ear (see Case U8).

Question 5: What are the common presenting symptoms and signs of perilymphatic fistula?

Answer 5: Common presenting symptoms and signs of perilymphatic fistula include sensorineural hearing loss that is often fluctuating, but may be constant or progressive, and tinnitus.[2] Vestibular symptoms are usually nonspecific, and include mild unsteadiness and disequilibrium. Occasionally, patients with perilymphatic fistula report vertigo, especially during Valsalva maneuvers (coughing, sneezing, bending, lifting, or straining at stool). Perilymphatic fistula should be considered in patients (usually children) with a history of recurrent meningitis or progressive sensorineural hearing loss following an episode of otitis media.[3] Although it is possible that perilymphatic fistula can cause a pure vestibular syndrome without auditory or aural symptoms, the prevalence of this entity is controversial. Because it is not possible to diagnose a perilymphatic fistula solely on the presence of vestibular symptoms, most clinicians require a history of a traumatic inciting event and clear localization of the affected ear by the presence of hearing loss to consider the diagnosis of a perilymphatic fistula.

Question 6: What are the causes of perilymphatic fistula?

Answer 6: Perilymphatic fistula can be iatrogenic, traumatic, erosive, spontaneous, and congenital. Traumatic perilymphatic fistula can be a result of direct penetrating injury, indirect injury following blunt head trauma, which probably accounts for this patient's perilymphatic fistula, or barotrauma.[4–6] Erosive perilymphatic fistula usually is caused by chronic middle ear and mastoid infection with cholesteatoma (see Case C19) or rarely neoplasia. Spontaneous perilymphatic fistulas are highly controversial unless a congenital inner ear malformation is present.[7] Perilymphatic fistula related to a congenital inner ear malformation can occur spontaneously or more commonly after minor head trauma or forced Valsalva maneuver.

This patient was given a diagnosis of *perilymphatic fistula.*

TREATMENT/MANAGEMENT

A suspected perilymphatic fistula can be initially treated with a period of bed rest and reduced activity. Persistence of symptoms or deterioration of hearing are indications for surgical middle ear exploration. Because this patient also had evidence for a ossicular chain dislocation, a middle ear exploration was performed without delay.

Middle ear exploration is usually performed under local anesthesia. Using an operating microscope, the tympanic membrane is reflected open and the ossicular chain and oval and round window membranes are inspected directly. Perilymphatic fistula can be confirmed by visualizing a tear, rupture, or fracture of one of the inner ear membranes. In the past, the observation of clear fluid "pooling" around the inner ear membranes had been considered evidence of a perilymphatic fistula. However, it is now known that this sign is highly inaccurate. Several of specific assays for detecting perilymph are under development, the most promising being the beta-2 transferrin assay.[8,9]

In this patient, the incus was found to be severely dislocated; the annular ligament of the stapes was torn and the stapes was partially subluxed into the vestibule. Repair was performed by first removing the incus. The stapes was then lifted back into proper position and a fascial graft was used to seal the ruptured annular ligament. The incus was then repositioned in the middle ear to reconstruct the ossicular chain.

After this procedure, the patient had complete restoration of the conductive component of her hearing loss, and she has had no further vertigo.

SUMMARY

A 42-year-old woman complained of dizziness following blunt head trauma. The patient had associated mild hearing loss and tinnitus in the left ear. Examination suggested damage to the ossicular chain and possible perilymphatic fistula. Laboratory testing demonstrated a mixed conductive and sensorineural hearing loss and a vestibular reduction on the left. The patient underwent middle ear exploration with repair of an oval window fistula and ossicular chain reconstruction.

TEACHING POINTS

1. **Peripheral vestibular-related symptoms following head trauma** can be caused by labyrinthine concussion, post-traumatic endolymphatic hydrops, and perilymphatic fistula.
2. **A perilymphatic fistula** is an abnormal connection between the middle and inner ear spaces, specifically between the air-filled middle ear and the perilymphatic space of the inner ear. A perilymphatic fistula can result from a microfissure of the bony labyrinth, a rupture of the oval window, or a rupture of the round window.

3. **Symptoms and signs of perilymphatic fistula** include sensorineural hearing loss that is often fluctuating but can be constant or progressive, and tinnitus. Vestibular symptoms are usually nonspecific, including mild unsteadiness and disequilibrium. Occasionally, patients with perilymphatic fistula report vertigo, especially during Valsalva maneuvers (coughing, sneezing, bending, lifting, or straining at stool).

4. **The causes of perilymphatic fistula** include iatrogenic, traumatic, erosive, congenital, and spontaneous varieties. The most common sites of iatrogenic perilymphatic fistula include bony fistula of the horizontal and posterior semicircular canals during mastoid surgery and rupture of the oval window during surgery for middle ear cholesteatoma and otosclerosis. Traumatic perilymphatic fistula can be a result of direct penetrating injury, indirect injury following blunt head trauma, or barotrauma. Erosive perilymphatic fistula usually is caused by chronic middle ear and mastoid infection with cholesteatoma or, rarely, neoplasia. Both oval window and round window fistulas are not uncommonly observed in association with congenital inner ear malformations. Congenitally related perilymphatic fistula can occur spontaneously or more commonly after minor head trauma or forced Valsalva maneuver. The occurrence of spontaneous perilymphatic fistulas is highly controversial unless a congenital inner ear malformation is present. Perilymphatic fistula should be considered in patients (usually children) with a history of recurrent meningitis or progressive sensorineural hearing loss following an episode of otitis media.

5. **The treatment of a suspected perilymphatic fistula** includes a trial of bed rest and reduced activity to allow natural healing of the fistula. Persistence of symptoms or deterioration of hearing are indications for surgical middle ear exploration. The purposes of surgical exploration are to confirm the presence of a fistula and to repair the fistula using fascial grafts.

REFERENCES

1. Bhansali, SA: Perilymph fistula. Ear Nose Throat 68:11–26, 1989.
2. Hughes, GB, Sismanis, A, and House, JW: Is there consensus in perilymph fistula management? Otolaryngol Head Neck Surg 102:111, 1990.
3. Bluestone, CD: Otitis media and congenital perilymphatic fistula as a cause of sensorineural hearing loss in children. Pediatr Infect Dis J 7:S141–S145, 1988.
4. Emmett, JR, and Shea, JJ: Traumatic perilymph fistula. Laryngoscope 90:1513–1520, 1980.
5. Glasscock, ME, McKennan, KX, and Levine, SC: Persistent traumatic perilymph fistulas. Laryngoscope 97:860–864, 1987.
6. Pullen, FW: Perilymphatic fistula induced by barotrauma. Am J Otol 13:270–272, 1992.
7. Schuknecht, HF: Mondini dysplasia: A clinical and pathological study. Ann Otol Rhinol Laryngol 89 (Suppl):3–23, 1980.
8. Bassiouny, M, et al: Beta 2 transferrin application in otology. Am J Otol 13:552–555, 1992.
9. Skedros, DG, et al: Sources of errors in use of beta 2 transferrin analysis for diagnosing perilymphatic and cerebral spinal fluid leaks. Otolaryngol Head Neck Surg 109:861–864, 1993.
10. Glasscock, ME, et al: Handbook of Vertigo. New York: Raven Press, 1990.

C24

Autoimmune Inner Ear Disease

HISTORY

A 33-year-old woman who worked in a day-care center presented with a chief complaint of hearing loss and disequilibrium gradually worsening over 14 months. The patient noted that her symptoms were more or less constant with periodic exacerbations. Her dizziness was characterized by lightheadedness and a sense of disequilibrium exacerbated by rapid head movements and ambulation. She also noted that her hearing in both ears was impaired and her hearing would periodically worsen only subsequently to improve, but sometimes not to her baseline. The patient had no significant past medical history. There were no complaints of abnormal strength or sensation. Aside from some blurred vision during episodes of extreme dizziness, there were no visual complaints. The family history was negative. Meclizine had been prescribed with no benefit.

Question 1: Based on the patient's history, what are the diagnostic considerations?

Answer 1: This patient has a history consistent with a peripheral vestibulopathy. Based on the complaints of bilateral hearing loss, the patient may be suffering from bilateral otologic disease. Given the information available from the history, the differential diagnosis for the patient's condition is broad. However, the progressive nature of the illness and the associated complaints of bilateral hearing loss render some diagnoses more likely than others. Meniere's disease (see Cases T3, T9, C10, C14, C16), ototoxicity (see Case C6), neurosyphilis, HIV infection, Lyme disease, autoimmune inner ear disease, bilateral acoustic neuroma associated with neurofibromatosis, and otosclerosis (see Case C20) are all possible.

PHYSICAL EXAMINATION

The patient's general examination was normal. Neurologic examination revealed a left-beating nystagmus on left gaze. There were no other abnormalities of cranial nerves.

Motor examination, sensation, and coordination were normal. The patient had a very wide based and unsteady gait. Romberg's test was negative, but the patient was unable to stand on a compliant surface even with her eyes open. She demonstrated some difficulty understanding speech during the interview, especially when lip reading was prevented. On tuning fork examination, Weber's test was midline and the Rinne test was positive bilaterally. Neuro-otologic examination revealed left-beating nystagmus with Frenzel glasses in the primary position that was worsened by left lateral gaze.

Question 2: Does the physical examination help to establish a diagnosis? What laboratory testing should be ordered to rule out other diagnostic possibilities?

Answer 2: The physical examination indicates a vestibular imbalance and the patient notes a bilateral hearing impairment. These findings support the idea of bilateral otologic disease. Laboratory testing should be performed to document the extent of hearing loss and the extent of vestibular involvement. An MRI scan should be obtained with special attention to the internal auditory canals. Blood studies should include rheumatologic studies, a serum FTA-ABS, and an HIV and a Lyme titer.

Laboratory Testing

Vestibular Laboratory Testing

ELECTRONYSTAGMOGRAPHY:	Ocular motor function was normal with the exception of a left-beating spontaneous vestibular nystagmus. There was a direction-fixed left-beating positional nystagmus of 6° per second. Alternate binaural bithermal caloric responses were absent bilaterally. A minimal response to ice water irrigation was apparent on the right and responses were absent on the left.
ROTATIONAL TESTING:	Rotational testing revealed markedly reduced responses and a left-directional preponderance
POSTUROGRAPHY:	Posturography indicated excessive sway on conditions 4, 5, and 6, that is, a surface dependence pattern.

Audiometric Testing: Audiometric testing revealed a bilateral flat sensorineural hearing loss of a moderate to severe degree. Word recognition score was 60 percent in the right ear and 80 percent in the left ear (Fig. C24–1).

Imaging: MRI scan of the brain was normal.

Other: Serum FTA-ABS, HIV, and Lyme titers were all negative. The erythrocyte sedimentation rate was slightly elevated; serum immunoglobulin levels, antinuclear antibody, rheumatoid factor, circulating immune complexes, and C_3, C_4 were all normal.

DIAGNOSIS/DIFFERENTIAL DIAGNOSIS

Question 3: Based on the history, physical examination, and laboratory results, what is the most likely diagnosis?

Answer 3: This patient's diagnosis is uncertain. She clearly has bilateral otologic disease impairing both cochlear and vestibular function. Autoimmune inner ear disease is an appropriate provisional diagnosis because there is no evidence for ototoxic drug exposure, little evidence for an infectious process, and no family history or imaging evidence for neurofibromatosis.

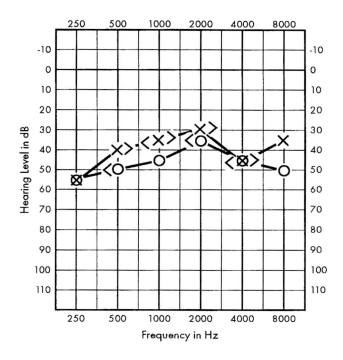

Figure C24-1
Audiogram.

Word Recognition Score			Right	Left
	Air	unmasked	O———O	X———X
		masked	△———△	□———□
Right : 60%				
Left : 80%	Bone	unmasked	←- - -<	>- - -→
		masked	E- - -[	]- - -]

Question 4: What is autoimmune inner ear disease? What are its manifestations? Are there any diagnostic tests that can confirm the diagnosis of autoimmune inner ear disease?

Answer 4: Autoimmune inner ear disease is a disorder characterized by auditory and vestibular dysfunction that most often is bilateral and is thought to be produced by damage mediated by both cellular and humoral immune mechanisms.[1,2] Autoimmune inner ear disease is usually bilateral, but it can begin unilaterally and rapidly progress to involve both sides. In its early stages, autoimmune disease may present in a fashion similar to endolymphatic hydrops. The typical patient is a middle-aged woman.[2]

There are currently no well-accepted diagnostic tests that can confirm the diagnosis of autoimmune inner ear disease, although a positive rheumatologic battery or elevated sedimentation rate may be suggestive. The diagnosis is usually one of exclusion and rests on clinical criteria and response to treatment (see later text). Several experimental tests are being studied that include testing patients' serum against inner ear antigens using Western blot analysis, the lymphocyte transformation test, and the migration inhibition test. These tests show some promise of detecting an autoimmune inner ear disorder. A positive test result is thought to predict a positive response to steroid treatment. Development of more antigen-specific tests is likely to increase the sensitivity and specificity of blood testing for autoimmune inner

TABLE C24–1
Systemic Autoimmune Diseases Associated with
Inner Ear Manifestations

Systemic lupus erythematosus
Rheumatoid arthritis
Vasculitides
    Polyarteritis nodosa
    Wegener's granulomatosis
    Cogan's syndrome
    Behçet's disease
Ulcerative colitis

Source: Adapted from Barna, GB, and Hughes, BP: Autoimmunity
    and otologic disease: Clinical and experimental aspects. Clin Lab
    Med 8:389, 1988.[12]

ear disease.[3–5] For example, Yoo[6] has reported the detection of autoantibodies to type II collagen in autoimmune inner ear disease, and animal studies have furthered the current concepts involving autoimmune inner ear disease.[7–9] Thus, patients with suspected autoimmune disease of the ear should undergo blood tests similar to those used for the evaluation of systemic rheumatologic disease. Moreover, because autoimmune inner ear disease is a feature of Cogan's syndrome, which is characterized by autoimmune inner ear disease and nonsyphilitic interstitial keratitis, slit lamp evaluation to search for interstitial keratitis should be undertaken.

Question 5: What are the cochleovestibular manifestations of systemic rheumatologic disease?

Answer 5: Several rheumatologic diseases have been associated with cochleovestibular dysfunction. The nature of this dysfunction is not well characterized but may include both unilateral and bilateral disease. Hearing loss is better documented than vestibular involvement. Table C24–1 lists those disorders in which cochleovestibular findings have been reported.

Question 6: What treatments have been advocated for autoimmune inner ear disease?

Answer 6: The most widely accepted treatment of autoimmune inner ear disease includes corticosteroids such as prednisolone 1 mg/kg per day for 1 to 2 weeks followed by a tapering dose. Cytotoxic agents such as azathioprine and cyclophosphamide have also been advocated as an adjunct to steroid therapy.[10] Lastly, plasmapheresis has been proposed.[11] Each of these treatments is variably successful. Often, patients require long-term treatment to prevent relapse.

The patient was given the diagnosis of *autoimmune inner ear disease.*

TREATMENT/MANAGEMENT

The patient was treated with steroids in the form of oral prednisolone 60 mg daily for 2 weeks. During this time, she experienced a slight improvement in her hearing, especially in her ability to understand speech and slight improvement in balance. After the 2-week course of high-dose steroids, the steroid dose was slowly tapered. When dosage reached 5 mg daily, the patient noticed worsening of her hearing and balance. The steroid dose was then increased to 20 mg every other day, after which hearing stabilized. The patient was enrolled in a vestibular rehabilitation program and noticed gradual improvement of balance.

SUMMARY

A 33-year-old woman presented with bilateral hearing loss and disequilibrium that had both gradually worsened over 14 months. On examination, the patient was found to be have bilateral hearing loss and spontaneous vestibular nystagmus. Laboratory testing revealed bilateral sensorineural hearing loss, bilateral vestibular loss with a vestibular asymmetry, and a normal MRI. Blood studies did not show evidence of an infectious process. Rheumatologic parameters were normal, with the exception of a mildly elevated erythrocyte sedimentation rate. On the basis of the patient's clinical presentation and positive response to a trial of steroids, the diagnosis of autoimmune inner ear disease was made. Treatment consisted of high-dose corticosteroids and vestibular rehabilitation. The patient's hearing loss and vestibular symptoms stabilized.

TEACHING POINTS

1. **Bilateral otologic disease** can cause dizziness symptoms consistent with peripheral vestibular dysfunction in conjunction with bilateral hearing loss. The differential diagnosis for this clinical situation includes bilateral Meniere's disease, ototoxicity, neurosyphilis, HIV infection, Lyme disease, autoimmune inner ear disease, bilateral acoustic neuroma associated with neurofibromatosis, and otosclerosis.
2. **Autoimmune inner ear disease** is a disorder characterized by auditory and vestibular dysfunction that most often is bilateral and is thought to be produced by damage mediated by both cellular and humoral immune mechanisms. Autoimmune inner ear disease is usually bilateral but may begin unilaterally and rapidly progress to involve both sides.
3. **A diagnosis of autoimmune inner ear disease is difficult to confirm.** A positive rheumatologic battery or elevated sedimentation rate may be suggestive. Thus, patients with suspected autoimmune inner ear disease should undergo blood tests similar to those used for the evaluation of systemic rheumatologic disease. Also, slit lamp evaluation to search for interstitial keratitis, a component of Cogan's syndrome, should be undertaken. Autoimmune inner ear disease is often a diagnosis of exclusion and frequently depends on clinical criteria and response to a trial of corticosteroid therapy.
4. **Rheumatologic diseases can be associated with cochleovestibular dysfunction.** Table C24–1 lists those systemic autoimmune diseases in which cochleovestibular findings have been reported.
5. **Treatment of autoimmune inner ear disease** usually includes corticosteroids, such as prednisolone, 1 mg/kg per day 1 to 2 weeks, followed by a tapering dose and maintenance dose if a positive response has occurred. Cytotoxic agents such as azathioprine and cyclophosphamide have also been advocated as an adjunct if the disease stops responding to steroid therapy. Plasmapheresis may be effective.

REFERENCES

1. Veldman, JE, et al: Autoimmunity and inner ear disorders: An immune-complex mediated sensorineural hearing loss. Laryngoscope 94:501, 1984.
2. Griffith, AJ: Biological and clinical aspects of autoimmune inner ear disease. Yale J Biol Med 65:17–28, 1992.
3. Moscicki, RA, et al: Serum antibody to inner ear proteins in patients with progressive hearing loss. JAMA 272:611–616, 1994.
4. Yamanobe, S, and Harris, JP: Inner ear–specific antibodies. Laryngoscope 103:319–326, 1993.
5. Hughes, GB, et al: Predictive value of laboratory tests in "autoimmune" inner ear disease: Preliminary report. Laryngoscope 96:502–505, 1986.
6. Yoo, TJ: Etiopathogenesis of Meniere's disease: A hypothesis. Ann Otol Rhinol Laryngol 93 (Suppl 113):6–12, 1984.
7. Soliman, AM: Experimental autoimmune inner ear disease. Laryngoscope 99:188–194, 1989.
8. Yoo, TJ, et al: Type II collagen-induced autoimmune endolymphatic hydrops in guinea pig. Science 222:65–67, 1983.
9. Harris, JP: Immunologic mechanisms in disorders of the inner ear. Otolaryngol Head Neck Surg, Update 1, Chapter 26, 1989, pp 380–395.
10. McCabe, BF: Autoimmune inner ear disease: Therapy. Am J Otolaryngol 10:196–197, 1989.
11. Luetje, CM: Theoretical and practical implications for plasmapheresis in autoimmune inner ear disease. Laryngoscope 99:1137–1146, 1989.
12. Barna, GB, and Hughes, BP: Autoimmunity and otologic disease: Clinical and experimental aspects. Clin Lab Med 8:389, 1988.

C25

Recurrent Vestibulopathy

HISTORY

A 51-year-old man complained of episodic dizziness. The patient stated that he had three discrete episodes of dizziness during the last 3 years. The most recent had been 6 weeks before evaluation. He related that during his episodes he experienced severe vertigo associated with nausea and vomiting. He was bedridden for each of these episodes for several hours and had great difficulty with ambulation for several additional hours. For the first 1 to 2 days following each episode, he had a mild sense of disequilibrium but was able to return to his work as a field service representative. He had no associated hearing loss, tinnitus, or fullness in the ears. Also, he had no loss of vision, double vision, numbness, weakness, or alteration in level of consciousness. The patient required an emergency room visit for two of these three episodes for control of nausea and vomiting. He was asymptomatic between episodes. There was no history of migraine headaches and no significant past medical history. The patient had no family history of otologic or neurologic disease, including migraine. An MRI scan requested by the patient's primary care physician was within normal limits.

Question 1: Based on the patient's history, what are the diagnostic considerations?

Answer 1: The clinical syndrome demonstrated by this patient consists of multiple episodes of vertigo lasting minutes to hours (not days to weeks) without auditory or neurologic symptoms. This syndrome has been termed *recurrent vestibulopathy*. Other diagnostic considerations include a vestibular-only form of endolymphatic hydrops (see Cases T3, T9, C10, C14, and C16), recurrent vestibular neuritis (see Cases T5 and C1), migraine-related vestibulopathy (see Cases C4, C12, U12, and U16), and benign positional vertigo (see Cases T1, C9, C15, and U17). This patient has little to suggest a central nervous system abnormality because of the isolated nature of the patient's vertigo. However, vertebrobasilar insufficiency (see Case C5), although unlikely, should be considered in the differential diagnosis. Other considerations include perilymphatic fistula (see Cases C19 and C23), panic disorder (see Case C2), and a seizure disorder (see Case U7).

PHYSICAL EXAMINATION

Physical examination was entirely normal, including general, neurologic, otologic, and neuro-otologic evaluation.

Laboratory Testing

Vestibular Laboratory Testing

ELECTRONYSTAGMOGRAPHY: Ocular motor, caloric, and positional testing were normal.

ROTATIONAL TESTING: Not performed

POSTUROGRAPHY: Not performed

Audiometric Testing: The audiogram was normal.

Imaging: Not performed

Other: Not performed

DIAGNOSIS/DIFFERENTIAL DIAGNOSIS

Question 2: This patient's symptoms are characteristic of the syndrome termed recurrent vestibulopathy. How can this diagnosis be confirmed?

Answer 2: The diagnosis of recurrent vestibulopathy cannot be confirmed and is both a provisional diagnosis and a diagnosis of exclusion.[1,2] As noted previously, recurrent vertigo can be seen in endolymphatic hydrops, recurrent vestibular neuritis, benign positional vertigo, perilymphatic fistula, migraine-related vestibulopathy, vertebrobasilar insufficiency, panic disorder, and seizure disorder. These entities can usually be ruled out by a careful history and physical examination. However, some of these entities, such as recurrent vestibular neuritis, migraine-related vestibulopathy, and endolymphatic hydrops, are difficult to rule out definitively. This uncertainty is reflected in the fact that in approximately 30 percent of patients with a provisional diagnosis of recurrent vestibulopathy, another specific diagnosis will become clear over time, most commonly endolymphatic hydrops, benign positional vertigo, or migraine-related vestibulopathy.[2]

Question 3: What is the cause of recurrent vestibulopathy?

Answer 3: The cause of recurrent vestibulopathy is not known, and the nonspecific name was originally chosen to reflect the unknown underlying pathophysiology. The signs and symptoms that typify recurrent vestibulopathy are most similar to those of vestibular neuritis, except that patients with vestibular neuritis have more prolonged vertigo (days versus minutes to hours) and chronic vestibular symptoms (weeks to months versus days) than patients with recurrent vestibulopathy. Thus, it has been hypothesized that recurrent vestibulopathy represents a milder form of vestibular neuritis. Although the precise mechanism of vestibular neuritis is unknown, there is evidence to support viral-induced injury to the vestibular nerve (see Cases T5 and C1). Given the similarities of vestibular neuritis and recurrent vestibulopathy, similar viral-related mechanisms may be involved in both clinical syndromes.[3-5]

This patient was given a diagnosis of *recurrent vestibulopathy*.

TREATMENT/MANAGEMENT

There is no specific treatment for recurrent vestibulopathy. Antinausea and antiemetic agents should be prescribed to prevent a needless hospital visit. Agents such as oral promethazine and prochlorperazine suppositories should be in the patient's possession and used when appropriate.

SUMMARY

A 51-year-old man presented with recurrent vertigo without hearing loss, tinnitus, ear fullness, or any neurologic complaints. There was no past medical history or family history to suggest a particular disorder such as migraine or panic attacks. The patient had normal laboratory studies, including brain imaging and caloric testing. He was given the provisional diagnosis of *recurrent vestibulopathy* and given prescriptions for antinausea agents to be used only on an as-needed basis.

TEACHING POINTS

1. **Recurrent vestibulopathy** is a clinical syndrome that consists of multiple episodes of vertigo lasting minutes to hours without auditory or neurologic signs or symptoms.
2. **Recurrent vestibulopathy is a diagnosis of exclusion.** Several other disorders that can cause recurrent vertigo such as endolymphatic hydrops, recurrent vestibular neuritis, benign positional vertigo, perilymphatic fistula, migraine-related vestibulopathy, vertebrobasilar insufficiency, panic disorder, and seizure disorder should be excluded before diagnosing recurrent vestibulopathy.
3. **Recurrent vestibulopathy may be a provisional diagnosis.** Approximately 30 percent of patients given a diagnosis of recurrent vestibulopathy develop a condition that warrants a more specific diagnosis, most commonly endolymphatic hydrops, benign paroxysmal vertigo, or migraine-related vestibulopathy.
4. **The cause of recurrent vestibulopathy** is not known. A reversible viral or immune-related injury to the vestibular nerve has been hypothesized.
5. **Treatment for recurrent vestibulopathy** is nonspecific. Antinausea and antiemetic agents should be prescribed for the patient to have on hand in the event of an episode of acute vertigo.

REFERENCES

1. LeLiever, WC, and Barber, HO: Recurrent vestibulopathy. Laryngoscope 91:1–6, 1981.
2. Rutka, JA, and Barber, HO: Recurrent vestibulopathy: Third review. J Otolaryngol 15:105–107, 1988.
3. Dix, MR, and Hallpike, CS: The pathology, symptomatology and diagnosis of certain common disorders of the vestibular system. Proc Roy Soc Med 45:15–28, 1952.
4. Coats, AC: Vestibular neuronitis. Acta Otolaryngol 251 (Suppl): 1–32, 1969.
5. Schuknecht, HF, and Kitamura, K: Vestibular neuritis. Ann Otol Rhinol Laryngol 78 (Suppl):1–19, 1981.

C26

Multiple Sclerosis

HISTORY

A 40-year-old woman presented with a chief complaint of blurred vision, lightheadedness, and imbalance. There was no complaint of hearing loss or tinnitus. The patient had a past medical history of multiple sclerosis with intermittent exacerbations. She had suffered from optic neuritis on several occasions. Additionally, she had suffered intermittent exacerbations characterized by weakness, incoordination, and urinary dysfunction. The patient recovered to a large extent from each of these episodes and was able to continue her work as a licensed practical nurse. One week before evaluation, the patient awoke with vertigo. She noticed a sense of disorientation worsened by head movement and had severe imbalance while attempting to walk. There was no change in any of her other neurologic functions. The patient's symptoms had decreased slightly during the week before evaluation. The family history was noncontributory.

Question 1: Based on the history, what is the likely cause of the patient's symptoms?

Answer 1: This patient's symptoms of vertigo and imbalance suggest a vestibular system abnormality. The multiple sclerosis could be an underlying cause of the patient's condition if there were a lesion in central vestibular tracts. Additionally, she could be suffering from a peripheral vestibular abnormality independent of her multiple sclerosis. In this case, the patient's central nervous system abnormalities might be interfering with recovery from a peripheral vestibular deficit (see Case C1).

PHYSICAL EXAMINATION

The patient's general examination was normal. Eye movement examination revealed a left-beating nystagmus on left gaze. With Frenzel glasses, the patient had a left-beating nystagmus in the primary position. There was no evidence of internuclear ophthalmoplegia or gaze paresis and no vertical nystagmus. The patient had normal strength and sensation. Coordination revealed abnormal finger-to-nose testing in the left upper extremity. Otherwise, there was no abnormality of coordination. Deep tendon reflexes were 3+ and symmetric. Plantar responses were flexor bilaterally. Gait was mildly ataxic with a negative Romberg's test. Otologic examination was normal. The patient was unable to stand on a compliant foam surface without assistance and fell to the right. The stepping test was wide-based and ataxic without significant rotation.

Question 2: Based on the history and physical examination, what is this patient's likely diagnosis?

Answer 2: The physical examination suggests the presence of a vestibular abnormality. The patient also had signs of central nervous system involvement with abnormal finger-to-nose testing on the left and gaze-evoked nystagmus on leftward gaze, which might have been the result of an accentuated vestibular nystagmus. The ataxic gait could be a result of either a vestibular system or cerebellar system abnormality or both. Thus, the patient has evidence of combined peripheral and central vestibular abnormalities.

Laboratory Testing

Vestibular Laboratory Testing

ELECTRONYSTAGMOGRAPHY:	A spontaneous left-beating nystagmus was recorded. There was a direction-fixed left-beating postional nystagmus. Caloric responses revealed a right reduced vestibular response of 50 percent.
ROTATIONAL TESTING:	Rotational testing revealed increased phase lead with a normal amplitude and symmetry of responses.
POSTUROGRAPHY:	Posturography indicated excessive sway on conditions 3, 5, and 6, that is, a combined vestibular deficit and visual dependence (see Chap. 2).

Audiometric Testing: Testing showed normal hearing in the left ear. The right ear showed a mild to moderate high-frequency sensorineural hearing loss. Word recognition scores were normal bilaterally (Fig. C26–1).

Imaging: An MRI scan of the head revealed a vestibular root entry-zone lesion on the right (Fig. C26–2). MRI scan also indicated numerous periventricular white matter hyperintensities on T_2-weighted images.

Other: None

DIAGNOSIS/DIFFERENTIAL DIAGNOSIS

Question 3: Based on the information from laboratory tests in addition to the information from the history and physical examination, what is this patient's likely diagnosis?

Answer 3: This patient has evidence for vestibular system involvement on history, physical examination, and vestibular laboratory testing. The MRI scan indicates a vestibular root entry-zone lesion. Thus, the patient is likely to have symptoms of dizziness and disequilibrium on the basis of multiple sclerosis, which can account for both the peripheral and central vestibular symptoms and signs.

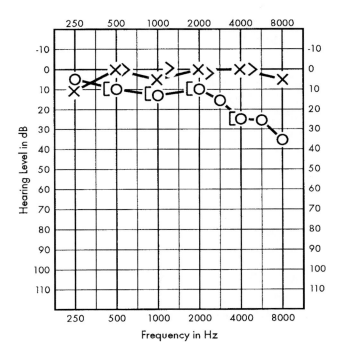

Figure C26-1
Audiogram.

Word Recognition Score		Air	unmasked	Right	Left

Word Recognition Score
Right : 100%
Left : 100%

		Right	Left
Air	unmasked	O——O	✕——✕
	masked	△——△	□——□
Bone	unmasked	←---<	>--->
	masked	E---[	]---]

Question 4: Should this patient's eighth nerve root entry-zone lesion be considered a peripheral or central vestibular abnormality?

Answer 4: A root entry-zone lesion should be considered a peripheral vestibular abnormality on the basis of *function* because damage is limited to afferent vestibular activity. *Structurally*, of course, a root entry-zone lesion, because it is intraparenchymal, is a central nervous system abnormality and thus could be labeled a central vestibular lesion. Moreover, patients with root entry-zone lesions on the basis of multiple sclerosis often have a much more prolonged recovery from their abnormality than patients with peripheral vestibular ailments. This prolongation of recovery probably results from lesions other than that at the root entry-zone that impair compensation, although there may be some inherent characteristic of a root entry-zone lesion that causes compensation to differ from that following lesions of the vestibular endorgan or vestibular nerve.

This patient was given the diagnosis of *demyelination of the vestibular nerve root entry zone* caused by *multiple sclerosis*.

Question 5: What are the common vestibular and ocular motor symptoms and signs associated with demyelinating disease?

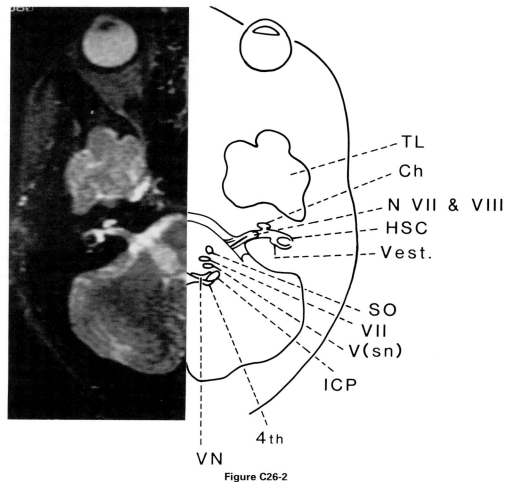

Figure C26-2

Axial magnetic resonance image showing high signal intensity typical of multiple sclerosis in the region of the eighth nerve root-entry zone. A line drawing showing the major anatomical structures of the brain stem is shown for comparison. TL = temporal lobe; Ch = cochlea; N VII & VIII = cranial nerves 7 and 8; HSC = horizontal semicircular canal; Vest. = labyrinthine vestibule; SO = superior olive; VII = facial nucleus; V(sn) = trigeminal nucleus and spinal-trigeminal tract; ICP = inferior cerebellar peduncle; 4th = fourth ventricle; VN = vestibular nuclei. (With permission from Furman JM, et al: Eighth nerve signs in a case of multiple sclerosis. Am J Otolaryngol 10:376–381, 1989.[2])

Answer 5: Demyelinating disease, most notably multiple sclerosis, can present with the acute onset of vertigo, as in this case. Statistically, about 5 percent of patients with multiple sclerosis suffer from vertigo as their first neurologic symptom, but most suffer from vertigo or disequilibrium at some time during the disease.[1] Patients with root entry-zone lesions often exhibit asymmetric vestibular function, including spontaneous nystagmus, a unilateral reduced vestibular response on caloric testing, and a directional preponderance on caloric and/or rotational testing. These patients often suffer from blurred vision. Patients with multiple sclerosis whose lesions do not affect the root entry zone may also have evidence of vestibulo-ocular, vestibulospinal, or balance system abnormalities as a result of brainstem and cerebellar lesions that affect central vestibular structures. Symptoms may be exacerbated by optic neuritis and posterior column disease, which may affect visual and somatosensory inputs important for balance.

Typical eye movement abnormalities associated with multiple sclerosis include internuclear ophthalmoplegia with dissociated nystagmus (see Cases T2 and U6), gaze-evoked nystagmus (see Case C3), vertical nystagmus (see Case C3), positional nystagmus (see Case C13), abnormal accuracy of saccades, and occasionally, pendular nystagmus (see Case C22) (see Grenman[1] for a review).

TREATMENT/MANAGEMENT

The patient was referred to a balance therapy program and given a short (2-week) trial of meclizine. Her dizziness and lightheadedness gradually resolved and her balance slowly improved, but she still had a wide-based gait.

SUMMARY

A 40-year-old woman with a history of multiple sclerosis complained of a vertiginous episode 1 week before evaluation, followed by persistent disequilibrium. Physical examination and vestibular laboratory testing suggested a combined peripheral and central vestibular abnormality. Magnetic resonance imaging disclosed a vestibular root entry-zone lesion, as well as numerous small areas of increased signal intensity. The patient was thought to have a vestibular system problem on the basis of multiple sclerosis with both peripheral and central features. Vestibular-suppressant medication, prescribed for a limited time of 2 weeks, produced a reduction of dizziness. A course of balance rehabilitation therapy provided the patient with a small but definite improvement in balance.

TEACHING POINTS

1. **Vertigo and imbalance in multiple sclerosis** may indicate a lesion in central vestibular tracts. A peripheral vestibular abnormality independent of multiple sclerosis should also be considered.
2. **A root entry-zone lesion,** because it is intraparenchymal, is a central nervous system abnormality and thus could be labeled a central vestibular lesion. However, a root entry-zone lesion should be considered a peripheral vestibular abnormality because damage is limited to afferent vestibular activity.
3. **Both peripheral and central vestibular** symptoms and signs can be seen in patients with multiple sclerosis if they have a lesion that includes the root entry zone in addition to other brainstem structures. In such cases, the vestibular symptoms and signs are a result of the interruption of vestibular afferents in the lateral brainstem that cause abnormalities indistinguishable from an end-organ lesion.
4. **A prolonged recovery** can be seen in patients with root entry-zone lesions caused by multiple sclerosis as compared to patients with vestibular end-organ lesions. This prolongation of recovery probably results from lesions other than those at the root entry zone that impair compensation.

5. **Multiple sclerosis can present with vestibular** and ocular motor symptoms and signs. About 5 percent with multiple sclerosis suffer from vertigo as their first neurologic symptom.
6. **Eye movement abnormalities** associated with multiple sclerosis include internuclear ophthalmoplegia, gaze-evoked nystagmus, vertical nystagmus, saccadic dysmetria, and pendular nystagmus.

REFERENCES

1. Grenman, R: Involvement of the audiovestibular system in multiple sclerosis. An otoneurologic and audiologic study. Acta Otolaryngol 420 (Suppl):1–95, 1985.
2. Furman, JM, et al: Eighth nerve signs in a case of multiple sclerosis. Am J Otolaryngol 10:376–381, 1989.

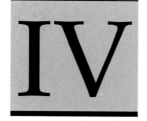

Unusual Disease
Case Studies

U1

Otolith-Ocular Reflex

HISTORY

A 68-year-old man presented with a chief complaint of constant double vision and vertigo. The patient was evaluated 1 day after the onset of symptoms. There was no complaint of hearing loss or tinnitus. There were no obvious exacerbating or remitting factors. Past medical history was significant for hypertension and diabetes. The patient's medication included a calcium-channel blocker and an oral hypoglycemic agent. The family history was noncontributory.

PHYSICAL EXAMINATION

The patient's general examination was normal. Cranial nerve examination revealed a skew deviation with a right hypertropia, a vertical ocular misalignment unaffected by gaze deviation. The remainder of the cranial nerve examination was normal except that the patient had a tilt of the head to the left. There were no abnormalities of strength or sensation and no limb dysmetria. The patient could not stand or walk without assistance. Otologic examination was normal.

Question 1: Based on the patient's history and physical examination, what is the likely diagnosis?

Answer 1: This patient's history and physical examination suggest a vestibular system abnormality because of the vertigo and inability to stand. The patient's double vision and skew deviation suggest a central nervous system lesion. Considering the risk factors of hypertension and diabetes, the patient has probably suffered from a brainstem infarction.

Question 2: What is the significance of this patient's skew deviation?

Answer 2: Skew deviation is thought to be a manifestation of abnormalities in the otolith-ocular pathways that create a left-right otolith-ocular imbalance.[1] This idea is somewhat controversial, however, considering that a vertical misalignment of the

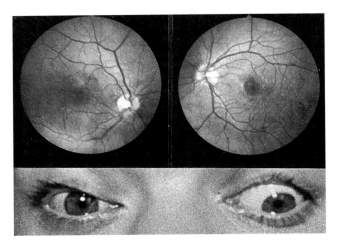

Figure U1-1
Photograph of ocular fundi and eyes of a patient with an ocular tilt reaction. Note the leftward torsion of the fundi and the left hypertropia indicating a leftward ocular tilt reaction. (With permission from Halmagyi, GM, et al: Tonic controversive ocular tilt reaction due to unilateral mesodiencephalic lesion. Neurology 40:1503–1509, 1990.[7])

eyes is never appropriate for frontal-eyed animals because such a misalignment always leads to a misalignment of the visual axes. However, there may be a vestigial pathway in the otolith-ocular system that causes a vertical misalignment, because lateral-eyed animals require such a vertical disconjugacy when the head is tilted.

A frequently unrecognized manifestation of an otolith-ocular reflex abnormality is misperception of the "subjective visual vertical," in which the world appears tilted or that only tilted objects appear vertical.[2]

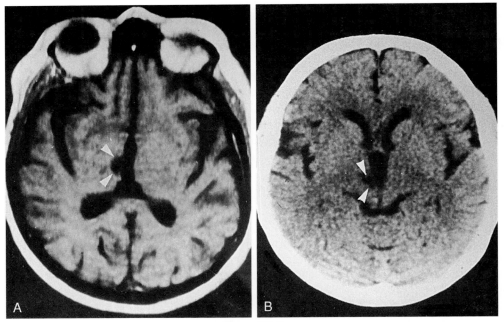

Figure U1-2
Magnetic resonance imaging scans of two patients with leftward ocular tilt reactions. Note that each scan shows a right paramedian meso-diencephalic lesion indicated by the arrowheads. (With permission from Halmagyi, GM, et al: Tonic controversive ocular tilt reaction due to unilateral mesodiencephalic lesion. Neurology 40:1503–1509, 1990.[7])

Question 3: What is the significance of the patient's head tilt? What is the ocular tilt reaction? In what disorders is the ocular tilt reaction commonly seen?

Answer 3: This patient's head tilt and skew deviation suggest a condition known as the "ocular tilt reaction,"[3] presumably as a result of damage to otolith-ocular connections in the brainstem. The ocular tilt reaction is the combination of head tilt, skew deviation, and ocular torsion, all in the same direction, presumably as a result of imbalance in tonic otolith-ocular drive. Figure U1–1 illustrates skew deviation and ocular torsion in a patient (not the individual in this case study) with the ocular tilt reaction. The ocular tilt reaction can be seen with acute peripheral vestibular abnormalities and with lesions of brainstem otolith-ocular pathways. Figure U1–2 provides two examples of the type of lesion that can produce an ocular tilt reaction. The images are not from the patient represented in this case study. Thus, brainstem infarctions, brainstem hemorrhages, and mass lesions are common causes of this condition. The ocular tilt reaction often goes unrecognized because: (1) severely ill bedridden patients may have an unnoticed head tilt, especially while supine; (2) ocular torsion can only be diagnosed objectively with fundus photography; and (3) the most obvious sign, skew deviation, is a subtle eye movement abnormality that requires a high index of suspicion and an experienced examination for diagnosis.

Laboratory Testing

Vestibular Laboratory Testing

ELECTRONYSTAGMOGRAPHY: Not performed

ROTATIONAL TESTING: Not performed

POSTUROGRAPHY: Not performed

Audiometric Testing: Not performed

Imaging: MRI scan of the brain demonstrated a lesion in the brainstem that was thought to be a small infarction.

Other: None

DIAGNOSIS/DIFFERENTIAL DIAGNOSIS

This patient was given the diagnosis of a *brainstem infarction*.

TREATMENT/MANAGEMENT

Treatment consisted of supportive care and control of the patient's hypertension and diabetes.

Question 4: What is the otolith-ocular reflex? What are manifestations of otolith-ocular reflex abnormalities?

Answer 4: The otolith-ocular reflex is that portion of the vestibulo-ocular reflex wherein linear acceleration or changes of the head with respect to gravity lead to eye movements.

The otolith-ocular reflex is best known through the phenomenon of *ocular counterrolling*, wherein a roll of the head, that is, a movement of ear to shoulder, is associated with a torsion of the eye about its visual axis in the opposite direction. Presumably, the otolith organs of the inner ear, specifically, the utricle and saccule, sense a change in orientation with respect to gravity and drive the eyes torsionally to counteract this tilt. With static tilts of the head, the amount of ocular counterrolling is far less than that required to entirely counteract the affect of head tilt on the orientation of the retina.[4,5] For example, a 45-degree head tilt is associated with approximately only a 9-degree ocular torsion (counterroll),[6] resulting in a tilt of the retina of about 40 degrees with respect to upright.

Other forms of the otolith-ocular reflex include eye movements generated by linear acceleration of the head such as that experienced in trains and motor vehicles. Linear motion along the interaural axis, that is, left and right, causes horizontal eye movement, whereas linear motion along the rostral-caudal body axis, that is, up and down, causes vertical eye movements. Because many movements of the head, for example, those that occur during walking, are a mixture of linear and rotational motion, the otolith-ocular reflex must combine with the semicircular canal–ocular reflex to maintain stable vision. Currently, there are no routine laboratory tests to assess the otolith-ocular reflex, although tilt suppression of postrotatory nystagmus is used in some specialized facilities to assess semicircular canal–otolith interaction (see discussion in Chap. 2 and Case C11).

SUMMARY

A 68-year-old man with hypertension and diabetes suffered from the acute onset of double vision and vertigo. The patient was found to have an ocular tilt reaction consisting of head tilt and skew deviation. Imaging revealed a small area of infarction in the brainstem. The patient was thought to have damage to central otolith-ocular pathways. Treatment consisted of supportive care and control of the patient's hypertension and diabetes.

TEACHING POINTS

1. **The otolith-ocular reflex** is that portion of the vestibulo-ocular reflex wherein linear acceleration or changes of head position with respect to gravity lead to eye movements. The best-known otolith-ocular phenomenon is ocular counterrolling, wherein a roll of the head, that is, a movement of ear toward the shoulder, is associated with torsion of the eyes about their visual axes in the opposite direction. Currently, there are no routine laboratory tests to assess the otolith-ocular reflex aside from tilt suppression of postrotatory nystagmus, which is used in some specialized facilities to assess semicircular canal-otolith interaction (see discussion in Chap. 2 and Case C11).
2. **The "ocular tilt reaction"** is the combination of head tilt and skew deviation in the same direction, for example, a rightward head tilt with a left hypertropia, presumably as a result of damage to otolith-ocular connections. The ocular tilt reaction can be seen with acute peripheral vestibular abnormalities and with lesions of brainstem otolith-ocular pathways.
3. **The ocular tilt reaction often goes unrecognized** because severely ill bedridden patients may have an unnoticed head tilt, especially while supine, and skew devi-

ation is a subtle eye movement abnormality that requires a high index of suspicion for diagnosis.

4. **Misperception of the "subjective visual vertical,"** in which the world appears tilted or that only tilted objects appear vertical, is a frequently unrecognized manifestation of an otolith-ocular abnormality.

REFERENCES

1. Leigh, RJ, and Zee, DS: The Neurology of Eye Movements, ed 2. Philadelphia: FA Davis Company, 1991.
2. Dieterich, M, and Brandt, M: Wallenberg's syndrome: Lateropulsion, cyclorotation, and subjective visual vertical in thirty-six patients. Ann Neurol 31:399–408, 1992.
3. Westheimer, G, and Blair, S: The ocular tilt reaction—a brainstem oculomotor routine. Invest Ophthalmol 14:833–839, 1975.
4. Collewijn, H, Van der, Steen J, Ferman, L, and Jansen, TC: Human ocular counterroll: Assessment of static and dynamic properties from electromagnetic scleral coil recordings. Exp Brain Res 59:185–196, 1985.
5. Vogel, H, Thumler, R, and Von Baumgarten, RJ: Ocular counterrolling. Acta Otolaryngol (Stockh) 102:457–462, 1986.
6. Fluur, E: A comparison between subjective and objective recording of ocular counterrolling as a result of tilting. Acta Otolaryngol 79:111–114, 1975.
7. Halmagyi, GM, et al: Tonic controversive ocular tilt reaction due to unilateral mesodiencephalic lesion. Neurology 40:1503–1509, 1990.

U2

Saccadic Fixation Instabilities

HISTORY

A 55-year-old man who worked as a shopkeeper complained of positional dizziness of 6 weeks' duration. The patient also complained of poor vision, especially when shifting his gaze from one point to another, constant disequilibrium, some tremulousness, chest palpitations, and a recent weight loss of several pounds. There was no complaint of hearing loss or tinnitus. The patient had no past medical history or family history of significance. He had recently been evaluated by his primary care physician, who could not establish a diagnosis. That evaluation included normal routine blood studies, a normal chest x-ray, and a normal electrocardiogram.

PHYSICAL EXAMINATION

The patient's general examination demonstrated a fine tremor of the head and limbs. He had a blood pressure of 150/100 and a heart rate of 95 with a regular rate and rhythm. The patient had no significant change in blood pressure or heart rate after standing for 3 and 5 minutes. His neurologic examination revealed full extraocular movements. He had no nystagmus. However, there was horizontal conjugate *ocular flutter* noted. Ocular flutter was apparent in bursts lasting 1 to 2 seconds. These bursts typically occurred immediately following refixation of gaze. The patient had normal strength and sensation. There was mild limb dysmetria on heel-knee-shin and finger-to-nose testing. The patient's gait was wide-based and he could not walk without assistance. Romberg's test could not be performed because the patient could not stand without assistance with feet together. Otologic examination was normal. Dix-Hallpike maneuvers were negative.

Question 1: What is ocular flutter? What are some other forms of saccadic oscillations? How does opsoclonus differ from ocular flutter?

Answer 1: Ocular flutter, unlike nystagmus, consists of a to-and-fro movement of the eyes wherein *both* components are rapid, that is, saccadic. Whereas nystagmus is defined as a to-and-fro movement of the eyes where at least one of the directions of movement is slow, (less than about 40° per second), for saccadic fixation instabilities, of which ocular flutter is one type, both leftward and rightward movements are rapid. Saccadic fixation instabilities include ocular flutter, opsoclonus, square-wave jerks (see Case U3), macro-square-wave jerks, and macrosaccadic oscillations[1-3] (Table U2–1).

     Whereas ocular flutter is limited to horizontal eye movements, opsoclonus includes horizontal, vertical, and torsional saccades that may occur separately or in combination such that the eyes move in quite erratic patterns. Like ocular flutter, the intersaccadic interval in opsoclonus is less than 200 milliseconds. Opsoclonus is considered a more severe form of saccadic fixation instability than ocular flutter. Some patients show different forms of saccadic fixation instabilities at different times in their illness. For example, ocular flutter can occur while a patient is recovering from opsoclonus.

Question 2: Based on the history and physical examination, what is the localization of this patient's problem?

Answer 2: Some of the patient's complaints are consistent with a vestibular abnormality. However, the patient's tremulousness and weight loss, coupled with the finding of ocular flutter on physical examination, clearly suggest a central abnormality. The patient's incoordination and severe gait instability strongly suggest that his problem includes an abnormality in the cerebellum. The ocular flutter suggests an abnormality in the pons, because this is the region of the brain important for the

TABLE U2–1
Types of Saccadic Fixation Instabilities

Category	Characteristics and Associated Ocular Motor Findings	Possible Pathophysiologic Substrate
Square-wave jerks	Small saccades (0.5–5 degrees) away from fixation and back with a 200-millisecond intersaccadic interval.	Can be normal, especially in the elderly. Common in cerebellar disease and progressive supranuclear palsy.
Macro-square-wave jerks	Saccadic intrusions (5–15 degrees) that take the eye away from fixation and return it within 70–150 milliseconds.	Multiple sclerosis and olivopontocerebellar atrophy.
Macrosaccadic oscillations	Oscillations *around* the fixation point that wax and wane. Intersaccadic interval of 200 milliseconds.	Lesions of dorsal vermis and fastigial nucleus.
Ocular flutter	Intermittent bursts of horizontal oscillations.	Saccadic oscillation without an intersaccadic interval.
Opsoclonus	Combined horizontal, vertical, and torsional oscillations.	Saccadic oscillations without an intersaccadic interval.

Source: Adapted from Leigh, RJ, and Zee, DS: The Neurology of Eye Movements, ed 2. Philadelphia: FA Davis, 1991, pp 380–381.[1]

generation of saccadic eye movements. The pons, however, receives powerful input from the cerebellum that may be used to trigger saccadic eye movements. In this way, a cerebellar abnormality can manifest itself as the abnormal occurrence of normally appearing saccadic eye movements. The patient's complaint of positional vertigo is unexplained.

Question 3: What are the diagnostic considerations for this patient?

Answer 3: The differential diagnosis for saccadic fixation instability is given in Table U2–2. The subacute onset of saccadic fixation instability can be caused by structural abnormalities of the pons or cerebellum, a viral brainstem encephalitis or cerebellitis, or a paraneoplastic syndrome. Some toxic agents and medications have been reported to cause saccadic fixation instability, but these would probably cause an acute onset of symptoms. Paraneoplastic-related saccadic fixation instability, typically in the form of opsoclonus, has been seen with carcinoma of the lung, especially oat cell carcinoma; carcinoma of the breast, especially ductal; and uterine carcinoma. In children, saccadic fixation instabilities, typically in the form of opsoclonus, are seen with postviral encephalitis and with neuroblastoma.[4]

Question 4: What additional laboratory testing would help in establishing the cause of this patient's condition?

Answer 4: Quantitative laboratory testing could further elucidate whether or not the patient is suffering from a vestibular abnormality and document the ocular flutter. MRI of the brain is critical to rule out a number of structural disorders. Because this patient may be suffering from a paraneoplastic syndrome, laboratory testing, including a CT or MRI of the chest, should entail a search for a remote carcinoma, especially of the

TABLE U2–2
Causes of Saccadic Fixation Instability

- Viral encephalitis
- Neuroblastoma
- Paraneoplasia
- Trauma (in association with hypoxia and sepsis)
- Meningitis
- Intracranial tumors
- Hydrocephalus
- Thalamic hemorrhage
- Multiple sclerosis
- Hypersmolar coma
- Viral hepatitis
- Sarcoid
- AIDS
- Side effects of drugs: lithium, amitriptyline, phenytoin and diazepam, phenelzine and imipramine, cocaine
- Toxins: chlordecone, thallium, strychnine, toluene, organophosphates
- As a component of the syndrome of myoclonic encephalopathy of infants (dancing eyes and dancing feet)
- As a transient phenomenon of healthy neonates

Source: Adapted from Leigh, RJ, and Zee, DS: The Neurology of Eye Movements, ed 2. Philadelphia: FA Davis, 1991, p 438.[1]

lung. A lumbar puncture may uncover a viral meningoencephalitis. Blood studies should include anti-Yo, anti-Hu, and anti-Ri antibody titers.

Laboratory Testing

Vestibular Laboratory Testing

ELECTRONYSTAGMOGRAPHY: Ocular motor testing revealed the presence of ocular flutter. Also, the patient had difficulty tracking a steadily moving target. There was a left-reduced vestibular response on caloric testing.

ROTATIONAL TESTING: Rotational testing revealed a left-directional preponderance.

POSTUROGRAPHY: Not performed

Audiometric Testing: Not performed

Imaging: An MRI scan of the brain was normal.

Other: A search for a remote carcinoma including a complete blood count and differential, urinalysis, and chest CT was negative. Cerebrospinal fluid examination was normal.

DIAGNOSIS/DIFFERENTIAL DIAGNOSIS

Question 5: Based on the additional information from laboratory testing, what is this patient's likely diagnosis?

Answer 5: Laboratory testing suggested both an ocular motor abnormality, namely ocular flutter, and a vestibular system abnormality. Imaging studies revealed no structural abnormality. The two most likely diagnoses for this patient's condition are the remote affects of a non–central nervous system neoplasm, that is, a paraneoplastic disorder, or a viral brainstem-cerebellar encephalitis. A toxic exposure is unlikely considering the lack of an appropriate history.

Question 6: What is the underlying pathophysiologic mechanism for saccadic fixation instability and how does this mechanism differ from the mechanism for the generation of nystagmus?

Answer 6: Saccadic fixation instabilities are presumably caused by an abnormality of the saccadic generation circuitry. The paramedian pontine reticular formation is particularly important for the generation of horizontal saccades.[1] The saccadic eye movement generation circuitry contains several types of cells, including the "burst" cells that fire during a saccade and "pause" cells that are active between saccades but shut off during saccades. The pause cells are thought to inhibit saccades. Presumably, inappropriate saccades occur when pause cells in the pons stop inappropriately, thereby allowing a rapid, that is, saccadic, eye movement to occur.[5] Because this triggering mechanism is premotor and does not involve the neural mechanism for generating conjugate eye movements, that is, the same eye movement in each of the two eyes, saccades caused by inappropriate pause cell behavior have normal velocity and are conjugate, even though they occur spontaneously at unwanted times. Also, the obligatory refractory period between two voluntary saccades (about 0.2 second) is violated by abnormal pause cell behavior. Whether saccadic fixation instabilities are a result of abnormal function of the pause cells themselves or of the triggers to the pause cells is uncertain. The triggers for the saccadic generation circuit are believed to reside in the superior colliculus and the frontal eye fields.

The patient was given the diagnosis of *ocular flutter of undetermined etiology*. A viral infection of the central nervous system or a paraneoplastic syndrome were both considered possibilities, despite negative laboratory studies. Additionally, the patient had a vestibular imbalance of uncertain etiology.

TREATMENT/MANAGEMENT

In the hope of reducing a central nervous system inflammatory response, the patient was treated with prednisone, 60 mg daily for 2 weeks, followed by a gradually tapering dose. He had significant symptomatic recovery with reduction of tremulousness and a resolution of his ocular flutter. He was enrolled in a vestibular rehabilitation program for gait and balance training with gradual resolution of his imbalance. One year after the initial presentation, the patient was asymptomatic. Despite such a response to steroids, the patient should be followed closely since subsequent manifestation of a tumor remote from the nervous system is possible.[6]

SUMMARY

A 55-year-old man presented with a 6-week history of dizziness, disequilibrium, and tremulousness. Physical examination revealed ocular flutter in addition to mild limb dysmetria and ataxic gait. Vestibular laboratory studies disclosed a vestibular asymmetry in addition to the saccadic instability. A definitive diagnosis could not be reached, but a viral syndrome or a remote effect of carcinoma was suspected. The patient was treated with prednisone. Symptoms resolved and the patient's balance improved during the subsequent 3 to 6 months. At 1-year follow-up, the patient was asymptomatic.

TEACHING POINTS
1. **Saccadic fixation instabilities**, unlike nystagmus, consist of a to-and-fro eye movement where both components are rapid, that is, saccadic. With nystagmus, at least one of the directions of movement is slow, that is, less than about 40° per second. Saccadic fixation instabilities include ocular flutter, opsoclonus, square-wave jerks, macro-square-wave jerks, and macrosaccadic oscillations (see Table U2–1).
2. **Opsoclonus**, which includes horizontal, vertical, and torsional saccades, is the most severe form of saccadic fixation instability. Ocular flutter, a purely horizontal form of saccadic fixation instability, is less severe and may occur while a patient is recovering from opsoclonus.
3. **Causes of ocular flutter and opsoclonus** include structural abnormalities of the pons or cerebellum, brainstem encephalitis or cerebellitis, a paraneoplastic syndrome, and several toxic agents and medications. In children, saccadic fixation instabilities, typically in the form of opsoclonus, can be seen with viral or postviral encephalitis and with neuroblastoma.
4. **The pathophysiology of saccadic fixation instability** is an abnormality of the

saccadic generation circuitry in the paramedian pontine reticular formation or a disorder of the triggering mechanisms for saccadic generation, which are believed to reside in the superior colliculus, the frontal eye fields, and in the cerebellum (possibly the dentate nucleus).

REFERENCES

1. Leigh, RJ, and Zee, DS: The Neurology of Eye Movements, ed 2. Philadelphia: FA Davis, 1991.
2. Sharpe, JA, and Fletcher, WA: Saccadic intrusions and oscillations. Can J Neurol Sci 11:426–433, 1984.
3. Abel, LA, et al: Square wave oscillation. Neuro-ophthalmology 4:21–25, 1984.
4. Digre, KB: Opsoclonus in adults. Arch Neurol 43:1165–1175, 1986.
5. Zee, DS, and Robinson, DA: A hypothetical explanation of saccadic oscillations. Ann Neurol 5:405–414, 1979.
6. Furman, JM, Eidelman, BH, and Fromm, GH: Spontaneous remission of paraneoplastic saccadic fixation instability. Neurology 38:499–501, 1988.

HISTORY

A 58-year-old woman who did not work outside the home complained of frequent falling. The patient's symptoms had begun several years previously, were gradually worsening, and did not fluctuate on a day-to-day basis. There was particular difficulty going down steps and stepping from the sidewalk to the street. The patient's spouse volunteered that she had some slowing of mentation and slurred speech. The patient had no complaint of vertigo or of hearing loss or tinnitus. There was no past medical history of significance and no family history of neurologic or otologic disease. The patient's primary physician had obtained a CT scan, which was normal, and had given the patient a diagnosis of Parkinson's disease. The patient had not responded to dopaminergic or anticholinergic agents.

Question 1: Based on the patient's history, what is the differential diagnosis?

Answer 1: This patient's history is most consistent with a progressive neurodegenerative syndrome, such as progressive supranuclear palsy, Parkinson's disease, striatonigral degeneration, or dementia with associated cerebellar signs. The differential diagnosis also includes multiple cerebral infarctions, hypothyroidism, CNS vasculitis, and a CNS neoplastic condition such as CNS lymphoma.

PHYSICAL EXAMINATION

The general examination revealed a disheveled woman who appeared to be depressed. A neurologic examination revealed limitation of vertical gaze, especially downward gaze during voluntary eye movements. There was severe slowing of vertical saccades and minimal slowing of horizontal saccades. Square-wave jerks were noted. There was saccadic pursuit. There was abnormal convergence. Doll's eyes (oculocephalic reflexes) revealed a full range of extraocular motion vertically and horizontally. The patient had a masked facies with a decreased blink rate. There was a hyperactive gag reflex. Motor system examination revealed increased tone with increased deep tendon reflexes that were symmetric. The plantar response was equivocal bilaterally. Sensation was normal. Coordination revealed slowing of alternating movements and slowing of finger-to-nose testing without dysrhythmia. Romberg's test was negative. Evaluation of the patient's gait revealed a widened base, stiff legs, and retropulsion. The otologic examination was normal.

Question 2: Based upon the additional information from the physical examination, what is this patient's likely diagnosis? What laboratory testing is appropriate?

Answer 2: This patient is probably suffering from progressive supranuclear palsy because the results of her examination are characteristic of this condition. Because of the poor prognosis for progressive supranuclear palsy and its poor response to treatment, an MRI scan should be performed before giving this diagnosis. Also, hematologic and thyroid blood studies and an erythrocyte sedimentation rate should be obtained.

Laboratory Testing

Vestibular Laboratory Testing

ELECTRONYSTAGMOGRAPHY: Not performed

ROTATIONAL TESTING: Not performed

POSTUROGRAPHY: Not performed

Audiometric Testing: Not performed

Imaging: An MRI of the brain was suggestive of midbrain atrophy (Fig. U3–1)

Other: A complete blood count was normal.

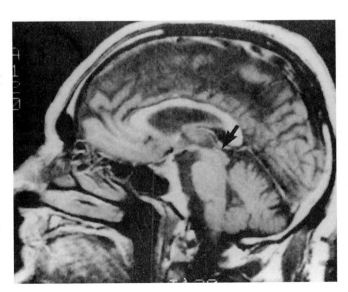

Figure U3-1
Sagittal MRI of a patient with progressive supranuclear palsy. Note the flattened quadrigeminal plate indicated by the arrow. (With permission from Scully RE, et al: Weekly clinicopathological exercises. N Engl J Med 329:1560, 1993.[6])

DIAGNOSIS/DIFFERENTIAL DIAGNOSIS

This patient was given a diagnosis of *progressive supranuclear palsy*.

Question 3: What are the manifestations of progressive supranuclear palsy?

Answer 3: The manifestations of progressive supranuclear palsy are given in Table U3–1.

Question 4: What is the pathophysiology of progressive supranuclear palsy?

Answer 4: Progressive supranuclear palsy is characterized by cell loss in many locations including the midbrain (substantia nigra, red nucleus, superior colliculus), the corpus striatum (especially the globus pallidus), and dentate nucleus of the cerebellum.[1,2]

Question 5: What is the role of the midbrain in the vestibulo-ocular and ocular motor system?

Answer 5: The midbrain is important for vertical and torsional eye movements in much the same way as the pons is important for horizontal eye movements. A premotor center in the midbrain important for vertical saccades is the rostral interstitial nucleus of the medial longitudinal fasciculus.[3] It is comparable to the paramedian pontine reticular formation, which is important for horizontal saccades. Other structures that are important for the vertical and torsional vestibulo-ocular reflex include the posterior commissure; the interstitial nucleus of Cajal, which is thought to be critical for *vertical* velocity storage (see Case U9); the third and fourth cranial nerve nuclei; and the medial longitudinal fasciculus, which carries signals from the medulla and the pons to the midbrain.[3,4]

TABLE U3–1
Manifestations of Progressive Supranuclear Palsy

Decreased cognitive ability
Abnormal ocular motor function
  Square-wave jerk
  Limitation of vertical eye movement
  Slow or absent vertical saccades
  Hypometric horizontal saccades
  Saccadic pursuit
  Abnormal convergence
  Normal oculocephalic reflexes
  Bell's phenomenon typically absent
Masked facies
Dysarthria
Dysphagia
Rigidity
Abnormal gait
Midbrain atrophy on CT

Question 6: What are the vestibulo-ocular, ocular-motor, and balance abnormalities that can be caused by midbrain lesions?

Answer 6: Midbrain lesions can cause limitation of vertical eye movements, vertical nystagmus, skew deviation, abnormal vergence, and an abnormal vertical and/or torsional vestibulo-ocular reflex.

Question 7: What disease states are associated with midbrain dysfunction?

Answer 7: Disorders that affect the midbrain include degenerative disorders, such as progressive supranuclear palsy; mass lesions, such as pinealoma; infarction, such as the "top of the basilar syndrome"; midbrain hemorrhage; hydrocephalus; and encephalitis.

TREATMENT/MANAGEMENT

The patient was treated with a course of bromocryptine. This provided minimal symptomatic relief for several months, after which time the patient began a progressive and relentless decline.

SUMMARY

A 58-year-old woman presented with a chief complaint of frequent falling, slowed cognition, blurred vision, and personality change. Examination revealed marked limitation of down-gaze square-wave jerks and retropulsion of gait. MRI scan suggested midbrain atrophy. The patient was given the diagnosis of progressive supranuclear palsy. She had been unresponsive to dopaminergic and anticholinergic agents. A course of bromocryptine provided minimal benefit.

TEACHING POINTS

1. **The gradual onset and worsening of imbalance** in the absence of vertigo suggests a progressive neurologic disorder. The differential diagnosis includes: (1) a neurodegenerative process such as progressive supranuclear palsy, (2) multiple cerebral infarctions, (3) hypothyroidism, (4) CNS vasculitis, and (5) a CNS neoplastic condition such as CNS lymphoma.
2. **Progressive supranuclear palsy** is a disorder characterized by the gradual onset of cognitive decline and poor balance. The manifestations of the condition are listed in Table U3–1. Progressive supranuclear palsy is caused by cell loss in many locations including the midbrain (substantia nigra, red nucleus, superior colliculus), the basal ganglia (especially the globus pallidus), and dentate nucleus of the cerebellum.
3. **The midbrain is important for vertical and torsional eye movements.** Thus, midbrain lesions can cause limitation of vertical eye movements, vertical nystagmus, skew deviation, and an abnormal vertical and/or torsional vestibulo-ocular reflex.
4. **Disorders that affect the midbrain** include degenerative disorders, such as progressive supranuclear palsy; mass lesions, such as pinealoma; infarction, such as

the top of the basilar syndrome; midbrain hemorrhage; hydrocephalus; and encephalitis.

REFERENCES

1. Steele, JC, Richardson, JC, and Olszewski, J: Progressive supranuclear palsy. Arch Neurol 10:333–359, 1964.
2. Behrman, S, Carroll, JD, Janota, I, and Matthews, WB: Progressive supranuclear palsy. Brain 92:663–678, 1969.
3. Buttner-Ennever, JA (ed): Neuroanatomy of the Oculomotor System. Amsterdam: Elsevier, 1988.
4. Leigh, RJ, and Zee, DS: The Neurology of Eye Movements, ed 2. Philadelphia: FA Davis, 1991.
5. Caplan, L: Top of the basilar syndrome. Neurology 30:72–79, 1980.
6. Scully RE, et al: Weekly clinicopathological exercises. N Engl J Med 329:1560, 1993.)

C A S E
U4

Vascular Supply of the Labyrinth

HISTORY

A 60-year-old man who worked as a building custodian presented with the acute onset of vertigo, tinnitus in the left ear, facial weakness, and disequilibrium. The patient experienced blurred vision and mild nausea. There was no complaint of loss of strength, but he complained of great difficulty ambulating and noted veering to the left. Past medical history was significant for hypertension. Family history was not contributory. The patient's family rushed him to a local emergency room, where a CT scan of the head was interpreted as within normal limits.

Question 1: Based upon the patient's history, where is this patient's lesion located and what is the differential diagnosis?

Answer 1: The patient's complaints of vertigo and hearing loss suggest an acute peripheral vestibular lesion. However, the facial weakness and disequilibrium suggest a *central* abnormality. Diagnostic possibilities include brainstem or cerebellar infarction or hemorrhage, an infectious process, and a peripheral vestibular ailment.

PHYSICAL EXAMINATION

The patient's general examination was normal aside from an elevated blood pressure of 150/100. The cranial nerve examination revealed an inability to gaze to the left. He had left facial weakness affecting the entire left side of the face, and decreased sensation on the left side of the face. Strength was normal. There was left upper and lower extremity dysmetria. Sensation was reduced for pain and temperature in the right arm and leg. He could not stand or walk unassisted. Otoscopy was normal. On tuning-fork testing, Weber's test lateralized to the right and the Rinne test was positive bilaterally indicating diminished sensorineural hearing in the left ear. Right-beating nystagmus was seen with Frenzel glasses.

Question 2: Based on the history and physical examination, what is this patient's likely diagnosis and what further diagnostic studies would be helpful?

Answer 2: This patient's examination is consistent with a lesion of the brainstem and cerebellum. However, the vertigo, tinnitus, hearing loss, and spontaneous nystagmus suggest a peripheral otologic lesion. The most likely diagnosis is an infarction in the territory of the anterior-inferior cerebellar artery, because this artery supplies the inner ear, lateral pons, and middle cerebellar peduncle.[1,2] Further diagnostic information should be obtained from an MRI scan. Audiometric and vestibulo-ocular testing would also help in confirming this diagnosis.

Laboratory Testing

Vestibular Laboratory Testing

ELECTRONYSTAGMOGRAPHY:	There was an inability to gaze to the left. A right-beating nystagmus was seen during loss of visual fixation. Caloric responses were absent on the left.
ROTATIONAL TESTING:	Not performed
POSTUROGRAPHY:	Not performed

Audiometric Testing: Testing revealed complete deafness on the left and normal hearing on the right.

Imaging: An MRI of the brain showed evidence of infarction in the territory of the anterior-inferior cerebellar artery.

Other: None

DIAGNOSIS/DIFFERENTIAL DIAGNOSIS

This patient was given the diagnosis of an *infarction in the territory of the anterior-inferior cerebellar artery.*

Question 3: What arteries supply the vestibular system, including the peripheral labyrinth, and central vestibular structures, including the vestibulocerebellum?

Answer 3: The arterial supply of the labyrinth arises from the labyrinthine artery, which arises from the anterior-inferior cerebellar artery, the first branch of the basilar artery (Fig. U4–1A). Figures U4–1B and C indicate that the vestibular nerve, the vestibular root-entry zone, and the cerebellar flocculus are all supplied by the anterior-inferior cerebellar artery.[3] The vestibular nuclei, deep cerebellar nuclei, and inferior vermis are supplied by the posterior-inferior cerebellar artery[4] (see Case T4).

Question 4: How does the lateral medullary syndrome differ from the anterior-inferior cerebellar artery syndrome?

Answer 4: The lateral medullary syndrome (i.e. Wallenberg's syndrome) (see Case T4) results from infarction in the territory of the posterior-inferior cerebellar artery,

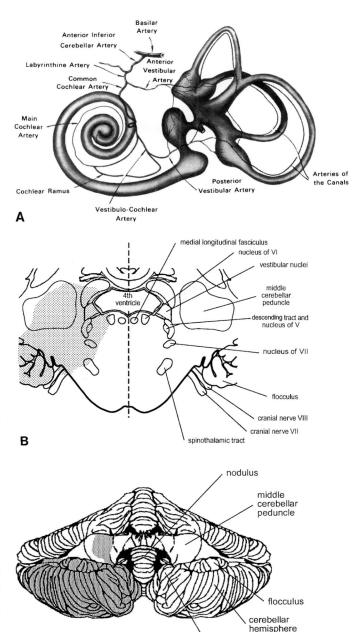

Figure U4-1

Vascular distribution of the anterior inferior cerebellar artery (AICA). (*A*) Arterial supply to the inner ear. (*B*) Line drawing of an axial section through the brainstem showing the major anatomical structures of the brainstem supplied by the AICA. The shaded region represents the region of the brainstem supplied by the AICA. (*C*) Line drawing of an anterior view of the cerebellum. Shaded areas represent regions supplied by AICA. *A* Modified by permission of the publisher from Schuknecht, HF: Pathology of the Ear. Cambridge, MA: Harvard University Press, Copyright 1974 by the President and Fellows of Harvard College, p 62.[5] *B* and *C* modified with permission from Oas, JG, and Baloh, RW: Vertigo and the anterior inferior cerebellar artery syndrome. Neurology 42:2274–2279, 1992, p 2276.[1])

which supplies a different region of the brain than the anterior-inferior cerebellar artery. Although some of the presenting symptoms and signs of the lateral medullary syndrome and the anterior-inferior cerebellar artery syndrome are the same, there are distinct and significant differences. Table U4–1 lists these similarities and differences and their origin pathophysiologically.[1–4]

TABLE U4–1
Comparison of Posterior-Inferior Cerebellar Artery (PICA) and Anterior-Inferior Cerebellar Artery (AICA) Syndromes

	Seen in Both PICA and AICA Syndromes	Typically Seen Only in PICA Syndrome	Typically Seen Only in AICA Syndrome
Symptoms	Vertigo, lateropulsion, unusual visual illusions, facial numbness, limb numbness, disequilibrium, dysphagia, and incoordination	Hoarseness	Tinnitus, hearing loss, and facial weakness
Signs	Vestibular nystagmus, decreased facial sensation ipsilaterally, dissociated sensory loss to pain and temperature contralaterally, dissociated sensory loss of the limbs contralaterally, Horner's syndrome, ipsilateral limb ataxia, and gait ataxia	Saccadic lateropulsion, skew deviation, and vocal cord paralysis	Hearing loss, facial weakness, and gaze palsy
Laboratory Abnormalities	Abnormal imaging, spontaneous nystagmus, and decreased hearing	Saccadic lateropulsion	Caloric reduction ipsilaterally
Pathophysiology	Damage of fifth nerve nucleus, spinothalamic tract, and vestibular nuclei	Damage of nucleus ambiguus and dorsal motor nucleus	Damage of inner ear, eighth cranial nerve, seventh cranial nerve, seventh and eighth cranial nerve root-entry zones, sixth nerve nucleus, flocculus, and middle cerebellar peduncle

TREATMENT/MANAGEMENT

The patient was treated with supportive measures, antihypertensive agents, and aspirin as an antiplatelet agent.

SUMMARY

A 60-year-old man presented with the acute onset of vertigo, left-sided tinnitus, facial weakness, and disequilibrium. Past medical history was significant for hypertension. Physical examination indicated left-sided hearing loss, an inability to move the eyes to the left, and abnormal sensation on the left side of the face and in the right arm and leg. MRI indicated infarction in the territory of the anterior-inferior cerebellar artery, which was thought to account for the patient's symptoms in entirety. Treatment consisted of supportive measures and an antiplatelet agent.

TEACHING POINTS

1. **The arterial supply of the inner ear** arises from the labyrinthine artery, which arises from the anterior-inferior cerebellar artery, the first branch of the basilar artery. The vestibular nuclei, deep cerebellar nuclei, and inferior vermis are supplied mostly by the posterior-inferior cerebellar artery.

2. **The anterior-inferior cerebellar artery** supplies the inner ear, the vestibular nerve, the vestibular root-entry zone, the lateral pons, the middle cerebellar peduncle, and the cerebellar flocculus.

3. **Infarction in the territory of the anterior-inferior cerebellar artery** produces a syndrome of acute vertigo, tinnitus, and hearing loss because of interruption of the vascular supply to the inner ear and its nerves. Neurologic abnormalities including ipsilateral facial nerve paralysis, contralateral reduced pain and temperature sensation, and ipsilateral upper- and lower-extremity dysmetria consistent with a lesion of the brainstem and cerebellum.

4. **The anterior-inferior cerebellar artery syndrome** shares many of the clinical features of the lateral medullary syndrome (that is, Wallenberg's syndrome), which results from infarction in the territory of the posterior-inferior cerebellar artery. Although some of the presenting symptoms and signs of the lateral medullary syndrome and the anterior-inferior cerebellar artery syndrome are the same, there are distinct and significant differences (Table U4–1).

REFERENCES

1. Oas, JG, and Baloh, RW: Vertigo and the anterior inferior cerebellar artery syndrome. Neurology 42:2274–2279, 1992.
2. Amarenco, P, et al: Anterior inferior cerebellar artery territory infarcts. Arch Neurol 50:154–161, 1993.
3. Amarenco, P, and Hauw, J-J: Cerebellar infarction in the territory of the anterior and inferior cerebellar artery. Brain 113:139–155, 1990.
4. Gilman, S, Bloedel, JR, and Lechtenberg, R (eds): Disorders of the Cerebellum. Contemporary Neurology Series. Philadelphia: FA Davis, 1981.
5. Schuknecht, HF: Pathology of the Ear. Cambridge, MA: Harvard University Press, 1974.

U5

Vascular Compression Syndrome of the Eighth Cranial Nerve

HISTORY

A 50-year-old man who worked as an accountant presented with a chief complaint of a sense of disequilibrium that was more or less constant but was particularly exacerbated by lying on his right side. The patient experienced a sense of motion while lying on his right side that was not paroxysmal. It would last for as long as he maintained that position and become worse until he could no longer stay in that position. The patient did not complain of hearing loss, but did note occasional noise and occasional sharp pain in his right ear. He had suffered from these symptoms for 2 years, and the onset had been gradual. His past history was significant for a 3-day episode of vertigo 5 years before evaluation that was diagnosed as "labyrinthitis." Several weeks after that episode of vertigo, the patient's symptoms had completely resolved and he became asymptomatic for approximately 3 years. There was no other past medical history of significance. He had used multiple medications including meclizine, diazepam, promethazine, lioresal, and amitriptyline with minimal or no benefit. The patient had been treated for presumed endolymphatic hydrops with a combination of hydrochlorothiazide and triamterene and a salt-restricted diet with no benefit. There was a family history of trigeminal neuralgia in the patient's mother. The patient was extremely troubled by his symptoms and had discontinued his work as an accountant.

Question 1: Based on the patient's history, what are the diagnostic possibilities?

Answer 1: This patient's history is unusual. The symptoms are positional but are not characterized by vertigo and are not paroxysmal. Thus, benign positional vertigo is unlikely (see Cases T1, C9, and C15). However, the patient's history is consistent with a peripheral vestibular ailment because of the ear pain, tinnitus, and past history of an acute vestibular syndrome. The vestibular abnormality is probably on the right, considering the laterality of the otologic symptoms and the exacerbation while lying on the right. Experience has shown that patients who can identify a side that elicits symptoms when dependent often have their abnormality on the ipsilateral side. The patient's history does not, however, fit into a common diagnostic category. Physical examination and laboratory testing hopefully will help to establish a diagnosis.

PHYSICAL EXAMINATION

The patient's general examination was normal. Neurologic examination was normal with the exception of mild instability during tandem walking and an inability to stand on a compliant foam surface with the eyes closed. The patient did not have spontaneous nystagmus. Paroxysmal positional testing (Dix-Hallpike maneuvers) revealed no paroxysmal positional nystagmus or vertigo. Static positional testing using Frenzel glasses revealed that the patient had a strong sense of disequilibrium while lying on his right side without observable nystagmus. Otologic examination was normal.

Laboratory Testing

Vestibular Laboratory Testing:

ELECTRONYSTAGMOGRAPHY:	Ocular motor function was normal. There was a low-amplitude left-beating nystagmus in the head right and right lateral positions of 4° per second. There was a 22 percent right reduced vestibular response during caloric testing.
ROTATIONAL TESTING:	Normal
POSTUROGRAPHY:	Posturography indicated excessive sway on conditions 5 and 6, that is, a vestibular pattern.

Audiometric Testing: A mild high-frequency sensorineural hearing loss in the right ear was revealed, with normal hearing in the left ear. Word recognition was excellent bilaterally with normal acoustic reflexes. Brainstem auditory-evoked responses were normal bilaterally.

Imaging: An MRI of the brain was normal.

Other: None

DIAGNOSIS/DIFFERENTIAL DIAGNOSIS

Question 2: Based on the patient's history, physical examination, and laboratory studies, what is the differential diagnosis?

Answer 2: This patient is likely to have a peripheral vestibulopathy on the right, possibly as a result of the viral syndrome and "labyrinthitis" 5 years before evaluation, which was probably a viral vestibular neuritis. The patient has evidence of an ongoing vestibulospinal abnormality and a very low-amplitude positional nystagmus, all consistent with an ongoing vestibular system abnormality. The precise nature of this patient's diagnosis cannot be stated with certainty. In light of the patient's family history of trigeminal neuralgia and history of atypical ear pain associated with chronic dizziness, the possibility of a vascular compression syndrome affecting the eighth cranial nerve should be considered.[1] The clinical description of this condition is controversial, with no agreed-upon set of diagnostic criteria. Indeed, in the minds of some experts, this condition does not even exist. However, recent histopathologic evidence suggests that the vestibular nerve can become demyelinated in small regions following an insult such as a viral infection, and this region could then become susceptible to irritation by adjacent blood vessels.[2,3] Vascular compression syndrome of the eighth cranial nerve has been called *disabling positional vertigo* by Jannetta[4] and *vestibular paroxysmia* by Brandt.[5]

This patient was given the diagnosis of *vascular compression syndrome of the eighth cranial nerve.*

TREATMENT/MANAGEMENT

Question 3: What treatments have been advocated for patients diagnosed with suspected vascular compression syndrome of the eighth cranial nerve?

Answer 3: Treatment of suspected vascular compression syndrome of the eighth cranial nerve includes medications known to be effective for other disorders thought to result from vascular compression, for example, tic douloureux and glossopharyngeal neuralgia. These agents include carbamazepine and baclofen.[5] Other medications that are often prescribed for this condition include vestibular suppressants, including diazepam. Numerous articles have been written about surgical treatment of suspected vascular compression syndrome of the eighth cranial nerve using microvascular decompression.[1–4] We advocate a trial of medical therapy before referring a patient for a surgical opinion.

This patient was treated with carbamazepine and was much improved symptomatically.

SUMMARY

A 50-year-old man presented with the chief complaint of a sense of disequilibrium that was exacerbated by prolonged recumbency with the right side down. The patient's past history was significant for an acute vestibular syndrome probably of viral origin 5 years previously. The patient had no signs or symptoms of paroxysmal positional nystagmus. Audiometric and vestibular testing suggested a right-sided peripheral vestibular lesion. MRI scan was negative. The patient was given a diagnosis of possible vascular compression syndrome of the eighth cranial nerve. The patient was treated with carbamazepine and had a nearly complete cessation of his symptoms.

TEACHING POINTS

1. **The vestibular nerve can become demyelinated in small regions** following an insult such as a viral infection, and this region could then become susceptible to irritation by adjacent blood vessels.
2. **Vascular compression syndrome of the eighth cranial nerve**, which has been called disabling positional vertigo and vestibular paroxysmia, refers to a cochleovestibular syndrome caused by compression of the eighth cranial nerve by blood vessels within the cerebellopontine angle.
3. **The clinical description of vascular compression syndrome** of the eighth cranial

nerve is controversial with no agreed-upon set of diagnostic criteria. Features of this syndrome include dizziness associated with head movements or particular head positions, tinnitus, hearing loss, and ear pain. A history of symptoms consistent with a vascular compression syndrome such as trigeminal neuralgia supports the diagnosis of vascular compression syndrome of the eighth cranial nerve.

4. **Treatment of vascular compression syndrome of the eighth cranial nerve** includes pharmacotherapy with carbamazepine or baclofen. Surgical treatment consists of microvascular decompression. We advocate a trial of medical therapy before referring a patient for a surgical opinion.

REFERENCES

1. Moller, MB, et al: Microvascular decompression of the eighth nerve in patients with disabling positional vertigo: Selection criteria and operative results in 207 patients. Acta Neurochir (Wien) 125:75–82, 1993.
2. Schwaber, MK, and Whetsell, WO: Cochleovestibular nerve compression syndrome. II. Vestibular nerve histopathology and theory of pathophysiology. Laryngoscope 102:1030–1036, 1992.
3. Colletti, V, Fiorino, FG, Carner, M, and Turazzi, S: Vestibular neurectomy and microvascular decompression of the cochlear nerve in Meniere's disease. Skull Base Surg 4:65–71, 1994.
4. Jannetta, PJ, Moller, MB, and Moller, AR: Disabling positional vertigo. N Engl J Med 310:1700–1705, 1984.
5. Brandt, TH: Vestibular paroxysmia: Vascular compression of the eighth nerve? Lancet 343:798–799, 1994.

C A S E

U6

Coma

HISTORY

A 65-year-old woman with a past history of coronary artery disease and hypertension presented with the acute onset of double vision and a depressed level of consciousness.

PHYSICAL EXAMINATION

The general physical examination was normal aside from lethargy. Blood pressure was 120/80 and pulse was 75 and regular. The patient was arousable and could follow simple commands. Cranial nerve examination revealed a horizontal ocular misalignment with the left eye abducted and the right eye in the primary position. When asked to gaze laterally, the patient was able to move her left eye fully to the left but only to the midline on right gaze. She could not move her right eye horizontally at all. Vertical gaze was full in each eye. There was left-beating nystagmus on the left gaze in the left eye. Corneal reflexes were reduced but present bilaterally. The patient had facial diplegia. The gag reflex was present but depressed. Motor examination revealed diminished strength throughout without a particular pattern of weakness. Tone was diminished. Deep tendon reflexes were depressed but present. Coordination revealed slowing of alternating movements and mild limb dysmetria bilaterally both in the upper and lower extremities. The patient's stance and gait could not be tested because she was unable to stand without assistance. Otologic examination was normal.

Question 1: What is the significance of this patient's eye movement examination? What is the probable cause?

Answer 1: This patient is exhibiting paralytic pontine exotropia,[1] also known as the *1½ syndrome*.[2] She is probably suffering from a lesion in the pons near the sixth cranial nerve nucleus. Figure U6–1 demonstrates the pathways that are damaged in patients with the 1½ syndrome. The syndrome gets its name from the fact that one eye cannot move at all horizontally (the ''1'') and the other eye can only move in one direction (the ''½''). This patient is probably suffering from a brainstem infarction, but

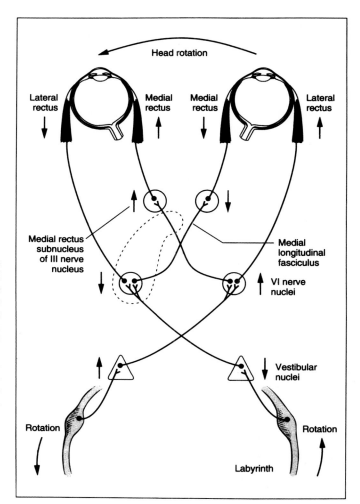

Figure U6-1

1½ syndrome. This diagram of the pathways subserving the horizontal vestibulo-ocular reflex indicates the region of damage that causes the 1½ syndrome (labeled "3"). This region includes both the sixth nerve nucleus and the ipsilateral medial longitudinal fasciculus. In this way, there is a conjugate gaze palsy in one direction and an inter-nuclear ophthalmoplegia on the ipsilateral side so that the only nor-mal eye movement is abduction of the contralateral eye. (Adapted from Furman, JM: Nystagmus and the vestibular system. In Podos, SM, and Yanoff, M (eds): Textbook of Ophthalmology. New York: Gower Medical Publishers, 1993.[3])

a pontine hemorrhage is also a consideration. A mass lesion is unlikely because of the strokelike onset of the patient's symptoms.

Question 2: What is the significance of the other abnormalities on neurologic examination?

Answer 2: The patient's facial diplegia suggests involvement of the facial nuclei or nerves; the limb dysmetria suggests involvement of cerebellar pathways.

Laboratory Testing

Vestibular Laboratory Testing

ELECTRONYSTAGMOGRAPHY:	Not performed
ROTATIONAL TESTING:	Not performed
POSTUROGRAPHY:	Not performed

Audiometric Testing: Not performed

Imaging: The patient's MRI scan revealed abnormal signal intensity in the pons consistent with the clinical presentation.

Other: None

Question 3: What are the eye movement abnormalities commonly seen in patients with a depressed level of consciousness?

Answer 3: Table U6–1 lists several eye movement abnormalities that can be seen in patients with coma. These include gaze palsies, tonic deviation of the eyes, roving eye movements, ocular bobbing, and "Ping-Pong" gaze. Each of these eye movement abnormalities suggests a lesion of the horizontal eye movement system, and in the case of ocular bobbing, the possibility of an abnormality of vertical eye movements as well.

There are several variations of ocular bobbing (Table U6–2); all of these movements have similar clinical significance, namely, damage of the pons or irritation of the midbrain.

Question 4: What are the typical vestibular findings in a patient with a depressed level of consciousness?

Answer 4: The vestibular findings in a patient with a depressed level of consciousness are usually assessed using oculocephalic reflexes also known as *dolls' eyes* and caloric irrigation at the bedside. Oculocephalic reflexes are performed by rotating the patient's head from side to side or chin to chest and observing horizontal and vertical eye movements, respectively. Patients in whom the vestibulo-ocular reflex pathways have been damaged may not have any eye movement in response to head movement. Patients with a depressed level of consciousness but intact vestibulo-ocular pathways exhibit dolls'-eyes movements. That is, during head movement the eyes move to maintain their line of sight. Thus, if the head is moved to the right, the eyes move to the left and vice versa; if the head is pitched up, the eyes move down, and vice versa. Patients with a depressed level of consciousness have an impaired ability to generate quick eye movements and thus do not develop vestibular nystagmus. Alert individuals typically suppress vestibular responses to some extent and may gaze in the direction of head movement, thereby appearing to have absent oculocephalic reflexes.

Patients with a depressed level of consciousness in whom oculocephalic movements are absent should undergo caloric irrigation at the bedside. Such testing

TABLE U6–1
Eye Movement Abnormalities in Patients with Coma

- Gaze palsies
- Tonic deviation—horizontal, vertical
- Roving eye movements
- Ocular bobbing
- Ping-Pong gaze
- Lack of vestibular (caloric) nystagmus

TABLE U6–2
Ocular Bobbing and Variations

- Bobbing: rapid down, slow up
- Inverse bobbing (dipping): slow down, rapid up
- Reverse bobbing: rapid up, slow down
- Converse (reverse dipping): slow up, rapid down

is often performed using ice water irrigation for 30 seconds using 5 mL of water. Although normal individuals develop a brisk nystagmus and patients with severe brainstem lesions that impair the vestibulo-ocular reflex display no response, patients with a depressed level of consciousness but normal vestibulo-ocular pathways show a tonic deviation of the eyes away from the ear that has been irrigated with ice water. The lack of nystagmus is probably the result of poor (saccade) quick component generation. Occasionally, patients have a monocular horizontal response to one or both irrigations. A failure of adduction suggests an internuclear ophthalmoplegia; a failure of abduction suggests a sixth nerve palsy. In patients with recent frontal lobe injury who have gaze deviation, caloric testing is almost always powerful enough to bring the patient's eyes across the midline.

DIAGNOSIS/DIFFERENTIAL DIAGNOSIS

This patient's diagnosis was the *1½ syndrome* on the basis of a pontine infarction.

TREATMENT/MANAGEMENT

The patient was treated with supportive measures and control of blood pressure. The patient's eye movement abnormality gradually resolved to some extent, but she was left with a bilateral internuclear ophthalmoplegia (see Case T2).

SUMMARY

A 65-year-old woman with a past history of a coronary artery disease and hypertension presented with the acute onset of double vision and a depressed level of consciousness. Examination revealed a paralytic pontine extratropia, mild facial diplegia, and limb dysmetria. MRI scan indicated ischemia in the pons. The patient was given the diagnosis of *1½ syndrome* and was treated with supportive measures.

TEACHING POINTS

1. **Coma** may be associated with numerous eye movement abnormalities, including gaze palsies, tonic deviation of the eyes, roving eye movements, ocular bobbing, and "Ping-Pong" gaze. Ocular bobbing, a spontaneous vertical rhythmic eye movement, indicates damage of the pons or irritation of the midbrain.
2. **Paralytic pontine exotropia**, also known as the *1½ syndrome*, refers to the inability to move one eye at all horizontally (the "1"), and an inability to move the

other eye medially (the "½"). This condition is caused by a unilateral lesion of the sixth nerve nucleus and the medial longitudinal fasciculus on the same side.

3. **Vestibular function in coma** can be assessed using oculocephalic reflexes, also known as *dolls' eyes*, and caloric irrigation at the bedside. Patients with a depressed level of consciousness and intact vestibulo-ocular pathways exhibit dolls' eyes, that is, during head movement, the eyes will counterrotate in the orbit. During caloric irrigation, such patients may demonstrate a tonic deviation of their eyes because of an impaired ability to generate vestibular nystagmus.

4. **Tonic gaze deviation** caused by recent frontal lobe injury usually can be overcome temporarily during caloric irrigation. Tonic gaze deviation caused by brainstem lesions usually cannot be overcome by caloric irrigation.

REFERENCES

1. Sharpe, JA, et al: Paralytic pontine exotropia. Neurology 24:1076–1081, 1974.
2. Pierrot-Deseilligny, C, et al: The "one-and-a-half" syndrome. Brain 104:665–699, 1981.
3. Furman, JM: Nystagmus and the vestibular system. In Podos, SM, and Yanoff, M (eds): Textbook of Ophthalmology. New York: Gower Medical Publishers, 1993.

C A S E
U7

Epilepsy and Vertigo

HISTORY

A 52-year-old woman who worked as a schoolteacher presented with a chief complaint of episodic dizziness. The patient's first episode was 2 years before evaluation. She had had four other episodes that she could remember until the last month, when she had about one episode each week. Each episode included a feeling of vertigo and blurred vision lasting for at most a minute and followed by a feeling of lethargy. There was no positional sensitivity, associated hearing loss, or tinnitus. The patient's past medical history was significant for migraine headaches that had begun when she was a teenager and remitted after menopause, which had occurred approximately 2 years before presentation. She also had a past history of a generalized seizure disorder treated with phenobarbital, which she had not taken for as long as she could remember. She could not recall when she had last had a seizure. There was no family history of neurologic or otologic disease.

Question 1: Based on the patient's history, what is this patient's differential diagnosis?

Answer 1: This patient's complaints suggest a peripheral vestibular abnormality of uncertain etiology, considering the episodic vertigo. Other diagnostic considerations are vertebrobasilar insufficiency, panic disorder, cardiac arrythmia, hypoglycemia, and migraine-associated dizziness (see Cases C4, C12, U12, and U16). The history of a seizure disorder is interesting and possibly of clinical significance because vertigo is a rare manifestation of a seizure.

PHYSICAL EXAMINATION

The general, neurologic, otologic, and neuro-otologic examinations were entirely normal.

273

Laboratory Testing

Vestibular Laboratory Testing

ELECTRONYSTAGMOGRAPHY: Ocular motor testing, positional testing, and caloric testing were normal.

ROTATIONAL TESTING: Normal

POSTUROGRAPHY: Normal

Audiometric Testing: Not performed

Imaging: MRI of the brain was normal.

Other: Blood studies including a glucose tolerance test were normal. A Holter monitor was normal, although the patient did not have an episode while wearing the monitor.

Question 2: Based on the additional information from the patient's physical examination and laboratory studies, what is the differential diagnosis and what further testing should be ordered?

Answer 2: The physical examination and laboratory testing do not provide information to establish a definitive diagnosis, although they help to rule out a large number of diseases. A peripheral vestibulopathy or migraine-associated dizziness is still a likely diagnosis. A seizure disorder, which could account for the patient's episodic vertigo, should be considered further. An electroencephalogram (EEG) should be ordered.

ADDITIONAL LABORATORY TESTING

EEG was normal.

Question 3: Should the patient be treated?

Answer 3: The patient probably has a nonspecific vestibulopathy. Treatment with a vestibular suppressant will probably prove ineffective because of the brief duration of the patient's episodes unless she uses a medication daily. Close follow-up should be obtained, especially regarding symptoms during episodes. The family should be instructed to observe several episodes and determine the patient's level of consciousness during and after the episodes.

ADDITIONAL HISTORY

The patient returned in 2 weeks with her daughter and husband, who had both witnessed an episode of dizziness. During this episode, the patient had a depressed awareness of her surroundings but could converse and answer simple questions. Afterwards, she could not recall the nature of the conversation during her episode, despite the fact that she had participated in it.

Question 4: What does this additional history suggest, and what, if any, additional laboratory tests should be ordered?

Answer 4: The additional history suggests that the patient may have epilepsy, considering the disorientation during the episodes. Vertebrobasilar insufficiency, panic disorder, and a cardiac arrhythmia are still possibilities. Panic disorder is unlikely because the patient had no anxiety symptoms before, during, or after episodes and cardiac arrythmia is unlikely given the normal Holter monitor readings during an episode.

The patient should be scheduled for prolonged EEG monitoring with simultaneous video monitoring and simultaneous EKG.

FURTHER LABORATORY TESTING

During prolonged EEG monitoring, a vertiginous episode occurred, during which time the patient evidenced nystagmus that could be seen on the video monitor and on the frontal EEG leads. She had modest tachycardia during the episode. Her EEG during this episode showed rhythmic fast activity in the left posterior temporal region. An EKG obtained during the EEG monitoring was normal.

DIAGNOSIS/DIFFERENTIAL DIAGNOSIS

The patient was given the diagnosis of *vestibular epilepsy*, also known as *tornado epilepsy*.

Question 5: What is the pathophysiologic basis for vertigo during a seizure?

Answer 5: Vertigo during seizures is presumably a result of activation of cortical areas that are associated with the perception of motion.[1] These areas are difficult to specify with certainty. However, the posterior aspect of the superior temporal gyrus and the parietotemporal junction, that is, the angular gyrus, are probably the most consistent regions associated with vestibular perceptions.[2] Vertiginous sensations can occur as the aura before a seizure.[3]

Question 6: What is the pathophysiologic basis for epileptic nystagmus?

Answer 6: In adults, epileptic nystagmus is probably less common than vertigo during a seizure. However, there are many well-described cases of epileptic nystagmus,[4] some of these including electro-oculographic recordings. Nystagmus during seizures is of uncertain cause but may be the result of activation of pursuit tracking pathways that drives the eyes toward the side of the cerebral focus with quick components in the opposite direction.[5,6]

TREATMENT/MANAGEMENT

This patient was treated with carbamazepine with a marked reduction in the frequency of her vertiginous episodes to only a few per year. She was restricted from driving and advised to avoid activities where a vertiginous episode or seizure could be injurious.

SUMMARY

A 52-year-old woman presented with episodic vertigo without associated hearing loss or tinnitus. The patient had a past history of migraine headaches and a remote history of a generalized seizure disorder without seizures for 20 years. She had a normal physical examination, normal MRI, and normal vestibular laboratory testing. Additional history suggested a seizure disorder. Electroencephalopathy revealed a focal abnormality during a vertiginous episode that occurred while the patient was undergoing prolonged video electroencephalopathy. She was given the diagnosis of vertiginous epilepsy and treated successfully with carbamazepine.

TEACHING POINTS

1. **Vestibular epilepsy**, also known as *tornado epilepsy*, refers to a disorder in which vertigo occurs during seizures, presumably as a result of activation of cortical areas that are associated with the perception of motion.
2. **A diagnosis of vestibular epilepsy** should be a considered in any patient with a history of a seizure disorder who presents with vertigo of uncertain etiology. A careful inquiry regarding changes in level of consciousness during or following vertiginous episodes is essential. Prolonged video EEG monitoring may be required to capture an ictal episode.
3. **Nystagmus** may or may not be associated with vestibular epilepsy. When present during a seizure, nystagmus may indicate activation of ocular pursuit pathways.

REFERENCES

1. Kogeorgos, J, Scott, DF, and Swash, M: Epileptic dizziness. Br Med J 282:687–689, 1981.
2. Smith, BH: Vestibular disturbances in epilepsy. Neurology 10:465–469, 1960.
3. Nielsen, JM: Tornado epilepsy simulating Meniere's syndrome. Neurology 9:794–796, 1959.
4. Stolz, SE, Chatrian, G-E, and Spence A: Epileptic nystagmus. Epilepsia 32:910–918, 1991.
5. Furman, JM, Crumrine, PK, and Reinmuth, OM: Epileptic nystagmus. Ann Neurol 27:686–688, 1990.
6. Tusa, RJ, Kaplan, PW, Hain, TC, and Naidu, S: Ipsiversive eye deviation and epileptic nystagmus. Neurology 40:662–665, 1990.

C A S E

U8

Congenital Inner Ear Malformations

HISTORY

A 16-year-old girl reported an acute onset of hearing loss, tinnitus, and disequilibrium. These symptoms began following a high school football game 7 days earlier. The patient, a majorette in the high school band, was seated in the grandstands in front of the bass drum. The football game was very exciting and the drummer had enthusiastically beaten his drum during the game. The patient had felt pain in her ears several times and then a full feeling in her right ear. Following the game, she noted bilateral loss of hearing, nonlocalized tinnitus, and unsteadiness. She claimed that she could not hear at all and that the world around her seemed to bounce or jiggle when she moved her head quickly.

There was a past history of a left-sided hearing loss of unknown etiology that was first noticed at age 5.

The following day, the patient was seen by an otolaryngologist who examined her ears and performed an audiogram that confirmed a profound loss of hearing in both ears. The otolaryngologist prescribed oral prednisone and referred the patient for further evaluation.

Question 1: What are the possible causes of this patient's new loss of hearing and of her vestibular symptoms?

Answer 1: The patient may have suffered from acoustic trauma or a temporary threshold shift (see later text) from the pounding of a bass drum close to her ears during an exciting football game.

Acoustic trauma generally refers to a single high-intensity *acoustic* event such as a firecracker or gun discharging near an unprotected ear. Acoustic trauma can damage hair cells within the cochlea, thereby causing an immediate and permanent sensorineural hearing loss that involves the midfrequency hearing range between 3 and 6 kHz and is typically centered at 4 kHz. Mild, temporary vestibular symptoms are not unusual in cases of acoustic trauma. In this patient's case, it is possible that a single note, aggressively played from the bass drum close to the patient's unprotected ear, caused acoustic trauma.

A temporary threshold shift is a temporary increase in auditory thresholds of 10 to 20 dB usually involving the mid to high frequencies (3 to 6 kHz). A temporary threshold shift often occurs after sustained exposure to high-intensity noise. Associated symptoms include high-pitched tinnitus and a sense of fullness in the ear. Vestibular symptoms are not generally noted during temporary threshold shifts. The symptoms of a temporary threshold shift are usually fully reversible over 12 to 24 hours and are thought to be the result of an acute overconsumption of essential metabolic factors within the inner ear. A permanent shift in hearing thresholds primarily affecting the high-frequency range can occur following repeated temporary threshold shifts and is referred to as *noise-induced hearing loss*. The incidence of both temporary threshold shifts and noise-induced hearing loss have increased recently in teenagers, primarily because of noise exposure at rock concerts and from the use of personal musical devices at high loudness levels.

Because this patient's hearing loss did not resolve and she has vestibular symptoms, she is probably suffering from the results of acoustic trauma caused by the proximity to a loud bass drum rather than from a temporary threshold shift.

Question 2: What are the possible causes of this patient's pre-existing unilateral hearing loss?

Answer 2: The differential diagnosis for hearing loss discovered during childhood is summarized in Table U8–1. Most disorders that cause an inherited or congenital hearing loss present with bilateral profound sensorineural hearing loss at birth. Although the incidence of vestibular abnormalities in congenitally deaf individuals is unknown, symptoms of vestibular dysfunction are rarely reported. A few reports of vestibular laboratory testing performed in conjunction with cochlear implantation

TABLE U8–1
Summary of the Differential Diagnosis of Sensorineural Hearing Loss in Children

Inherited
  Congenital
  Noncongenital
Acquired
  Prenatal
    Infectious
    Inner ear malformations
  Perinatal
    Infectious
    Hyperbilirubinemia
    Prematurity, birth trauma, anoxia
    Persistent fetal circulation
  Postnatal
    Infectious
    Head trauma
    Acoustic trauma
    Noise-induced
    Perilymphatic fistula
    Endolymphatic hydrops

suggest that many profoundly deaf individuals have decreased or absent vestibular function. The lack of vestibular symptoms despite abnormal vestibular function may be a result of substitution of other sensory modalities for the abnormal vestibular function. Also, patients with bilateral vestibular loss rarely have vertigo (see Cases C6 and C21).

Inherited hearing loss that develops beyond infancy may be associated with other nonotologic abnormalities such as kidney disease (e.g., Alport's syndrome), ocular disease (e.g., Usher's syndrome), pigmentary disorders (e.g., Waardenburg's syndrome), bony abnormalities (e.g. osteogenesis imperfecta), and mucopolysaccharide storage disease (e.g., Hurler's syndrome and Hunter's syndrome).

Inherited noncongenital hearing loss may or may not be associated with vestibular abnormalities. There are many patterns of hearing loss and vestibular function; they vary in the relative affliction of hearing versus balance and in severity, age of onset, and rate of progression. For example, Usher's syndrome, Type I, an inherited autosomal recessive disorder characterized by severe to profound hearing loss and retinitis pigmentosa, is associated with absent vestibular responses. Mixed X-linked progressive deafness with stapes fixation, a condition in which males show progressive moderate to severe mixed hearing loss, is also associated with abnormal vestibular function. Female carriers of this disorder have only mild hearing loss and normal vestibular function.

Acquired prenatal hearing loss, whether infectious or a result of inner malformations (dysplasias or dysgenesis), may cause vestibular dysfunction. Many patients with inner ear malformations have other abnormalities that comprise a syndrome, such as Klippel-Feil syndrome, Pendred's syndrome, trisomy syndrome, and DiGeorge's syndrome.

A spectrum of inner ear malformations can occur ranging from total agenesis to various combinations of bony and membranous abnormalities of the cochlea and semicircular canals.[2,3] Examples include Mondini dysplasia, the enlarged vestibular aqueduct syndrome, and cochlear-saccular dysgenesis (i.e., Sheibe dysplasia). Individuals with inner ear dysplasias may present with sudden or progressive hearing loss in childhood or young adulthood. The hearing loss may be unilateral or bilateral. Vestibular symptoms are frequently noted but generally are mild, although acute vertigo may occasionally be the most prominent symptom of an inner ear malformation. A bump on the head, a strong sneeze, or straining during a bowel movement may worsen the hearing or vestibular symptoms associated with inner ear malformations.

Inner ear dysplasias can also be associated with an abnormal communication between the middle ear space and the cerebrospinal fluid space, that is, a perilymphatic fistula (see Cases C19 and C23). Children with this condition are at risk for recurrent meningitis.[4]

The perinatal causes of hearing loss are listed in Table U8–1. These abnormalities can usually be ruled out by reviewing the child's history of perinatal hospitalization or complications at birth.

The postnatal causes of childhood hearing loss include infection, such as bacterial or viral meningitis. Mumps labyrinthitis is the most common cause of unilateral hearing loss. Head trauma, acoustic trauma, and noise-induced hearing loss are common causes of hearing loss, especially affecting teenagers, and should be sought out in the patient interview.[5] Perilymphatic fistula can cause both hearing loss and vestibular disturbances.[6] The presence of inner malformations or head trauma may contribute to the formation of a perilymphatic fistula (see Cases C19 and C23).

Endolymphatic hydrops can occur in childhood and produces a symptom complex of recurrent vertigo, fluctuating hearing loss, tinnitus, and aural fullness similar to that seen in adults[7] (see Cases T3, T9, C10, C14, and C16).

ADDITIONAL HISTORY

Further history revealed no known familial hearing loss or history of consanguinity. The patient was a full-term infant and there were no reported maternal complications of pregnancy or delivery. The parents reported two episodes of high fever of unknown cause during childhood. There was no history of head trauma or noise exposure.

Question 3: What is the most likely cause of this patient's prior hearing loss? How does this relate to the likely cause of this patient's new hearing loss?

Answer 3: The negative maternal and perinatal history do not reveal the cause of the prior left-sided profound hearing loss first noticed at age 5. It is possible that the hearing loss may have been related to a viral labyrinthitis during one of the episodes of high fever. The prior hearing loss may also have been caused by an occult inner ear malformation.[8] This idea is supported by the sudden loss of hearing in the contralateral ear precipitated by acoustic trauma, which is suggestive of a bilateral inner ear malformation.

PHYSICAL EXAMINATION

General examination was normal. Neurologic examination was normal. There was no nystagmus even with Frenzel glasses. Otoscopic examination was normal. No nystagmus or vertigo was noted during pressure changes in the external auditory canal induced by a pneumatic otoscope. The patient had a normal Romberg's test but could not stand on a compliant foam pad with her eyes open or closed. A stepping test revealed a significant 90 degree deviation to the right side.

Question 4: How should the possibility of an inner ear malformation be evaluated with laboratory testing?

Answer 4: Audiometric and vestibular testing can help to define the extent of audiovestibular abnormalities including severity and laterality. A high-resolution CT scan of the temporal bones is most frequently used to diagnose an inner ear anatomic malformation. Because most inner ear malformations include some degree of bony labyrinthine abnormalities, they are easily detected and characterized by CT imaging, which provides bony detail of the inner ear superior to that of MRI. However, recent advances in MR imaging have led to visualization of the labyrinthine fluid spaces in sufficient detail to characterize many inner ear malformations.

Laboratory Testing

Vestibular Laboratory Testing

ELECTRONYSTAGMOGRAPHY:	Ocular motor and positional testing were normal. Caloric testing indicated absent response to bithermal stimulation and minimal responses to ice water irrigation, that is, a severe bilateral vestibular reduction.
ROTATIONAL TESTING:	Rotational testing revealed severely reduced gain and increased phase lead.

POSTUROGRAPHY: Posturography indicated excessive sway on conditions 4, 5, and 6, that is, a surface-dependent pattern.

Audiometric Testing: An audiogram (Fig. U8–1) showed a profound sensorineural hearing loss in the left ear. The right ear showed a flat severe sensorineural hearing loss. Word recognition was 0 in the left ear and 66 percent in the right ear.

Imaging: CT imaging of the temporal bones showed the presence of a bilateral inner ear malformation consistent with the enlarged vestibular aqueduct syndrome (Fig. U8–2).

Other: None.

DIAGNOSIS/DIFFERENTIAL DIAGNOSIS

This patient was given the diagnosis of *enlarged vestibular aqueduct syndrome.*

Question 5: What is the enlarged vestibular aqueduct syndrome?

Answer 5: The enlarged vestibular aqueduct syndrome is a congenital malformation of the temporal bone in which the vestibular aqueducts are abnormally enlarged. The vestibular aqueduct syndrome predisposes children to develop progressive sensorineural hearing loss and vestibular dysfunction at a relatively early age.[2,3,4] An

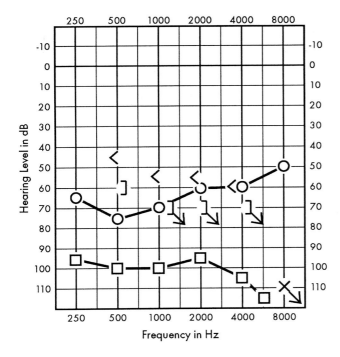

Word Recognition Score		
Right : 66%		
Left : 0%		

		Right	Left
Air	unmasked	o——o	x——x
	masked	△——△	□——□
Bone	unmasked	◄---<	>---►
	masked	⊏---⊏	⊐---⊐

Figure U8-1
Audiogram.

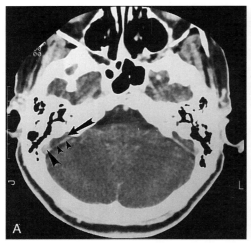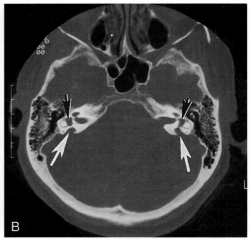

Figure U8-2

Axial computed tomographic images showing bilateral dilated vestibular aqueducts. (A) Soft-tissue algorithm shows the dilated endolymphatic sac (large arrow), seen here better on the left side. The sac is a fluid-density structure adjacent to the contrast-enhanced sigmoid sinus (large arrowhead). Enhancing dura defines the medial border of the sac (small arrowheads). (B) Bone algorithm demonstrates the osseous anatomy of the inner ear. The osseous vestibular aqueduct is markedly enlarged (white arrows). The labyrinthine vestibules (highlighted arrows) are slightly dysplastic. (With permission from Hirsch, BE, et al: Magnetic resonance imaging of the large vestibular aqueduct. Arch Otolaryngol Head Neck Surg 118:1124–1127, 1992.[10])

abnormally large vestibular aqueduct can occur as an isolated finding or it can accompany more widespread congenital malformations of the cochlea and semicircular canals. The vestibular aqueduct syndrome is more common than Mondini dysplasia by a ratio of 4 to 1.

Question 6: What is the mechanism whereby acoustic trauma or barotrauma (a gradual but large, rather than an abrupt but modest, change in external auditory canal pressure) causes or exacerbates hearing loss and vestibular dysfunction in patients with inner ear malformations?

Answer 6: Although the exact mechanism of hearing loss and vestibular dysfunction as a result of acoustic trauma or barotrauma in patients with inner ear malformations is unknown, two theories are most commonly proffered: (1) hearing and vestibular dysfunction may result from an abnormal susceptibility to rupture of the membranous labyrinth, or (2) hearing and vestibular dysfunction may result from a perilymphatic fistula. In addition to avoiding acoustic trauma, that is, exposure to excessively loud sounds and barotrauma, patients and their parents should be counseled concerning avoidance of activities such as weightlifting, contact sports, or scuba diving, which increase intrathoracic and cerebrospinal fluid pressure, thereby increasing the likelihood of either rupture of inner ear membranes or the development of a perilymphatic fistula.

TREATMENT/MANAGEMENT

The possibility of exploring the right ear for a perilymphatic fistula was discussed with the patient and her family. It was decided that the patient complete a 2-week course of oral prednisone at a dose of 1 mg/kg per day and remain at bed rest with minimal activity for 2 weeks in case the recent worsening of symptoms was a result of a pressure-induced membrane rupture. The patient's symptoms stabilized. One month later, she resumed normal activities and was counseled regarding avoidance of contact sports, straining, or lifting heavy objects. She was fitted with a hearing aid in the right ear and asked to enroll in a lip-reading class to help improve her communication skills. At 6-week follow-up, the patient reported no further vertigo or disequilibrium and some subjective improvement in hearing. Follow-up audiometric testing showed that word recognition scores had increased to 85 percent, although pure tone thresholds were unchanged.

SUMMARY

A 16-year-old girl presented with disequilibrium and a loss of hearing and tinnitus in an only-hearing ear following acoustic trauma. A congenital bilateral inner ear malformation was subsequently discovered by CT scanning. Treatment included consideration of middle ear exploration for repair of a possible perilymphatic fistula, a short course of steroids, and 2 weeks of bed rest. Surgery was not performed. The patient's vestibular symptoms resolved, and she had recovery of some of her hearing. She was fitted with a hearing aid and counseled to avoid strenuous activities and contact sports. The patient also was enrolled in a lip-reading class in order to improve her communication skills and to prepare her for the possibility of future bilateral profound hearing loss.

TEACHING POINTS

1. **Acoustic trauma** refers to a single high-intensity acoustic event such as a firecracker or gun discharging near an unprotected ear. Acoustic trauma can damage hair cells within the cochlea, thereby causing an immediate and permanent sensorineural hearing loss that is typically centered at 4 kHz. Mild and temporary vestibular symptoms are not unusual in cases of acoustic trauma.

2. **A temporary threshold shift** is a temporary increase in auditory thresholds of 10 to 20 dB, primarily involving the mid to high frequencies. A temporary threshold shift often occurs following sustained exposure to high-intensity noise. Associated symptoms include high-pitched tinnitus and a sense of fullness in the ear. Vestibular symptoms are not generally noted during temporary threshold shifts. The symptoms of a temporary threshold shift are usually fully reversible over 12 to 24 hours and are thought to be caused by an acute overconsumption of essential metabolic factors within the inner ear. A permanent shift in hearing thresholds primarily affecting the high-frequency range can occur following repeated temporary threshold shifts and is referred to as noise-induced hearing loss.

3. **Hearing loss discovered during childhood** has many causes. The differential diagnosis is summarized in Table U8–1.

4. **Inner ear dysplasia** may present with sudden or progressive hearing loss in childhood or young adulthood. The hearing loss can be unilateral or bilateral. Vestibular symptoms are frequently noted but generally are mild, although acute vertigo may occasionally be the most prominent symptom of an inner ear malformation. A bump on the head, a strong sneeze, or straining during a bowel movement may worsen

the hearing or vestibular symptoms associated with inner ear malformations. Inner ear dysplasias can also be associated with a perilymphatic fistula.

5. **Inner ear malformations** often include some degree of bony labyrinthine abnormalities. They are easily detected and characterized by CT imaging. MRI scan lacks the ability to visualize the bony detail necessary to characterize inner ear malformations.

6. **The enlarged vestibular aqueduct syndrome** is a congenital malformation of the temporal bone in which the vestibular aqueducts are abnormally enlarged. The enlarged vestibular aqueduct syndrome predisposes children to develop progressive sensorineural hearing loss and vestibular dysfunction at a relatively early age. An abnormally large vestibular aqueduct can occur as an isolated finding or can accompany more widespread congenital malformations of the cochlea and semicircular canals.

7. **The mechanism of acoustic trauma–induced or barotrauma-induced otologic dysfunction** in patients with congenital inner ear malformations is unknown. In addition to avoiding acoustic trauma and exposure to barotrauma, patients with congenital inner ear malformations and their parents should be counseled concerning avoidance of activities such as weightlifting, contact sports, or scuba diving, which increase intrathoracic and cerebrospinal fluid pressure, thereby increasing the likelihood of either rupture of inner ear membranes or the development of a perilymphatic fistula.

8. **Treatment for an acute worsening** of hearing loss and acute vestibular symptoms associated with congenital inner ear malformations should include consideration of middle ear exploration for repair of a possible perilymphatic fistula, a short course of corticosteroids, and a period of reduced activity and bedrest. Surgery directed at the endolymphatic sac should not be performed.

REFERENCES

1. Meyerhoff, WL, et al: Progressive sensorineural hearing loss in children. Otolaryngol Head Neck Surg 110:569–579, 1994.
2. Schuknecht, HF: Mondi dysplasia: A clinical and pathological study, Part 2. Ann Otol Rhinol Laryngol 89 (Suppl 65):3–23, 1980.
3. Jackler, RK, and De La Cruz, A: The large vestibular aqueduct syndrome. Laryngoscope 99:1238–1243, 1989.
4. Parisier, SC, and Birken, EA: Recurrent meningitis secondary to idiopathic oval window CSF leak. Laryngoscope 86:1503–1515, 1976.
5. Brookhouse, PE, Worthington, DW, and Kelly, WJ: Noise-induced hearing loss in children. Laryngoscope 102:645–655, 1992.
6. Supance, JS, and Bluestone, CD: Perilymph fistulas in infants and children. Otolaryngol Head Neck Surg 91:663–671, 1983.
7. Meyerhoff, WL, Paparella, MM, and Shea, D: Meniere's disease in children. Laryngoscope 88:1504–1511, 1978.
8. Jackler, RK, and Dillon, WP: Computed tomography and magnetic resonance imaging of the inner ear. Otolaryngol Head Neck Surg 99:494–504, 1988.
9. Levenson, MJ, Parisier, SC, Jacobs, M, and Edelstein, DR: The large vestibular aqueduct syndrome in children. Arch Otolaryngol Head Neck Surg 115:54–58, 1989.
10. Hirsch, BE, et al: Magnetic resonance imaging of large vestibular aqueduct. Arch Otolaryngol Head Neck Surg 118:1124–1127, 1992.

U9

Wernicke's Encephalopathy

HISTORY

A 54-year-old woman who did not work outside the home presented with a chief complaint of 2 weeks of forgetfulness, "wandering eyes," and very poor balance. The patient's past history was significant for left hemiglossectomy and left radical neck dissection 6 months before presentation. The patient had no complaints of vertigo or hearing loss and no tinnitus. There was no prior history of balance disorder. The family history was negative.

Question 1: Based on the patient's history, what are the diagnostic considerations?

Answer 1: The patient's history is consistent with a wide differential diagnosis that includes a vestibular system abnormality because of imbalance. However, abnormal eye movements and impaired cognition suggest a central nervous system disorder. A single condition that includes all three of this patient's signs and symptoms: eye movement abnormalities, mental status change, and ataxia, is *Wernicke's encephalopathy*. Many other conditions can account for one or two of these signs and symptoms, and these should be considered. Because Wernicke's encephalopathy is a result of vitamin B_1 deficiency, further history from the patient regarding nutrition is extremely important. Also, further details should be obtained regarding the patient's recent mental status. Physical examination and laboratory testing should also help to establish the diagnosis.

ADDITIONAL HISTORY

This patient had become depressed following recent surgery for head and neck cancer and had limited her caloric intake severely. For the month before evaluation, she had consumed ethanol as her sole caloric intake. During the last 2 weeks, the patient had become increasingly forgetful and confused and was brought in for evaluation by her family when she became disoriented.

PHYSICAL EXAMINATION

The patient was an emaciated woman with a supine blood pressure of 100/60. Neurologic examination revealed that she was not oriented to person, place, or time. She was unable to remember any objects at 1 minute during memory testing. Cranial nerve examination revealed upbeating nystagmus in the primary position that was *diminished* with up-gaze and *increased* with down-gaze, the reverse of that expected from Alexander's law (see Case T3). The patient could not move her eyes horizontally when asked to do so. There was facial asymmetry and an inability to protrude the tongue, both presumably caused by the radial neck dissection and hemiglossectomy. Coordination testing revealed a severe dysmetria of upper and lower extremities. The patient could not perform heel-knee-shin testing. The deep tendon reflexes were normal. Sensation could not be assessed reliably. Romberg's test could not be performed because the patient could not stand with her eyes open without assistance. Her gait was severely ataxic. Otoscopic examination was normal.

Laboratory Testing

Vestibular Laboratory Testing

ELECTRONYSTAGMOGRAPHY:	Ocular motor testing revealed upbeating nystagmus that was not changed when the patient was placed in darkness. Caloric testing revealed bilaterally reduced responses; there was minimal response to ice water irrigations bilaterally.
ROTATIONAL TESTING:	Rotational testing revealed reduced responses with markedly increased phase lead.
POSTUROGRAPHY:	Not performed

Audiometric Testing: Not performed

Imaging: Magnetic resonance imaging of the brain was normal. Cerebrospinal fluid evaluation was normal.

Other: None

DIAGNOSIS/DIFFERENTIAL DIAGNOSIS

Question 2: Based on the patient's history, physical examination, and laboratory tests, what is the likely diagnosis?

Answer 2: This patient is suffering from Wernicke's encephalopathy. Table U9–1 lists the clinical features of this condition, which is a result of hypovitaminosis B_1. The

TABLE U9–1
Clinical Features of Wernicke's Encephalopathy

Ocular motor abnormalities such as nystagmus and gaze palsy
Ataxia
Global confusional state
Vestibular paresis
Hypotension
Hypothermia

TABLE U9–2
Conditions Associated with
Wernicke's Encephalopathy

Alcoholism
Prolonged intravenous feeding
Intravenous hyperalimentation
Hyperemesis gravidarum
Anorexia nervosa
Prolonged fasting
Refeeding after starvation
Gastric plication

characteristic clinical features of this condition include eye movement abnormalities, mental status change, and gait ataxia. An additional commonly seen feature of this condition is vestibular paresis, either unilaterally or bilaterally, as assessed by caloric testing.[1] This patient had each of these four features. Presumably, the patient's head and neck surgery and her depression contributed to her poor nutritional habits and vitamin B_1 deficiency.

Question 3: In what clinical settings is Wernicke's encephalopathy seen?

Answer 3: Table U9–2 indicates the conditions that predispose to Wernicke's encephalopathy. Alcoholism is the most common of these conditions.

Question 4: This patient's vestibular laboratory testing demonstrated markedly increased phase lead on rotational testing. What is the basis of this abnormality? What determines the dynamics of the vestibulo-ocular reflex? In what disorders are vestibulo-ocular reflex dynamics abnormal?

Answer 4: This patient's abnormal phase lead on rotational testing suggests an abnormality in the so-called velocity storage system.[2] Velocity storage refers to a central nervous system circuit that maintains vestibular information beyond the cessation of activity of the eighth nerve afferents induced by vestibular stimulation. Thus, following a brief acceleratory stimulus, eighth nerve afferent activity will return to baseline in 5 to 7 seconds, whereas vestibular-induced eye movements may persist for about three to four times that duration, that is, 15 to 30 seconds. A possible purpose of the velocity storage system is to improve the function of the vestibulo-ocular reflex, especially for slow head movements. The velocity storage system is also critical for the generation of optokinetic nystagmus, and thus probably plays a role during exposure to prolonged moving visual stimuli such as during walking.[3]

The central nervous system structures important for the velocity storage mechanism include the vestibular nucleus and the cerebellar uvula and nodulus.[4] Thus, abnormalities in these structures or their interconnections can impair velocity storage. However, despite its central nervous system localization, abnormalities of velocity storage are also seen with damage to the peripheral vestibular system.[5]

Abnormalities of the velocity storage system appear as increased phase lead during sinusoidal rotation, and a shortened vestibulo-ocular reflex time constant, that is, an increased rate of decay of postrotatory nystagmus following abrupt changes in head velocity. There are no clinical correlates that are specific for abnormalities of the velocity storage system. Many different disorders can cause abnormalities in the velocity storage mechanism. Abnormal vestibulo-ocular reflex dynamics indicative of abnormal velocity storage are a sensitive but nonspecific indicator of vestibular system damage.

Question 5: What is the basis of this patient's caloric reduction and abnormal vestibulo-ocular reflex dynamics?

Answer 5: Wernicke's encephalopathy leads to reduced vestibular sensitivity, presumably because of damage to the vestibular nuclei in the medulla.[1] Abnormalities of vestibulo-ocular reflex dynamics, that is, abnormal velocity storage, are probably caused by vestibular nucleus or cerebellar damage.[2]

This patient was given a diagnosis of *Wernicke's encephalopathy*.

TREATMENT/MANAGEMENT

This patient was treated with intravenous thiamine. Her nystagmus resolved, and she became less confused but had a persistent memory deficit. The gait ataxia persisted, though at a somewhat lessened degree. The patient's vestibular sensitivity improved so that bithermal responses were reduced, but not absent. Vestibulo-ocular reflex *dynamics* remained abnormal as evidenced by an increased phase lead of eye movements induced by sinusoidal rotation.

SUMMARY

A 54-year-old woman presented with forgetfulness and abnormal eye movements several months following hemiglossectomy for head and neck cancer. The patient was found to have poor memory, upbeating nystagmus, and gait ataxia. Laboratory testing revealed bilaterally reduced vestibular responses. Brain imaging was normal. The patient was given the diagnosis of *Wernicke's encephalopathy*. Treatment consisted of intravenous thiamine. The patient improved somewhat but was left with a persistent deficit in memory and balance.

TEACHING POINTS

1. **Wernicke's encephalopathy**, which is caused by vitamin B_1 deficiency, is characterized by the combination of abnormal eye movements, mental status change, and ataxia. Wernicke's encephalopathy is associated with the conditions listed in Table U2–9. The most common condition in which Wernicke's encephalopathy is seen is alcoholism.
2. **Eye movement abnormalities in Wernicke's encephalopathy** include various types of nystagmus and gaze palsies.
3. **Vestibular paresis**, either unilaterally or bilaterally, probably as a result of damage to the vestibular nuclei in the medulla, is a feature of Wernicke's encephalopathy that is often not appreciated.
4. **Abnormal vestibulo-ocular reflex dynamics**, for example, increased phase lead on rotational testing, suggests dysfunction of the so-called velocity storage system,

a circuit that maintains the central nervous system response to activity of the eighth nerve afferents induced by vestibular stimulation. The velocity storage system is also critical for the generation of optokinetic nystagmus. Although many different disorders can cause abnormalities in the velocity storage mechanism, there are no clinical correlates that are specific for abnormalities of the velocity storage system.

REFERENCES

1. Ghez, C: Vestibular paresis: A clinical feature of Wernicke's disease. J Neurol Neurosurg Psychiatry 32:132–139, 1969.
2. Furman, JM, and Becker, JT: Vestibular responses in Wernicke's encephalopathy. Ann Neurol 26:669–674, 1989.
3. Cohen, B, Matsuo, V, and Raphan, T: Quantitative analysis of the velocity characteristics of optokinetic nystagmus and optokinetic after-nystagmus. J Physiol 270:321–344, 1977.
4. Waespe, W, Cohen, B, and Raphan, T: Dynamic modification of the vestibulo-ocular reflex by the nodulus and uvula. Science 288:199–202, 1985.
5. Zee, D, Yee, R, and Robinson, D: Optokinetic responses in labyrinthine-defective human beings. Brain Res 113:423–428, 1976.

U10

Dysautonomia

HISTORY

A 50-year-old man who worked as an electronics repairman complained of constant dizziness and lightheadedness that had gradually worsened over several years. He rarely experienced vertigo. Rather, the patient's symptoms included a sense of disequilibrium and a feeling of generalized weakness and faintness. These symptoms were especially noticeable on first arising and on standing for more than several minutes in one place. The patient had no complaint of hearing loss, tinnitus, paresthesias, air hunger, palpitations, fear, or anxiety. The family history was positive for adult-onset diabetes mellitus and negative for neurologic or otologic disease. The patient stated that he had recently been tested for abnormal blood sugar and that this was normal. The patient was not using medications.

Question 1: What are the diagnostic considerations for this case? What additional history should be obtained? What special maneuvers, if any, should be performed during physical examination?

Answer 1: This patient's history provides little information for establishing a definitive diagnosis of a peripheral or central vestibular disorder. In fact, the symptoms of faintness and presyncope suggest a *nonvestibular* cause for the patient's dizziness. Disorders to be considered include hypotension, especially orthostatic hypotension, intermittent hyperventilation associated with anxiety and/or a chronic anxiety state, hypoglycemia, anemia, hyperthyroidism or hypothyroidism, and medication side effects.

   The patient also has little to suggest an anxiety disorder. He indicated that he had been checked for hypoglycemia and that this was negative. The patient should be specifically questioned as to whether or not he had undergone blood studies for anemia and hypothyroidism. During physical examination, blood pressure and pulse should be measured with the patient seated and at 1, 3, and 5 minutes after standing.

ADDITIONAL HISTORY

The patient indicated that a complete blood count, thyroid and adrenocortical steroid function tests, and a screening electrolyte battery were normal.

290

PHYSICAL EXAMINATION

The patient's examination revealed a blood pressure of 130/85 while he was seated with a pulse of 70. After 1 minute of standing, his blood pressure was 90/60 and pulse was 90. The patient stated that he was experiencing his typical symptoms of faintness and requested that he be permitted to sit down. He felt less symptomatic almost immediately on sitting. The remainder of the neurologic examination was normal except that the patient had a somewhat wide-based gait. During Romberg's test, the patient complained of feeling lightheaded but did not fall with his eyes closed and was able to stand on a compliant foam surface without difficulty. The otologic examination was normal.

DIAGNOSIS/DIFFERENTIAL DIAGNOSIS

Question 2: Based on the patient's history and physical examination, what is the probable diagnosis?

Answer 2: This patient has orthostatic hypotension. There is no evidence from the physical examination for vestibular system disease. Blood studies ruled out several other diagnostic possibilities.

Laboratory Testing

Not performed

Question 3: What are the characteristics of nonvestibular dizziness and how do they differ from the symptoms of vestibular-induced dizziness?

Answer 3: Patients with vestibular dizziness often complain of vertigo that may include spinning or tilting and a sense of being off balance, whereas patients with nonvestibular dizziness often complain of lightheadedness, a floating sensation, a swimming sensation, or giddiness. Vestibular dizziness is often episodic, whereas nonvestibular dizziness is often constant. Vestibular dizziness is often produced or exacerbated by rapid head movements and certain changes in position, such as rolling over in bed. Symptoms associated with vestibular disorders can include nausea, vomiting, unsteadiness, tinnitus, hearing loss, impaired vision, and oscillopsia, whereas nonvestibular dizziness may be associated with perspiration, palpitation, paresthesias, syncope or presyncope, difficulty concentrating, and malaise.[1]

This patient was given the diagnosis of *idiopathic orthostatic hypotension.*

Question 4: What is the physiologic basis for the nausea and malaise associated with vestibular system ailments?

Answer 4: The vestibular system has powerful influences on the autonomic nervous system, particularly the sympathetic nervous system, and on respiration.[2–4] Vestibular activity can alter blood pressure and heart rate and can influence the baroreflex. Vestibular inputs that are excessive or in conflict with other sensory inputs can produce motion sickness,[5] wherein individuals have a sense of malaise associated with nausea, diaphoresis, and sometimes vomiting.

The mechanism whereby vestibular abnormalities and excessive vestibular stimulation induce motion sickness is unknown. Moreover, the purpose of motion sickness is unknown. It is interesting that symptoms of postural hypotension mimic some of the symptoms of vestibular system dysfunction. Possibly, the vestibuloautonomic pathways are responsible for this overlap in symptoms.

TREATMENT/MANAGEMENT

This patient was treated with support stockings, increased dietary salt intake, and fludrocortisone 0.1 mg twice daily. He was also advised that, when changing from a seated to a standing position he should do so slowly, and once upright, begin ambulation as soon as possible to avoid standing in one place for more than a very brief time.

The patient responded favorably to this treatment but still experienced some dizziness and lightheadedness when standing.

SUMMARY

A 50-year-old man presented with the chief complaint of dizziness, especially when standing, associated with a sense of faintness and lower-extremity weakness. The patient's examination revealed postural hypotension without evidence of vestibular system abnormality. The patient was treated with support stockings and fludrocortisone and experienced a reduction in symptoms.

TEACHING POINTS

1. **Dizziness of vestibular origin** is often produced or exacerbated by rapid head movements and certain changes in position such as rolling over in bed. Patients with dizziness of vestibular origin often complain of episodic vertigo that may include spinning or tilting and a sense of being off balance, whereas patients with nonvestibular dizziness often complain of constant lightheadedness, a floating sensation, a swimming sensation, or giddiness.
2. **Symptoms associated with vestibular disorders** include nausea, vomiting, unsteadiness, tinnitus, hearing loss, impaired vision, and oscillopsia, whereas nonvestibular dizziness is more likely to be associated with perspiration, palpitation, paresthesias, syncope or presyncope, difficulty concentrating, and malaise.
3. **Symptoms of faintness and presyncope** should suggest a nonvestibular cause for a patient's dizziness, such as postural hypotension, intermittent hyperventilation associated with anxiety, hypoglycemia, anemia, hypothyroidism, or medication side effects.
4. **Vestibuloautonomic pathways** may underlie the mechanism whereby vestibular abnormalities cause malaise, nausea, and vomiting. These pathways are thought to underlie the ability of vestibular activity to alter blood pressure and heart rate.

REFERENCES

1. Baloh, RW, and Honrubia, V: Clinical Neurophysiology of the Vestibular System, ed 2. Philadelphia: FA Davis, 1990.
2. Yates, BJ: Vestibular influences on the sympathetic nervous system. Brain Res Rev 17:51–59, 1992.
3. Yates, B, Jakus, J, and Miller, A: Vestibular effects on respiratory outflow in the decerebrate cat. Brain Res 629:209–217, 1993.
4. Yates, BJ, and Miller, AD (eds): Vestibular Autonomic Regulation. Boca Raton: CRC Press (in press).
5. Crampton, GH (ed): Motion and Space Sickness. Boca Raton: CRC Press, 1990.

Ramsay Hunt Syndrome

HISTORY

A 55-year-old male physician presented with ear pain, hearing loss, vertigo, and progressive facial paralysis. The symptoms began 3 days before evaluation with the acute onset of severe left ear pain. Two days before evaluation, he had noticed distortion of hearing in the left ear, tinnitus, and disequilibrium when he moved quickly. By that evening, he had severe vertigo, nausea and vomiting, and a definite loss of hearing in the left ear. He also noticed that he could not fully close his left eye, his smile was asymmetric, his voice had become slightly hoarse, and his swallowing felt "funny." Worried about a possible stroke, he went to the emergency room for evaluation. The patient's past medical history and family history were negative.

Question 1: What is the differential diagnosis for this patient's combination of symptoms?

Answer 1: The combination of hearing loss, vertigo, facial paralysis, and bulbar symptoms suggests brainstem dysfunction, possibly as a result of cerebrovascular disease or encephalitis. Another possibility is a cranial polyneuropathy.

PHYSICAL EXAMINATION

General examination was normal. Cranial nerve examination revealed full extraocular movements. Saccadic and pursuit movements were normal. A right-beating jerk-nystagmus was present with Frenzel glasses. There was no nystagmus present with visual fixation. Facial sensation to light touch and pinprick was normal. Corneal reflexes were intact. There was weakness of the right side of the face; the patient was unable to raise his eyebrow or fully close his eye; he had only a slight amount of movement of his levator labii. His facial tone appeared to be normal. Facial function was graded as House-Brackmann level 4.[1] Tuning-fork examination revealed a positive Rinne test bilaterally and a midline Weber's test with 512-Hz and 1024-Hz tuning forks. The gag reflex was intact. However, visualization of the larynx revealed a left vocal cord paralysis, suggesting a lesion of the left vagus nerve. The patient had normal strength during shoulder shrug and was able to lift his arms over his head. However, his right sternocleidomastoid muscle appeared to be weak.

The patient had normal strength and muscle tone in all extremities. Romberg's test demonstrated increased sway without falls. He could stand on a foam pad with his eyes closed. Gait was within normal limits, although the patient tended to veer slightly to the left when he made sharp turns. Stepping testing showed that he deviated 90 degrees to the left.

Examination of the pinna, external auditory canal, and eardrum revealed multiple vesicles in the concha and external ear canal and a few on the ear drum. The drum appeared to be slightly reddened, but there was no evidence of acute otitis media. Examination of the oral cavity revealed a number of small vesicles on the left buccal mucosa.

Question 2: Based on the results of the physical examination, what is this patient's most likely diagnosis?

Answer 2: The presence of vesicles on the auricle and in the mouth is highly suggestive of an acute viral process, most likely herpes zoster. J. Ramsay Hunt[2] described a syndrome consisting of facial paralysis, inner ear disturbances, and painful herpetiform blisters of the auricle in 1907. The cause of the syndrome has been confirmed to be herpetic infection involving the seventh and eighth cranial nerves.[3] Thus, this patient's most likely diagnosis is Ramsey Hunt syndrome, also known as herpes zoster oticus. Facial paralysis is seen in about 60 percent of patients, and eighth nerve dysfunction, consisting of either sensorineural hearing loss or vertigo, appears in about 40 percent of patients with herpes zoster oticus. Histopathologic studies have confirmed the direct involvement of the seventh nerve by an inflammatory process marked by hemorrhage, extravasation of blood, inflammatory cell infiltration, and ultimately nerve fiber degeneration. It is not known if this effect is the result of an autoimmune phenomenon or to the viral infection itself. The histopathologic correlate of the eighth nerve disturbance has not been elucidated.

Laboratory Testing

Vestibular Laboratory Testing

ELECTRONYSTAGMOGRAPHY:	Ocular motor testing revealed a right-beating spontaneous vestibular nystagmus. Caloric testing revealed a reduced vestibular response on the left.
ROTATIONAL TESTING:	Rotational testing revealed a mild right directional preponderance.
POSTUROGRAPHY:	Posturography indicated excessive sway on conditions 5 and 6, that is, a vestibular pattern.

Audiometric Testing: An audiogram showed a high-frequency sensorineural hearing loss in the left ear; word recognition score was 80 percent in the left ear. The right ear was normal. A brainstem auditory-evoked potential revealed normal amplitudes and latencies in the right ear. However, the left ear showed a slight delay between waves 1 and 3 and a slight delay of wave 5. Otoacoustic emissions were normal bilaterally.

Imaging: An MRI scan of the head was performed and showed enhancement of the seventh and eighth cranial nerves within the internal auditory canal suggestive of an inflammatory neuritis (Fig. U11–1). No mass lesions or other abnormalities were noted.

Other: None

Question 3: How does the laboratory testing help to localize the site of viral involvement?

Answer 3: The abnormal audiogram and loss of caloric function in the left ear suggest involvement of both the vestibular and cochlear subdivisions of the inner ear or eighth cranial nerve on the left. The otoacoustic emissions were normal, suggesting that the hearing loss is a result of neural rather than sensory dysfunction. The brainstem auditory-evoked potential suggests a lesion between the spiral ganglion and the brainstem. As in this case, inflammatory cranial neuritis, which may be of viral origin, can be demonstrated on MRI.[4]

Question 4: Can viruses other than herpes zoster cause neuritis leading to hearing loss or vestibular system disturbances? Can other infectious agents cause neuritis leading to hearing loss or vestibular system disturbances?

Answer 4: Several other viruses can cause hearing loss or vestibular disturbance, including rubella, rabies, mumps, cytomegalic viruses, and human immunosuppresive virus. In addition to the viral causes of neuritis, a number of bacterial infections can also produce inner ear disturbances, including tetanus, typhoid fever, leptospirosis, syphilis, diphtheria, and Lyme disease.

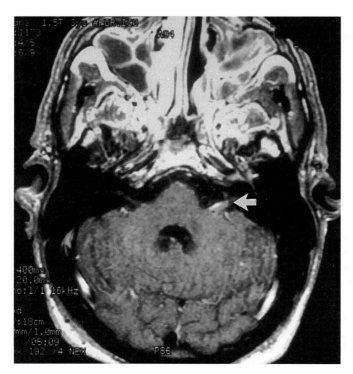

Figure U11-1
Axial magnetic resonance image of the head showing enhancement of the 7th and 8th cranial nerves within the internal auditory canal suggestive of an inflammatory neuritis. White arrow = vestibular cochlear nerve bundle within the internal auditory canal. [With permission from Hirsch, BE, et al: Localizing retrocochlear hearing loss. Am J Otol (submitted for publication).[8]]

Question 5: Can Lyme disease cause both facial nerve paralysis and inner ear disturbances?

Answer 5: Lyme disease, a systemic spirochetal (*Borrelia burgdorferi*) infection that follows the bite of an infected tick (*Ixodes dammini*), should be considered as a possible cause of any inflammatory polyneuritis.[5] Lyme disease is well known to cause facial paralysis, but it may also cause decreased hearing, tinnitus, and vertigo.

During the first stage of Lyme disease, erythema chronicum migrans, characterized by a small expanding papula that forms an annular lesion with a central clear zone and an erythematous outer border, is reported in 60 to 80 percent of patients. During stage 2 Lyme disease, about 15 to 20 percent of patients develop neurologic complications. Although facial paralysis is one of the most common neurologic signs, both hearing loss and vertigo are common. Krejcova[6] reported 44 percent of her patients with hearing abnormalities and 81 percent with vestibular abnormalities.

DIAGNOSIS/DIFFERENTIAL DIAGNOSIS

This patient was given the diagnosis of *herpes zoster oticus*.

TREATMENT/MANAGEMENT

This patient was treated with a combination of acyclovir given 4 g daily in divided doses and prednisone 1 mg/kg per day for 10 days.[7] Phenergan, 25 to 50 mg ID, was needed for 2 days to control nausea and vomiting. Ophthalmic ointments were prescribed because of exposure of the cornea as a result of the facial paralysis. The skin lesions of the auricle were treated with mupirocin ointment. There was no apparent secondary infection of the skin by staphylococcal or streptococcal bacteria, so no systemic antibiotic therapy was needed.

The patient was followed closely over the ensuing 2 weeks. No further progression of the cranial nerve deficits or significant side effects from the medications occurred. The ear pain and vesicles on the ear resolved within 2 weeks. The facial nerve never became completely paralyzed and recovered to nearly normal within 3 months. The tenth and eleventh cranial nerve abnormalities recovered completely. The patient reported the continued presence of a mild hearing impairment and unilateral tinnitus 6 months later.

SUMMARY

A 55-year-old man presented with ear pain, hearing loss, vertigo, and progressive facial paralysis. Physical examination suggested the diagnosis of a polyneuritis with involvement of cranial nerves 7, 8, 10, and 11. A vesicular eruption of the pinna along with facial paralysis and audiovestibular symptoms suggested Ramsay Hunt syndrome. Treatment consisted of acyclovir, steroids, skin care, eye care, and vestibular-suppressant medications. The patient recovered nearly completely with only a residual mild hearing impairment and tinnitus.

TEACHING POINTS

1. **Ramsay Hunt syndrome** consists of facial paralysis, inner ear disturbances, and painful herpetiform blisters of the auricle. It was first described in 1907. The cause of the syndrome has been confirmed to be herpetic infection involving the seventh and eighth cranial nerves. Occasionally, viral involvement of other cranial nerves also occurs.
2. **Viruses other than herpes zoster** can cause hearing loss and vestibular system disturbances. These viruses include rubella, rabies, mumps, cytomegalic viruses, and human immunodeficiency virus (HIV).
3. **Inflammatory cranial neuritis** may be demonstrated on MRI.
4. **The treatment of Ramsay Hunt syndrome** includes acyclovir given 4 g daily in divided doses and prednisone 1 mg/kg per day for 10 days. Vestibular suppressants may be required for nausea and vomiting. Ophthalmic ointments may be needed if exposure of the cornea occurs as a result of the facial paralysis. The skin lesions of the auricle can be treated with medicated ointments. Secondary infection of the skin by staphylococcal or streptococcal bacteria can occur in severe cases and should be treated appropriately.
5. **Bacterial infection** also may produce inner ear disturbances. Examples include tetanus, typhoid fever, leptospirosis, syphilis, diphtheria, and Lyme disease. In particular, Lyme disease causes both facial nerve paralysis and inner ear disturbances. Lyme disease is caused by a systemic spirochetal (*Borrelia burgdorferi*) infection that follows the bite of an infected tick (*Ixodes dammini*) and should be considered as a possible cause of any inflammatory polyneuritis.

REFERENCES

1. House, JW, and Brackmann, DE: Facial nerve grading system. Otolaryngol Head Neck Surg 93:146–147, 1985.
2. Hunt, JR: Herpetic inflammations of the geniculate ganglion: A new syndrome and its aural complications. Arch Otol 36:371–381, 1907.
3. Weller, TH: Varicella and herpes zoster: Changing concepts of the natural history, control, and importance of a not-so-benign virus. N Engl J Med 309:1434–1440, 1983.
4. Korzec, K, et al: Gadolinium-enhanced magnetic resonance imaging of the facial nerve in herpes zoster oticus and Bell's palsy: Clinical implication. Am J Otol 12:163–168, 1991.
5. Moscatello, AL, et al: Otolaryngologic aspects of Lyme disease. Laryngoscope 101:592–595, 1991.
6. Krejcova, H, et al: Otoneurological symptomatology in Lyme disease. Adv Otorhinolaryngol 42:210–212, 1988.
7. Dickins, JRE, Smith, JT, and Graham, SS: Herpes zoster oticus: Treatment with intravenous acyclovir. Laryngoscope 98:776–779, 1988.
8. Hirsch, BE, et al: Localizing retrocochlear hearing loss. Am J Otol (submitted for publication).

C A S E
U12

Syncope

HISTORY

A 15-year-old girl presented with a complaint of vertiginous attacks associated with fainting starting 6 months before evaluation. The patient described episodes occurring once or twice per month, characterized by the acute onset of leg weakness, vertigo, disorientation, and disequilibrium noticed occasionally, as were loss of vision and double vision. On several occasions, the patient was thought by her mother to have lost consciousness briefly. The family stated that, during her episodes, the patient did not respond normally and when she spoke sounded as if she were drunk. Following each episode, the patient had a sense of malaise and ataxia. These symptoms were followed some minutes later by headache and drowsiness. The symptoms were markedly reduced after sleep. The patient had occasional tinnitus with her episodes but had no complaint of hearing loss. She was not using medications. The family history was significant for her mother, who had suffered from similar episodes when an adolescent and, as an adult, suffered from migraine headaches accompanied by a sense of dizziness.

Question 1: Based on the patient's history, what are the diagnostic considerations?

Answer 1: This patient's history is consistent with a vestibular system abnormality that certainly involves central nervous system structures, considering the association of neurologic symptoms, especially loss of consciousness. The conditions that should be considered include basilar artery migraine (see later text), vertebrobasilar insufficiency (see Case C5), Chiari malformation (see Cases C3 and C18), posterior fossa neoplasm (see Case T6), and other causes of syncope such as loss of postural tone with brief loss of consciousness (Table U12–1).

PHYSICAL EXAMINATION

The patient had normal general, neurologic, otologic, and neuro-otologic examinations. There was no orthostatic hypotension.

299

TABLE U12–1
Causes of Syncope

Loss of circulatory blood volume
Hyperventilation
Hypoglycemia
Cardiopulmonary disease, such as cardiac arrhythmia
Orthostatic hypotension
Basilar artery migraine
Reflex (vasovagal) syncope
Raised intrathoracic pressure
Seizure disorder
Transient brainstem ischemia from structural lesions

Source: With permission from Johnson, RH, et al: The autonomic nervous system. In Joynt, RJ (ed): Clinical Neurology
(Vol. 4). Philadelphia: JB Lippincott, 1994.[5]

Laboratory Testing

Vestibular Laboratory Testing

ELECTRONYSTAGMOGRAPHY: Not performed

ROTATIONAL TESTING: Not performed

POSTUROGRAPHY: Not performed

Audiometric Testing: Not performed

Imaging: MRI of the brain and a magnetic resonance angiogram were normal.

Other: Complete blood count, electrolyte, metabolic screen, EEG, and Holter monitor were all normal.

Question 2: What are the clinical characteristics of basilar artery migraine?

Answer 2: Basilar artery migraine is a condition described by Bickerstaff[1] that is associated with symptoms referable to the region supplied by the basilar artery. The diagnosis of basilar artery migraine is somewhat controversial in that many of the symptoms of migraine of any type can be ascribed to territory supplied by the basilar artery, and in this sense all migraine is basilar artery migraine. Nonetheless, basilar artery migraine is a well-defined, distinct, diagnostic entity that should be considered in patients with recurrent neurologic symptoms referable to the vertebrobasilar system followed by headache in a patient with a strong family history of migraines.[2]

The clinical manifestations of basilar artery migraine include: (1) visual symptoms, for example, tunnel vision and hallucinations; (2) ataxia, vertigo, and sometimes tinnitus; and (3) parathesias of the face and limbs. Other symptoms that may be found include nystagmus, double vision, internuclear ophthalmoplegia, and cranial neuropathy.[2]

DIAGNOSIS/DIFFERENTIAL DIAGNOSIS

Because other causes for both drop attacks and loss of consciousness were ruled out, the patient was given the diagnosis of *basilar artery migraine.*

TREATMENT/MANAGEMENT

The patient was treated with dietary restriction of possible migraine-triggering foods and instructed to keep a diary so that precipitant factors could be identified.[3,4] Additionally, she was treated with propranolol. The patient experienced a decrease in the frequency of attacks to one every 2 or 3 months.

SUMMARY

A 15-year-old girl presented with episodes of abrupt loss of postural tone followed by vertigo, disequilibrium, and poor balance. A reduced level of consciousness occurred with some of the episodes. These symptoms were followed by severe headaches and were relieved by sleep. The patient had a family history of migraine headaches. Laboratory studies appropriate for the evaluation of syncope were all normal. She was given the diagnosis of basilar artery migraine. Treatment consisted of dietary restrictions and propranolol. The patient had a reduction in the frequency of her episodes.

TEACHING POINTS

1. **Syncope, that is, a brief loss of consciousness**, may be associated with symptoms suggestive of a vestibular disorder. However, syncope that is caused by impaired central nervous system function cannot be the result of a peripheral vestibular abnormality alone.
2. **Causes of syncope** are listed in Table U12–1. Basilar artery migraine, vertebrobasilar insufficiency, Chiari malformation, and posterior fossa neoplasm are the causes most likely to have vestibular symptoms as part of their presentation.
3. **Basilar artery migraine**, which can be associated with syncope, refers to a condition that includes: (1) visual symptoms, such as tunnel vision and hallucinations; (2) ataxia, vertigo, and sometimes tinnitus; and (3) parathesias of the face and limbs. Other symptoms that can be found include nystagmus, double vision, internuclear ophthalmoplegia, and cranial neuropathy.

REFERENCES

1. Bickerstaff, E: Basilar artery migraine. Lancet 1:15–17, 1961.
2. Hockaday, JM (ed): Migraine in Childhood. London: Butterworths, 1988.
3. Burlet, P: Headache. In Nicholson, B and Schmidt, EB (eds): Harvard Health Letter: A Special Report. Cambridge: Harvard Medical School Health Publications Group, 1992.
4. American Council for Headache Education, Constantine, LM, and Scott, S: Migraine: The Complete Guide. New York: Dell, 1994.
5. Johnson, RH, et al: The autonomic nervous system. In Joynt, RJ (ed): Clinical Neurology (Vol. 4). Philadelphia: JB Lippincott, 1994.

U13

Chronic Fatigue Syndrome

HISTORY

A 28-year-old male accountant complained of a constant sense of lightheadedness, dizziness, and spatial disorientation that he dated to a flulike illness accompanied by fever, chills, and a sore throat 9 months before evaluation. He did not experience vertigo or disequilibrium. Symptoms of disequilibrium were first noticed several weeks after the flulike illness. These were accompanied by a sense of fatigue and decreased "energy." The patient had little fluctuation on a day-to-day basis but noted that symptoms could be exacerbated by fatigue, exertion, stress, and emotional upset. He did not describe true vertigo or exacerbation of symptoms with rapid head movement. He had a sense of weakness in the legs but no complaint of hearing loss or tinnitus. There was no significant past medical history. The family history was negative for neurologic or otologic disease.

The patient's primary care physician had obtained an MRI scan, which was normal. The patient had reduced his workload as an accountant from full time to part time.

Question 1: Based on the patient's history, what are the diagnostic considerations?

Answer 1: This patient's history is quite nonspecific and gives little indication of a vestibular disorder, especially of a peripheral vestibular abnormality. A nonvestibular cause of dizziness should be considered (see Case U10). The role of the patient's flulike illness is uncertain.

PHYSICAL EXAMINATION

The general examination was normal. Neurologic examination was normal with the exception of a slightly wide-based gait. The patient's sway during Romberg's test was

302

somewhat increased, but he did not fall. He also swayed but did not fall while standing on a compliant foam surface with his eyes either open or closed. Otologic examination was normal.

Question 2: How does the physical examination add to the diagnostic considerations? What laboratory testing, if any, would be helpful in establishing a diagnosis?

Answer 2: The physical examination provides little additional information regarding diagnostic possibilities. Laboratory testing may provide additional help in establishing a diagnosis. Vestibular laboratory testing in particular is appropriate because of this patient's complaint of spatial disorientation and disequilibrium. Screening blood studies are appropriate. The patient's complaint of chronic fatigue and decreased energy level suggests the possibility of a persistent viral infection, such as with the Epstein-Barr virus.

Laboratory Testing

Vestibular Laboratory Testing

ELECTRONYSTAGMOGRAPHY:	Ocular motor function was normal. There was no static or paroxysmal positional nystagmus. Caloric irrigations were normal.
ROTATIONAL TESTING:	Normal
POSTUROGRAPHY:	Posturography indicated excessive postural sway in a nonspecific pattern.

Audiometric Testing: Not performed

Imaging: Not performed

Other: Blood studies suggest a reactivated Epstein-Barr virus infection.

DIAGNOSIS/DIFFERENTIAL DIAGNOSIS

Question 3: Based on the additional information from laboratory studies, what are the diagnostic possibilities?

Answer 3: This patient's laboratory testing suggests a nonspecific disorder that may or may not involve the vestibular system, considering the isolated nonspecific abnormalities on posturography. Possibly, the patient's flulike illness 9 months before evaluation was related to the Epstein-Barr virus, and his persistent symptoms are in some way related to this previous virus infection.

Question 4: What is chronic fatigue syndrome? What are the balance symptoms associated with chronic fatigue syndrome? What is the relationship, if any, between Epstein-Barr virus infection and chronic fatigue syndrome?

Answer 4: Chronic fatigue syndrome is a disorder characterized by fatigue, malaise, decreased "energy," and disequilibrium.[1,2] Some patients experience depression.[2] The cause is unknown. Patients with this syndrome may have elevated Epstein-Barr virus antibody titers.[3] Two studies have documented nonspecific postural sway abnormalities in patients with chronic fatigue syndrome.[4,5] A vestibular origin for this disequilibrium is uncertain.[5]

This patient was given a diagnosis of *chronic fatigue syndrome.*

TREATMENT/MANAGEMENT

The patient was treated with vestibular rehabilitation. Several mild vestibular suppressants, including meclizine and diazepam, were prescribed but worsened symptoms. The patient did not benefit from a trial of amitriptyline. During an 18-month period following evaluation, the patient gradually recovered from his symptoms and was able to return to his work as an accountant on a full-time basis.

SUMMARY

A 28-year-old male accountant presented with a constant sense of dizziness, disequilibrium, and lightheadedness that had persisted for 9 months. The patient dated the onset of his symptoms to a flulike illness unaccompanied by vertigo. The physical examination revealed only increased postural sway during standing. The MRI was normal. Vestibular laboratory testing indicated increased postural sway without obvious vestibular system involvement. Blood studies indicated an elevated Epstein-Barr virus titer consistent with a previous infection. The patient was given the diagnosis of *chronic fatigue syndrome.* The significance of the elevated Epstein-Barr virus titer was considered questionable. Treatment consisted of a trial of vestibular-suppressant medications, which were not helpful, and balance therapy. The patient gradually improved during the 18 months following evaluation.

TEACHING POINTS

1. **Chronic fatigue syndrome** is a disorder characterized by fatigue, malaise, decreased "energy," and, not uncommonly, disequilibrium.
2. **Disequilibrium associated with chronic fatigue syndrome** is of uncertain etiology. Nonspecific postural sway abnormalities are commonly observed that do not aid in the localization of this disorder.
3. **The cause of chronic fatigue syndrome** is unknown. Although it has been suggested that patients with chronic fatigue syndrome are more likely to have elevated Epstein-Barr virus titers, this finding has not been substantiated in the literature.
4. **Treatment of chronic disequilibrium associated with chronic fatigue syndrome** consists of a trial of vestibular-suppressant medications and vestibular rehabilitation (see C18 for the treatment of nonspecific vestibulopathy). Gradual improvement with periods of waxing and waning of symptoms may be expected.

REFERENCES

1. Schluederberg, A, et al: Chronic fatigue syndrome research. Ann Intern Med 117:325–331, 1992.
2. Komaroff, AL: Clinical presentation of chronic fatigue syndrome. In Bock, GR, and Whelan, J (eds): Chronic Fatigue Syndrome. New York: Wiley, 1993, pp 43–61.

3. Komaroff, AL: Experience with sporadic and ''epidemic'' cases. In Dawson, DM, and Sabin, TD (eds): Chronic Fatigue Syndrome. Boston: Little, Brown, 1993.
4. Furman, JM: Testing of vestibular function: An adjunct in the assessment of chronic fatigue syndrome. Rev Infect Dis 13 (Suppl 1): S109–S111, 1991.
5. Ash-Bernal, R, et al: Vestibular function test anomalies in patients with chronic fatigue syndrome. Acta Otolaryngol (Stockh) 115(1):9–17, 1995.

C A S E
U14

Mal de Débarquement Syndrome

HISTORY

A 45-year-old woman who worked as a molecular biologist complained of persistent dizziness after a 1-week pleasure cruise in the Caribbean 6 weeks before evaluation. The patient had no prior history of dizziness or disequilibrium and used no medications. During her vacation, she had a sense of malaise and motion sickness while on board ship. These symptoms were mild, not associated with vomiting, and treated successfully by the ship's doctor with medication (most likely scopolamine) that she wore as a patch behind her ear. The patient noted that, while returning home she was bothered by motion sickness during air travel. She had not experienced air sickness previously. Following arrival home, the patient noted a persistent rocking sensation. She had no complaints of hearing loss, tinnitus, or fullness in the ears. The patient had no significant family history. Meclizine had been prescribed, but was not helpful. An MRI scan, requested by the patient's primary care physician, was normal.

Question 1: Based on the patient's history, what are the diagnostic considerations?

Answer 1: This patient has persistent complaints referable to the vestibular system following a sea voyage. Diagnostic considerations include a vestibulopathy or some other balance disorder that coincidentally began during the patient's travel or an unusual syndrome known as *mal de débarquement*. Mal de débarquement has been defined as "sensations of motion experienced on return to stable land after adaptation to motion lasting from hours to days for normal individuals."[1]

PHYSICAL EXAMINATION

The patient had a normal general, neurologic, otologic, and neuro-otologic examination.

Laboratory Testing

Vestibular Laboratory Testing

ELECTRONYSTAGMOGRAPHY: Ocular motor testing, positional testing, and caloric testing were normal.

ROTATIONAL TESTING: Normal

POSTUROGRAPHY: Normal

Audiometric Testing: Not performed

Imaging: An MRI scan of the brain, which the patient received prior to evaluation, was normal.

Other: None

DIAGNOSIS/DIFFERENTIAL DIAGNOSIS

This patient was given the diagnosis of *mal de débarquement syndrome*.

Question 2: What is the pathophysiologic basis of mal de débarquement syndrome?

Answer 2: Mal de débarquement syndrome probably results from the capability of the vestibular system to adapt to various motion environments that include combinations of vestibular and visual stimuli. Animal studies have suggested that even vestibular-induced nystagmus can continue beyond the cessation of a repetitive stimulus.[2] The existence of a rare ocular motor disorder known as periodic alternating nystagmus suggests that the human vestibular system can oscillate indefinitely. Possibly, patients with mal de débarquement syndrome have adapted to an environment that is no longer present and cannot "unadapt." That is, they have adapted to the environment on board ship, and this is no longer appropriate for dry land. The precise origin of mal de débarquement syndrome is uncertain. Such factors as the otolith organs, hormonal factors, and central nervous system abnormalities have been postulated but not proved to be related to the syndrome.[3]

TREATMENT/MANAGEMENT

Question 3: What treatments should be considered for mal de débarquement syndrome?

Answer 3: Considerations for treatment of mal de débarquement syndrome include vestibular suppressants such as meclizine and promethazine, anxiolytics such as diazepam, antidepressants such as amitriptyline, and the carbonic anhydrase inhibitor acetazolamide.[3]

Before evaluation, the patient failed treatment with meclizine. Low-dose diazepam, 2 mg PO bid, was prescribed with some benefit. The patient was also enrolled in a course of balance rehabilitation therapy. Over the course of the subsequent 3 to 6 months, her symptoms gradually declined.

SUMMARY

A 45-year-old woman presented with the complaint of 6 weeks of persistent dizziness and disequilibrium characterized by a sense of rocking and imbalance that began following a 1-week sea voyage. The patient did not gain relief from meclizine. Physical examination, brain imaging, and vestibular laboratory testing were all normal. Low-dose diazepam and a vestibular rehabilitation program provided some relief. The patient's symptoms gradually declined over 3 to 6 months.

TEACHING POINTS

1. **Mal de débarquement syndrome** is an unusual disorder defined as a sensation of motion experienced on return to stable land and after adaptation to motion, lasting from hours to days for normal individuals.
2. **The pathophysiology of mal de débarquement syndrome** is probably related to the capability of the vestibular system to adapt to various motion environments that include combinations of vestibular and visual stimuli. Possibly, patients with mal de débarquement syndrome have adapted to an environment that is no longer present and cannot "unadapt." That is, they have adapted to the environment on board ship, and this is no longer appropriate for dry land. The precise origin of mal de débarquement syndrome is uncertain. Such factors as the otolith organs, hormonal factors, and central nervous system abnormalities have been postulated but not proven to be related to the syndrome.
3. **Treatments for mal de débarquement syndrome** include vestibular suppressants such as meclizine and promethazine, anxiolytics such as diazepam, antidepressants such as amitriptyline, and the carbonic anhydrase inhibitor acetazolamide. Most cases of mal de débarquement syndrome resolve spontaneously within weeks to months.

REFERENCES

1. Brown, JJ, and Baloh, RW: Persistent mal de débarquement syndrome: A motion-induced subjective disorder of balance. Acta Otolaryngol 8:219–222, 1987.
2. Von Baumgarten, RJ: Plasticity in the nervous system at the unitary level. In Schmitt, FO (ed): The Neurosciences: Second Study Program, New York: Rockefeller University, 1970.
3. Murphy, TP: Mal de débarquement syndrome: A forgotten entity? Otolaryngol Head Neck Surg 109:10–13, 1993.

U15

Prion Disease

HISTORY

A 50-year-old sales representative presented with a chief complaint of dizziness of 2 months' duration. The patient noted that his symptoms were constant, characterized by a sense of lightheadedness and disequilibrium, associated with poor balance. Additional symptoms included some difficulty with vision and poor concentration. The patient's symptoms had been slowly progressive following a subacute onset. He had no complaint of hearing loss or tinnitus. There was no family history of neurologic or otologic disease. The patient had no important past medical history and used no medications.

Question 1: Based on the patient's history, what are the diagnostic considerations?

Answer 1: This patient has a very nonspecific history consistent with both vestibular and nonvestibular causes of dizziness. His condition appears to be progressive, and the complaints of poor vision and difficulty with concentration, although consistent with a vestibular system abnormality, are more likely to be symptoms of a central nervous system abnormality. Physical examination and appropriate laboratory testing are required to further define this patient's problem.

PHYSICAL EXAMINATION

The patient had a normal general examination except that he was disheveled. He was cooperative and oriented to person and place, but was unsure of the date. He was unable to recall any of three objects at 3 minutes. His blood pressure was normal. There was some slowing of speech with mild dysarthria but no aphasia. Eye movement examination revealed poor upgaze and poor convergence, with gaze-evoked nystagmus. There were no other cranial nerve abnormalities. Coordination testing revealed mild dysmetria both of the upper and lower extremities. Strength and sensation were normal. The patient had a wide-based gait and could not tandem walk. He had great difficulty standing with his feet together even with his eyes open, and could not stand with his eyes closed without assistance. Otologic examination was normal.

Question 2: Based on the history and physical examination, what are the diagnostic considerations and what laboratory testing, if any, would be appropriate?

Answer 2: This patient's history and physical examination are consistent with a central nervous system abnormality apparently affecting the cerebellum and possibly the midbrain given poor upgaze and poor convergence. There is little to suggest a vestibular system abnormality. Laboratory testing should certainly include brain imaging and routine blood studies. A lumbar puncture should be considered.

Laboratory Testing

Vestibular Laboratory Testing

ELECTRONYSTAGMOGRAPHY: Not performed

ROTATIONAL TESTING: Not performed

POSTUROGRAPHY: Not performed

Audiometric Testing: Not performed

Imaging: MRI scan of the brain was normal. Cerebrospinal fluid examination was normal.

Other: Blood tests, including a complete blood count, electrolytes, metabolic parameters, thyroid function tests, and rheumatologic parameters were negative.

ADDITIONAL HISTORY

No firm diagnosis was established and the patient was treated with a course of steroids without benefit. The patient's clinical status progressively declined in terms of both balance and cognitive function. Several weeks after the initial evaluation, he was noted to have intermittent myoclonic jerks. He underwent electroencephalography, which revealed diffuse slowing with some sharp waves.

The patient had a relentless course and died 3 months after evaluation. Neuro-pathologic evaluation was consistent with a spongiform encephalopathy.

Question 3: With the laboratory results and additional history, what are the diagnostic considerations?

Answer 3: The differential diagnosis includes spinocerebellar degeneration (see Case C11) with an associated cognitive deficit, paraneoplastic cerebellar degeneration (see Case U2), Alzheimer's disease, an unusual central nervous system neoplasm such as lymphoma, AIDS, progressive multifocal leukoencephalopathy, and the ataxic form of Creutzfeldt-Jakob disease. The last disorder is the most likely because of the constellation of symptoms and signs and the rate of progression.

Question 4: What are the clinical features of Creutzfeldt-Jakob disease? What are the particular features of the ataxic form of Creutzfeldt-Jakob disease? What is the pathophysiology of this condition?

Answer 4: The typical clinical characteristics of Creutzfeldt-Jakob disease include subacute onset of difficulty with memory and concentration. Patients may suffer from disequilibrium, double vision, incoordination, dysarthria, and tremor. Most patients go on to develop myoclonus, including startle-myoclonus, and can also develop corticospinal tract and extrapyramidal symptoms.

Patients with the ataxic form of Creutzfeldt-Jakob disease typically present with abnormalities of gait and limb incoordination. Dysarthria and nystagmus occur early in the course. With time, patients with the ataxic form develop the other symptoms of Creutzfeldt-Jakob disease noted above. Patients deteriorate over a period of weeks to months with a relentless decline in neurologic function.[1,2]

Creutzfeldt-Jakob disease, including the ataxic form, is thought to be caused by an "unconventional virus."[3] Such agents have been called "slow viruses," which cause "slow infections." These agents are called *prions*. Prion is loosely an acronym for a "small proteinaceous infectious particle that resists inactivation by procedures that modify nucleic acids."[4] The agent that causes Creutzfeldt-Jakob disease is thought to be related to the agent or agents that cause other dementing illnesses such as kuru and the Gerstmann-Straussler syndrome.[4,5]

Neuropathologically, there is loss of granule cells with relative sparing of the Purkinje cells in the cerebellum.[2,6] Spongy degeneration, neuronal loss, gliosis, and amyloid plaques also affect vestibular nuclei,[7] the inferior olive, and the dentate nucleus.[8]

DIAGNOSIS/DIFFERENTIAL DIAGNOSIS

This patient's diagnosis was the *ataxic form of Creutzfeldt-Jakob disease*.

SUMMARY

A 50-year-old man presented with a 2-month progressive course of dizziness, disequilibrium, and poor concentration. The patient had no significant past medical history and was using no medications. Incoordination suggested cerebellar system abnormalities. Eye movement abnormalities suggested a cerebellar and possibly a midbrain abnormality. The patient had normal brain imaging. A course of steroids was not helpful. The patient's clinical condition worsened; he developed dementia and myoclonus. An electroencephalogram was diffusely abnormal. The patient died 3 months after evaluation, at which time a neuropathologic evaluation indicated spongiform encephalopathy. The patient's clinical course suggested that he had the ataxic form of Creutzfeldt-Jakob disease.

TEACHING POINTS

1. **Creutzfeldt-Jakob disease** is an unusual neurologic disorder that presents with the subacute onset of difficulty with memory and concentration, disequilibrium, double vision, incoordination, dysarthria, and tremor. Most patients go on to develop myoclonus, including startle-myoclonus, and can also develop corticospinal tract and extrapyramidal symptoms.
2. **An "ataxic form" of Creutzfeldt-Jakob disease** affects a subgroup of patients with this disorder, who present with poor balance, ataxia, and limb incoordination. Dysarthria and nystagmus also may occur early in the course of the disease. With time, patients develop the other typical symptoms of Creutzfeldt-Jakob disease. They deteriorate over a period of weeks to months with a relentless decline in neurologic function.

3. **The cause of Creutzfeldt-Jakob disease**, including its ataxic form, is thought to be caused by an "unconventional virus." Such agents, called *prions*, also have been called "slow viruses," which cause "slow infections."
4. **The balance abnormalities seen in Creutzfeldt-Jakob disease** can be explained by the neuropathologic findings of a loss of granule cells in the cerebellum and spongy degeneration, neuronal loss, gliosis, and amyloid plaques in the inferior olive and dentate nucleus.

REFERENCES

1. Gomori, AJ, Partnow, MJ, and Horoupian, DS: The ataxic form of Creutzfeldt-Jakob disease. Arch Neurol 29:318–323, 1973.
2. Brownell, B, and Oppenheimer, DR: An ataxic form of subacute presenile polioencephalopathy (Creutzfeldt-Jakob disease). J Neurol Neurosurg Psychiatry 28:350–361, 1965.
3. Bale, JF: Disorders caused by unconventional agents. In Joynt, RJ (ed): Clinical Neurology, vol 2. Philadelphia: JB Lippincott, 1994.
4. Prusiner, SB: Prions and neurodegenerative diseases. N Engl J Med 317:1571–1581, 1987.
5. Yee, RD, et al: Abnormal eye movements in Gerstmann-Straussler-Scheinker disease. Arch Ophthalmol 110:68–74, 1992.
6. Lafarga, M, et al: Cytology and organization of reactive astroglia in human cerebellar cortex with severe loss of granule cells: A study of the ataxic form of Creutzfeldt-Jakob disease. Neuroscience 40:337–352, 1991.
7. Manolidis, LS, and Balojannis, SJ: Ultrastructural alterations of the vestibular nuclei in Jacob-Creutzfeld disease. Acta Otolaryngol 95:508–521, 1983.
8. Dow, RS, Kramer, RE, and Robertson, LT: Disorders of the cerebellum. In Joynt, RJ (ed): Clinical Neurology, vol 3. Philadelphia: JB Lippincott, 1994.

C A S E
U16

Drop Attacks

HISTORY

A 36-year-old woman who worked as a librarian presented with a complaint of episodic loss of balance. These attacks had occurred intermittently for 2 years before evaluation. They were stereotyped and characterized by an abrupt loss of balance, causing the patient to feel as if she were being pulled to the ground. There was no associated vertigo or nausea. The patient was unaware of any precipitating factors. Episodes occurred approximately once a month. No episodes has occurred while the patient was driving. However, on several occasions, she fell and suffered bruises.

The patient was evaluated by her primary care physician, who was unable to reach a diagnosis. That evaluation included a negative MRI scan of the brain and negative blood studies including hematologic, metabolic, and rheumatologic parameters.

Question 1: What are the possible explanations for this patient's attacks and what further historical information would be helpful?

Answer 1: The patient's attacks of loss of postural tone could be an indication of brief episodes of loss of consciousness. Thus, detailed questioning of the patient and her family regarding evidence of loss of consciousness is essential. If the patient is suffering from episodic loss of consciousness, her attacks should be labeled as *syncope*, whose differential diagnosis is discussed in Case U12.

If the patient does not lose consciousness during her episodes, the attacks should be labeled as *drop attacks*, abrupt loss of postural tone without loss of consciousness.[1]

Because the patient's attacks occur monthly, any association with menses should be ascertained. Additional important information includes past medical history, especially of any otologic or neurologic abnormality, past or present medication use, and family history.

ADDITIONAL HISTORY

The patient and her family were adamant that the patient did not lose consciousness during these episodes. Despite the abrupt onset and seemingly immediate result of the patient finding herself on the floor, she remembered each episode and was alert, oriented, and conversant immediately following each episode. There was no apparent postictal lethargy or confusion. The patient noted no association between her episodes and menses. Her family history was significant for her mother and sister, who suffered from typical migraine headaches. Also, the patient's past history was significant for "sick headaches" as a teenager, usually associated with menses. These headaches had stopped approximately 15 years before evaluation, when the patient was in her early twenties. She was not currently using any medications.

Question 2: What are the causes of drop attacks?

Answer 2: Drop attacks can be a manifestation of several disease states (Table U16–1), and their origin is often difficult to determine with certainty. In patients with endolymphatic hydrops (see Cases T3, T9, C10, C14, C16), drop attacks sometimes occur and have been labeled *Tumarkin's otolithic crisis*. Presumably, Tumarkin's otolithic crises result from abrupt alterations in otolithic function with concomitant changes in the vestibulospinal system and loss of postural tone without an alteration in level of consciousness. Drop attacks may also be a component of migraine (see Cases C4, C12, U12, and U16). Abrupt loss of postural tone could represent a migraine aura somewhat akin to so-called basilar artery migraine (see Case C12), although this is quite unusual. Another unlikely possibility for the underlying pathophysiology for this patient's drop attacks is a vascular cross-compression syndrome, that is, vascular compression syndrome of the eighth cranial nerve. As discussed in Case U5, this is a poorly understood condition whose very existence is controversial. Drop attacks also can be seen in patients with astatic seizures and in some patients with partial and generalized epilepsy. In addition to these possibilities, one should always be concerned that a patient thought to have drop attacks is actually suffering from syncopal episodes associated with a very brief duration of loss of consciousness. Thus, the conditions discussed in Case U12 should also be considered, especially vertebrobasilar insufficiency, postural hypotension, and simple "faints."

PHYSICAL EXAMINATION

The patient's physical examination was entirely normal, including general, neurologic, otologic, and neuro-otologic examinations.

Question 3: Based on the history and physical examination, what laboratory tests should be ordered?

Answer 3: Based on the discussion above, laboratory testing should include vestibular laboratory testing and an audiogram to search for subclinical hearing loss

TABLE U16–1
Causes of Drop Attacks

Tumarkin's otolithic crisis
Migraine
Vascular compression syndrome of the eighth cranial nerve
Epilepsy
Misrecognized syncope

that may suggest endolymphatic hydrops (see Cases T3, T9, C10, C14, and C16). Electrocochleography should also be considered to detect the presence of endolymphatic hydrops. The patient should also undergo electroencephalography and Holter monitoring.

Laboratory Testing

Vestibular Laboratory Testing

ELECTRONYSTAGMOGRAPHY: Normal

ROTATIONAL TESTING: Normal

POSTUROGRAPHY: Normal

Audiometric Testing: An audiogram and electrocochleography were normal.

Imaging: Not performed

Other: Electroencephalography and Holter monitoring were both normal.

DIAGNOSIS/DIFFERENTIAL DIAGNOSIS

Question 4: Based on the history, physical examination, and laboratory studies, what is this patient's most likely diagnosis?

Answer 4: The patient's diagnosis is uncertain. An unusual variant of migraine, an unusual presentation of endolymphatic hydrops, and vascular compression syndrome of the eighth cranial nerve are the most likely diagnostic considerations.

TREATMENT/MANAGEMENT

Question 5: Based on the differential diagnosis, what treatment, if any, should be instituted?

Answer 5: This patient should be treated for either endolymphatic hydrops, migraine, or vascular compression syndrome of the eighth cranial nerve. The risk-benefit ratio of each of these medications should be carefully considered. Treatment for migraine with a migraine prophylactic agent has little risk in this patient, who has no other medical problems; treatment for endolymphatic hydrops with a diuretic and salt restriction has little risk; treatment for vascular compression syndrome of the eighth cranial nerve has some risk if carbamazepine is selected. However, there is little risk if baclofen is prescribed.

FOLLOW-UP

The patient was advised to begin dietary restriction of foods known to provoke migraine (see Cases C4, C12, U12, and U16) and was treated with a combination of hydrochlorothiazide and triamterene and salt restriction for possible endolymphatic hydrops. She continued to suffer further episodes of loss of postural control for an additional 2 months. Diuretic therapy was discontinued and the patient was started on a calcium-channel blocking agent. She immediately noticed a reduction in the frequency of her attacks. The patient continued this medication for 6 months, during which the attacks tapered off completely. She then discontinued all medications and has done well ever since.

Based on the patient's response to therapy, she received the presumptive and uncertain diagnosis of *drop attacks secondary to migraine*.

SUMMARY

A 36-year-old woman presented with episodes of abrupt loss of postural tone without loss of consciousness. Episodes occurred approximately once a month but were not associated with menses. An extensive evaluation was unable to uncover any objectifiable abnormalities. The patient was treated presumptively for endolymphatic hydrops without success. She was then treated with a calcium-channel blocking agent such as an antimigrainous drug. Her episodes resolved. Following discontinuation of medication, the patient remained symptom-free.

TEACHING POINTS

1. **A "drop attack"** is an abrupt loss of postural tone without loss of consciousness. It is essential that patients with presumed drop attacks be questioned carefully about even brief episodes of loss of consciousness because this would suggest *syncope*, which has a different and more ominous differential diagnosis.
2. **Drop attacks can be a manifestation of several disease states** (see Table U16–1), and their cause is often difficult to determine with certainty.
3. **Tumarkin's otolithic crisis** refers to drop attacks in some patients with endolymphatic hydrops (Meniere's disease). Presumably, Tumarkin's otolithic crises result from abrupt alterations in otolithic function. If a patient is believed to have Tumarkin's otolithic crises, treatment for endolymphatic hydrops with a diuretic and salt restriction is the most appropriate initial therapy.

REFERENCE

1. Kubala, MJ, and Millikan, CH: Diagnosis, pathogenesis, and treatment of "drop attacks." Arch Neurol 11:107–113, 1964.

U17

Horizontal Semicircular Canal Benign Positional Vertigo

HISTORY

A 50-year-old man complained of 3 weeks of positional dizziness. He noted symptoms of brief vertigo that occurred only when rolling over in bed, either to the right or to the left. Otherwise, the patient, who worked as a design engineer, had no symptoms. His past medical history was significant for hypertension, which was treated with a diuretic. Ten years earlier, the patient had had 1 week of positional dizziness that resolved spontaneously. He had no significant family history.

Question 1: Based on the patient's history, what is the differential diagnosis?

Answer 1: This patient's history is highly suggestive of benign positional vertigo (see Cases T1, C9, and C15). Although he may have another cause for episodic vertigo, which has a broad differential diagnosis, benign positional vertigo is most likely.

PHYSICAL EXAMINATION

The patient's general, neurologic, and otologic examinations were normal. On neuro-otologic examination, the patient had a negative Dix-Hallpike maneuver. Also, no nystagmus was seen with Frenzel glasses when the patient was sitting. However, when he was asked to move from a supine to either lateral position or to turn his head to the right or left while his torso was supine, he became vertiginous for approximately 10 seconds and was noted to have horizontal nystagmus that lasted for the same duration as the vertigo. There was associated nausea but no vomiting. The nystagmus was noted

317

to be right-beating in the right-lateral and head-right positions and left-beating in the head-left and left-lateral positions. If the patient maintained a lateral or head-turned position, neither nystagmus nor vertigo persisted after they had decayed.

Laboratory Testing

Vestibular Laboratory Testing

ELECTRONYSTAGMOGRAPHY: Ocular motor function was normal. There was no vestibular nystagmus when the patient was seated, and caloric testing was normal. With static positional testing, however, the patient was noted to have 10 to 15 seconds of nystagmus that was right-beating in the head-right and right-lateral positions and left-beating in the head-left and left-lateral positions.

ROTATIONAL TESTING: Rotational testing was normal.

POSTUROGRAPHY: Posturography was normal.

Audiometric Testing: Not performed

Imaging: Not performed

Other: None

DIAGNOSIS/DIFFERENTIAL DIAGNOSIS

Question 2: Based on the patient's history, physical examination, and laboratory studies, what is the diagnosis?

Answer 2: This patient is suffering from horizontal semicircular canal benign positional vertigo.[1-3] This entity is thought to result from debris in the horizontal semicircular canal endolymph in much the same way that typical (posterior semicircular canal benign positional vertigo) results from debris in the posterior semicircular canal endolymph (see Cases T1, C9, and C15). Interestingly, it is not uncommon to see horizontal canal benign positional vertigo occur transiently after the particle repositioning maneuver for posterior canal benign positional vertigo or some time later after an episode of posterior canal benign positional vertigo.

Question 3: Because patients with horizontal benign positional vertigo experience vertigo and have nystagmus in both lateral positions, how can this condition be lateralized to one ear?

Answer 3: Based on the presumed pathophysiology for this condition (Fig. U17–1), the affected ear is determined by the lateral position that provokes the more intense vertigo and nystagmus.

This patient was given the diagnosis of *horizontal semicircular canal benign positional vertigo*.

TREATMENT/MANAGEMENT

Question 4: What is the treatment for patients with horizontal semicircular canal benign positional vertigo?

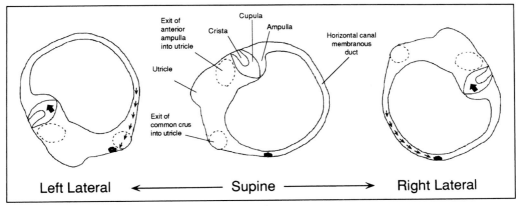

Exit of anterior ampulla into utricle

Cupula

Crista

Ampulla

Horizontal canal membranous duct

Utricle

Exit of common crus into utricle

Left Lateral ← **Supine** → **Right Lateral**

Figure U17-1

Schematic drawing showing presumed pathophysiology of horizontal semicircular canal benign positional vertigo. The right horizontal semicircular canal is illustrated in three panels: left lateral position, supine position, and right lateral position. Small arrows indicate movement of the debris within the endolymph. Large arrows indicate direction of cupula deviation. Movement of the head from the supine position to the right lateral position causes movement of debris in an ampulopedal direction, which causes excitation of the right horizontal semicircular canal and thus, right-beating horizontal nystagmus. Movement of the head from the supine position to the left lateral position causes movement of debris in an ampulofugal direction, which causes inhibition of the right horizontal semicircular canal ampulla and, thus, left-beating horizontal nystagmus. (With permission from Baloh RW, Jacobson K, and Honrubia V. Horizontal semicircular canal variant of benign paroxysmal vertigo. Neurology 43:2542–2549, 1993.[3])

Answer 4: Analogous to the treatment for typical benign positional vertigo, which affects the *posterior* semicircular canal, treatment for *horizontal* semicircular canal benign positional vertigo consists of a particle-repositioning maneuver, turning the patient in the appropriate manner to move the debris that is presumed to be floating in the endolymph of the horizontal semicircular canal into the vestibule. This movement of debris is accomplished by rolling the patient from the supine position toward the unaffected ear, then to the prone position, then to the side-down position with the affected ear down, then back to the supine position (see Fig. U17–1). The maneuver should be performed slowly.

SUMMARY

A 50-year-old male design engineer presented with 3 weeks of positional vertigo. Physical examination disclosed a negative Dix-Hallpike maneuver, but paroxysmal vertigo and nystagmus were elicited during static positional testing. Laboratory testing was negative aside from paroxysmal nystagmus induced by assuming the head-right, head-left, right-lateral, and left-lateral positions. The patient received the diagnosis of horizontal semicircular canal benign positional vertigo. Treatment consisted of a particle-repositioning maneuver, comparable to that used for the treatment of typical posterior semicircular canal benign positional vertigo. After this maneuver, the patient was asymptomatic.

TEACHING POINTS

1. **Horizontal semicircular canal benign positional vertigo** is a variant of typical benign positional vertigo. This entity is thought to result from debris in the en-

dolymph of the horizontal semicircular canal rather than in the posterior semi-circular canal as occurs in typical benign positional vertigo.

2. **The diagnosis of horizontal semicircular canal benign positional vertigo** can be made by turning a patient's head to the right and to the left while the patient is supine. The patient will become vertiginous for 10 to 30 seconds and a horizontal nystagmus will be observed for as long as the vertigo persists. The nystagmus is right-beating in the head-right position and left-beating in the head-left position. If the patient maintains a head-turned position, the direction of nystagmus may briefly reverse, then decay. The nystagmus and vertigo should not persist if the patient maintains the head position. Patients with horizontal semicircular canal benign positional vertigo have vertigo and nystagmus in both head-turned positions. However, when the affected ear is down, the vertigo and nystagmus that are provoked are more intense than those experienced with the unaffected ear down.

3. **Treatment for horizontal semicircular canal benign positional vertigo** consists of a particle-repositioning maneuver. The patient is turned in the appropriate manner to move the debris that is presumed to be floating in the endolymph of the horizontal semicircular canal into the vestibule. This movement of debris is accomplished by rolling the patient from the supine position toward the unaffected ear, then to the prone position and then to the side-down position with the affected ear down, then back to the supine position.

REFERENCES

1. McClure, JA: Horizontal canal BPV. J Otolaryngol 14:30–35, 1985.
2. Pagnini, P, Nuti, D, and Vannucchi, P: Benign paroxysmal vertigo of the horizontal canal. ORL J Otorhin-olaryngol Relat Spec 51:161–170, 1989.
3. Baloh, RW, Jacobson, K, and Honrubia, V: Horizontal semicircular canal variant of benign positional vertigo. Neurology 43:2542–2549, 1993.

Bibliography

Abel, LA, et al: Square wave oscillation. Neuro-ophthalmol 4(1):21–25, 1984.

Amarenco, P, and Hauw, J-J: Cerebellar infarction in the territory of the anterior and inferior cerebellar artery. Brain 113:139–155, 1990.

Amarenco, P, et al: Anterior inferior cerebellar artery territory infarcts. Arch Neurol 50:154–161, 1993.

American Council for Headache Education, Constantine LM, Scott S: Migraine: The complete guide. New York: Dell, 1994.

American Psychiatric Association: Diagnostic and Statistical Manual of Mental Disorders, ed 4. Washington, DC, 1994.

Arenberg, IK, et al: ECoG results in perilymphatic fistula: Clinical and experimental studies. Otolaryngol Head Neck Surg 99(5):435–443, 1988.

Ariyasu, L, et al: The beneficial effect of methylprednisolone in acute in acute vestibular vertigo. Arch Otolaryngol Head Neck Surg 116:700–703, 1990.

Ash-Bernal, R, et al: Vestibular function test anomalies in patients with chronic fatigue syndrome. Acta Otolaryngol (Stockh) 115(1):9–17, 1995.

Bale, JF: Disorders caused by unconventional agents. In Joynt, RJ (ed): Clinical Neurology, Vol 2, Philadelphia: JB Lippincott, 1994.

Baloh, RW: Dizziness, Hearing Loss, and Tinnitus: The Essentials of Neurotology. Philadelphia: FA Davis, 1984.

Baloh, RW: Otological aspects of cerebrovascular disease. In Tool, JF (ed): Handbook of Clinical Neurology, Vol 11(55): Vascular Diseases, Part III. New York: Elsevier Science Publishers B.V., 1989.

Baloh, RW: Bilateral vestibular deficits: Ototoxic, sequential, spontaneous. Clinical Management of Vestibular Disorders. Johns Hopkins University, Personal Communication, 1992.

Baloh, RW, Henn, V, and Jager, J: Habituation of the human vestibulo-ocular reflex by low frequency harmonic acceleration. Am J Otolaryngol 3:235, 1982.

Baloh, RW, and Honrubia, V: Clinical Neurophysiology of the Vestibular System, ed 2: Philadelphia: FA Davis, 1990.

Baloh, RW, Honrubia, V, and Jacobson, K: Benign positional vertigo: Clinical and oculographic features in 240 cases. Neurology 37:371–378, 1987.

Baloh, RW, Jacobson, K, and Honrubia, V: Horizontal semicircular canal variant of benign positional vertigo. Neurology 43:2542–2549, 1993.

Baloh, RW, Jacobson, KM, and Socotch, TM: The effect of aging on visual-vestibuloocular responses. Exp Brain Res 95:509–516, 1993.

Baloh, RW, et al: Quantitative vestibular testing. Otolaryngol Head Neck Surg 92:145–150, 1984.

Baloh, RW, and Spooner, JW: Downbeat nystagmus: A type of central vestibular nystagmus. Neurology 31(3):304–310, 1981.

Bance, M, et al: The changing direction of nystagmus in acute Meniere's disease: Pathophysiological implications. Laryngoscope 101:197–201, 1991.

Barber, HO, and Wright G: Positional nystagmus in normals. Adv Otolaryngol 19:276, 1973.

Barlow, D, and Freedman, W: Cervico-ocular reflex in the normal adult. Acta Otolaryngol (Stockh) 89:487–496, 1980.

Barna, GB, and Hughes, BP: Autoimmunity and otologic disease: Clinical and experimental aspects. Clin Lab Med 8(2):385–398, 1988.

Basser, L: Benign paroxysmal vertigo of childhood. Brain 87:141–152, 1964.

Bassiouny, M, et al: Beta 2 transferrin application in otology. Am J Otol 13(6):552–555, 1992.

Behrman, S, et al: Progressive supranuclear palsy. Brain 92:663–678, 1969.

Belal, A, and Glorig, A: Dysequilibrium of ageing (presbyastasis). J Laryngol Otol 100:1037–1041, 1986.

Bergstrom, B: Morphology of the vestibular nerve. II. The number of myelinated vestibular nerve fibers in man at various ages. Acta Otolaryngol (Stockh) 76:173–179, 1973.

Bhansali, SA: Perilymph fistula. Ear Nose Throat J 68:11–26, 1989.

Bickerstaff, E: Basilar artery migraine. Lancet 1:15–17, 1961.

Bienhold, H, and Flohr, H: Role of commissural connexions between vestibular nuclei in compensation following unilateral labyrinthectomy. J Physiol 284:178, 1978.

Biscaldi, GP, et al: Acute toluene poisoning. Electroneurophysiological and vestibular investigations. Toxicol Eur Res 3(6):271–273, 1981.

Black, FO, et al: Bilateral multiple otosclerotic foci and endolymphatic hydrops. Ann Otol Rhinol Laryngol 78:1062–1073, 1969.

Bluestone, CD: Otitis media and congenital perilymphatic fistula as a cause of sensorineural hearing loss in children. Pediatr Infect Dis J 7:S141–S145, 1988.

Brandt, T: Background, technique, interpretation, and usefulness of positional and positioning testing. In Jacobson, GP, Newman, CW, and Kartush, JM (eds): Handbook of Balance Function Testing. St. Louis: Mosby-Year Book, 1993.

Brandt, T: Vestibular paroxysmia: Vascular compression of the eighth nerve? Lancet 343:798–799, 1994.

Brandt, T, and Daroff, R: Physical therapy for benign paroxysmal positional vertigo. Arch Otolaryngol 106:484–485, 1980.

Brandt, T, and Daroff, R: The multisensory physiological and pathological vertigo syndromes. Ann Neurol 7:195–203, 1980.

Bronstein, A, and Hood, J: The cervico-ocular reflex in normal subjects and patients with absent vestibular function. Brain Res 373:399–408, 1986.

Brookhouse, PE, Worthington, DW, and Kelly, WJ: Noise-induced hearing loss in children. Laryngoscope 102:645–655, 1992.

Brown, DH, McClure, JA, and Downar-Zapolski, Z: The membrane rupture theory of Meniere's disease—Is it valid? Laryngoscope 98:599–601, 1988.

Brown, JJ, and Baloh, RW: Persistent mal de débarquement syndrome: A motion-induced subjective disorder of balance. Acta Otolaryngol (Stockh) 8:219–222, 1987.

Brownell, B, and Oppenheimer, DR: An ataxic form of subacute presenile polioencephalopathy (Creutzfeldt-Jakob disease). J Neurol Neurosurg Psychiatry 28:350–361, 1965.

Burlet, P: Headache. In Nicholson, B, and Schmidt, EB (eds): Harvard Health Letter: A Special Report. Cambridge: Harvard Medical School Health Publications Group, 1992.

Buttner-Ennever, JA (ed): Neuroanatomy of the Oculomotor System. Amsterdam: Elsevier, 1988.

Campbell, KCM, Harker, LA, and Abbas, PJ: Interpretation of electrocohleography in Meniere's disease and normal subjects. Ann Otol Rhinol Laryngol 101:496–500, 1992.

Cannon, SC, and Robinson, DA: The final common integrator is in the prepositus and vestibular nuclei. In Keller, EL, and Zee, DS (eds): Adaptive Processes in Visual and Oculomotor Systems. Oxford: Pergamon Press, 1986.

Caplan, L: Top of the basilar syndrome. Neurology 30:72–79, 1980.

Carl, JR, et al: Head shaking and vestibulo-ocular reflex in congenital nystagmus. Invest Ophthalmol Vis Sci 26(8):1043–1050, 1985.

Case Records of the Massachusetts General Hospital. N Engl J Med, Case 46-1993, 329(21):1560–1567, 1993.

Cass, SP: Role of medications in otological vertigo and balance disorders. Semin Hearing 12(3):257–269, 1991.

Cass, SP, et al: Migraine-related vestibulopathy. J Otolaryngol, 1995 (in press).

Cass, SP, Kartush, JM, and Graham, MD: Patterns of vestibular function following vestibular nerve section. Laryngoscope 102(4):388–394, 1992.

Causse, JR, et al: The enzymatic mechanism of the otospongiotic disease and NaF action on the enzymatic balance. Am J Otol 3:297, 1982.

Cawthorne, TE: Vestibular injuries. Proc R Soc Med 39:270–273, 1945.

Chambers, BR, and Gresty, MA: The relationship between disordered pursuit and vestibulo-ocular reflex suppression. J Neurol Neurosurg Psychiatry 46:61–66, 1983.

Coats, AC: Vestibular neuronitis. Acta Otolaryngol (Stockh) (Suppl)251:5–28, 1969.

Cody, DT, and Baker, HL: Otosclerosis: Vestibular symptoms and sensorineural hearing loss. Ann Otol 87:778–796, 1978.

Cohen, B, Matsuo, V, and Raphan, T: Quantitative analysis of the velocity characteristics of optokinetic nystagmus and optokinetic after-nystagmus. J Physiol 270:321–344, 1977.

Colletti, V, et al: Vestibular neurectomy and microvascular decompression of the cochlear nerve in Meniere's disease. Skull Base Surg 4:65–71, 1994.

Collewijn, H, et al: Human ocular counterroll: Assessment of static and dynamic properties from electromagnetic scleral coil recordings. Exp Brain Res 59:185–196, 1985.

Collins, WE: Arousal and vestibular habituation. In Kornhuber, HH (ed): Vestibular System, Part 2: Psychophysics, Applied Aspects and General Interpretations. Berlin: Springer-Verlag, 1974.

Cooksey, FS: Rehabilitation in vestibular injuries. Proc R Soc Med 39:275, 1945.

Crampton, GH (ed): Motion and space sickness. Boca Raton: CRC Press, 1990.

Cutrer, FW, and Baloh, RW: Migraine-associated dizziness. Headache 32(6):300–304, 1992.

Dandy, WE: Meniere's disease: Its diagnosis and methods of treatment. Arch Surg 16:1127–1152, 1928.

De Jong, PTV, et al: Ataxia and nystagmus induced by injection of local anesthetics in the neck. Ann Neurol 1(3):240–246, 1977.

Demer, JL, and Zee, DS: Vestibulo-ocular and optokinetic deficits in albinos with congenital nystagmus. Invest Ophthalmol Vis Sci 25:739–745, 1984.

Dickins, JRE, Smith, JT, and Graham, SS: Herpes zoster oticus: Treatment with intravenous acyclovir. Laryngoscope 98:776–779, 1988.

Dieterich, M, and Brandt, M: Wallenberg's Syndrome: Lateropulsion, cyclorotation, and subjective visual vertical in thirty-six patients. Ann Neurol 31(4):399–408, 1992.

Digre, KB: Opsoclonus in adults. Arch Neurol 43:1165–1175, 1986.

Dix, MR, and Hallpike, CS: The pathology, symptomology and diagnosis of certain common disorders of the vestibular system. Proc R Soc Med 45:341–354, 1952.

Dix, MR, and Hood, JD: Vestibular habituation: Its clinical significance and relationship to vestibular neuronitis. Laryngoscope 80:226–232, 1970.

Dizziness: Hope through research. Prepared by the Office of Scientific and Health Reports, NICDS, NIH Publication No. 86–76, pp 5–6, September 1986.

Dow, RS, Kramer, RE, and Robertson, LT: Disorders of the cerebellum. In Joynt, RJ (ed): Clinical Neurology, Vol 3. Philadelphia: JB Lippincott, 1994.

Drachman, DA, Diamond, ER, and Hart, CW: Posturally-evoked vomiting: Association with posterior fossa lesions. Ann Otol (86):97–101, 1977.

Drachman, DA, and Hart, CW: An approach to the dizzy patient. Neurology 22:323–334, 1972.

Duncan, P, et al: Functional reach: A new clinical measure of balance. J Gerontol 45:192–197, 1990.

Emmett, JR, and Shea, JJ: Traumatic perilymph fistula. Laryngoscope 90:1513–1520, 1980.

Engstrom, H, et al: Structural changes in the vestibular epithelia in elderly monkeys and humans. Adv Otorhinolaryngol 22:93–110, 1977.

Epley, JM: The canalith repositioning procedure: For treatment of benign paroxysmal positional vertigo. Otolaryngol Head Neck Surg 107:399–404, 1992.

Eviatar, L: Vestibular testing in basilar artery migraine. Ann Neurol 9:126–130, 1980.

Ferraro, JA, Arenberg, K, and Hassanein, S: Electrocochleography and symptoms of inner ear dysfunction. Arch Otolaryngol 111:71–74, 1985.

Fisher, CM: Vertigo in cerebrovascular disease. Arch Otolaryngol 85:529–534, 1967.

Fitz-Ritson, D: Assessment of cervicogenic vertigo. J Manipulative Physiol Ther 14(3):193–198, 1991.

Flohr, H, and Luneburg, U: Effects of ACTH on vestibular compensation. Brain Res 248:169–173, 1982.

Fluur, E: A comparison between subjective and objective recording of ocular counter-rolling as a result of tilting. Acta Otolaryngol (Stockh) 79:111–114, 1975.

Forster, FM, and Booker, HE: The epilepsies and convulsive disorders. In Joynt, RI (ed): Clinical Neurology, Vol 3. Philadelphia: JB Lippincott, 1994.

Fukuda, T: The stepping test. Acta Otolaryngol (Stockh) 50:95–108, 1959.

Furman, JM: Testing of vestibular function: An adjunct in the assessment of chronic fatigue syndrome. Rev Infect Dis (Suppl)1(13):S109–11, 1991.

Furman, JM: Nystagmus and the vestibular system. In Podos, SM, and Yanoff, M (eds): Textbook of Ophthalmology. New York: Gower Medical Publishers, 1993.

Furman, JM: Posturography: Uses and Limitations. Bailliere's Clinical Neurology 3(3):501–513, 1994.

Furman, JM, and Becker, JT: Vestibular responses in Wernicke's encephalopathy. Ann Neurol 26:669–674, 1989.

Furman, JM, Crumrine, PK, and Reinmuth, OM: Epileptic nystagmus. Ann Neurol 27:686–688, 1990.

Furman, JM, Durrant, JD, and Hirsch, WL: Eighth nerve signs in a case of multiple sclerosis. Am J Otolaryngol 10:376–381, 1989.

Furman, JM, Eidelman, BH, and Fromm, GH: Spontaneous remission of paraneoplastic saccadic fixation instability. Neurology 38(3):499–501, 1988.

Furman, JM, and Kamerer, DB: Rotational responses in patients with bilateral caloric reduction. Acta Otolaryngol (Stockh) 108:355–361, 1989.

Furman, JM, Wall III, C, and Pang, D: Vestibular function in periodic alternating nystagmus. Brain 113:1425–1439, 1990.

Gacek, RR: Transection of the posterior ampulary nerve for relief of benign paroxysmal positional vertigo. Ann Otol Rhinol Laryngol 83:596–605, 1974.

Gacek, RR: Singular neurectomy update II: Review of 102 cases. Laryngoscope 101:855–862, 1991.

Ghez, C: Vestibular paresis: A clinical feature of Wernicke's disease. J Neurol Neurosurg Psychiatry 32:132–139, 1969.

Gilman, S, Bloedel, JR, and Lechtenberg, R (eds): Disorders of the Cerebellum. Philadelphia: FA Davis, 1981.

Glasscock, ME, McKennan, KX, and Levine, SC: Persistent traumatic perilymph fistulas. Laryngoscope 97:860–864, 1987.

Gomori, AJ, Partnow, MJ, and Horoupian, DS: The ataxic form of Creutzfeldt-Jakob disease. Arch Neurol 29:318–323, 1973.

Grad, A, and Baloh, RW: Vertigo of vascular origin. Arch Neurol 46:281–284, 1989.

Grenman, R: Involvement of the audiovestibular system in multiple sclerosis: An otoneurologic and audiologic study. Acta Otolaryngol (Stockh) (Suppl)420:1–95, 1985.

Gresty, MA, et al: Assessment of vestibulo-ocular reflexes in congenital nystagmus. Ann Neurol 17:129–136, 1985.

Griffith, AJ: Biological and clinical aspects of autoimmune inner ear disease. Yale J Biol Med 65:17–28, 1992.

Gyntelberg, F, et al: Acquired intolerance to organic solvents and results of vestibular testing. Am J Ind Med 9:363–370, 1986.

Hain, TC, Fetter, M, and Zee, DS: Head-shaking nystagmus in patients with unilateral peripheral vestibular lesions. Am J Otolaryngol 8:36–47, 1987.

Hain, TC, Zee, DS, and Maria, BL: Tilt suppression of vestibulo-ocular reflex in patients with cerebellar lesions. Acta Otolaryngol (Stockh) 105:13–20, 1988.

Hall, SF, Ruby, RRF, and McClure, JA: The mechanics of benign paroxysmal vertigo. J Otolaryngol 8:151–158, 1979.

Halmagyi, GM, et al: Tonic contraversive ocular tilt reaction due to unilateral meso-diencephalic lesion. Neurology 40:1503–1509, 1990.

Halmagyi, G, and Curthoys, I: A clinical sign of canal paresis. Arch Neurol 45:737–739, 1988.

Hamid, M, Hughes, G, and Kinney, S: Criteria for diagnosing bilateral vestibular dysfunction. In Graham, MD, and Kemink, JL (eds): The Vestibular System: Neurophysiologic and Clinical Research. New York: Raven Press, 1987, pp 115–118.

Hamid, MA, et al: ENG-MRI correlates in cerebellar oculomotor dysfunction. Otolaryngol Head Neck Surg 99:302–308, 1988.

Harada, Y (ed): The Vestibular Organs. New York: Kugler and Guedini, 1988.

Harris, JP: Immunologic mechanisms in disorders of the inner ear. Otolaryngol Head Neck Surg, Update 1, Chapter 26, 1989, pp 380–395.

Herdman, SJ (ed): Vestibular Rehabilitation. Philadelphia: FA Davis, 1994.

Herr, RD, Zun, L, and Mathews, JJ: A directed approach to the dizzy patient. Ann Emerg Med 18(6):664/101–672/109, 1989.

Hillel, AD: History of stapedectomy. Am J Otolaryngol 4:131–140, 1983.

Hirsch, BE, et al: Localizing retrocochlear hearing loss. Am J Otol, 1995 (submitted for publication).

Hockaday, JM (ed): Migraine in Childhood. London: Butterworth Publishers, 1988.

Hodgson, MJ, et al: Encephalopathy and vestibulopathy following short-term hydrocarbon exposure. J Occup Med 31(1):51–54, 1989.

House, JW, and Brackmann, DE: Facial nerve grading system. Otol Laryngol Head Neck Surg 93:146–147, 1985.

Hughes, GB, et al: Predictive value of laboratory tests in "autoimmune" inner ear disease: Preliminary report. Laryngoscope 96:502–505, 1986.

Hughes, GB, Sismanis, A, and House, JW: Is there consensus in perilymph fistula management? Otolaryngol Head Neck Surg 102:111, 1990.

Hunt, JF: Herpetic inflammations of the geniculate ganglion: A new syndrome and its aural complications. Arch Otol 36:371–381, 1907.

Huygen, PLM, Verhagen, WIM, and Nicolasen, MGM: Cervico-ocular reflex enhancement in labyrinthine-defective and normal subjects. Exp Brain Res 87:457–464, 1991.

Hyden, D, et al: Impairment of visuo-vestibular interaction in humans. ORL J Otorhinolaryngol Relat Spec 45:262–269, 1983.

Igarashi, M: Physical exercise and acceleration of vestibular compensation. In Lacour, M, et al (eds): Vestibular Compensation. Amsterdam: Elsevier, 1989.

Jacker, RK, and Dillon, WP: Computed tomography and magnetic resonance imaging of the inner ear. Otolaryngol Head Neck Surg 99:494–504, 1988.

Jackler, RK, and De La Cruz, A: The large vestibular aqueduct syndrome. Laryngoscope 99:1238–1243, 1989.

Jackler, RK, et al: Endolymphatic sac surgery in congenital malformations of the inner ear. Laryngoscope 98:698–794, 1988.

Jackson, CG, Glasscock, ME, and Davis, WE: Medical management of Meniere's disease. Ann Otol 90:142–147, 1981.

Jacob, RG: Panic disorder and the vestibular system. Psychiatr Clin North Am 11:361–374, 1988.

Jacob, RG, Furman, JM, and Balaban, CD: Psychiatric aspects of vestibular disorders. In Baloh, RW, and Halmagyi, M (eds): Handbook of Neurotology/Vestibular System. New York: Oxford University Press (in press).

Jacob, RG, et al: Psychogenic dizziness. In Barber, HO, and Sharpe, JA (eds): The Vestibular Ocular Reflex, Nystagmus, and Vertigo. New York: Raven Press, 1993.

Jacob, RG, et al: Discomfort with space and motion: A possible marker of vestibular dysfunction assessed by the Situational Characteristics Questionnaire. J Psychopathol Beh Assessment 15:299–324, 1993.

Jacobson, GP, and Newman, CW: The development of the dizziness handicap inventory. Arch Otolaryngol Head Neck Surg 116:424–427, 1990.

Jacobson, GP, and Newman, CW: Handbook of Balance Function Testing. St. Louis: Mosby-Year Book, 1993.

Jannetta, PJ, Moller, MB, and Moller, AR: Disabling positional vertigo. N Engl J Med 310:1700–1705, 1984.

"JC": Living without a balancing mechanism. N Engl J Med 246:458–460, 1952.

Jenkins, HA, et al: Dysequilibrium of aging. Otolaryngol Head Neck Surg 100(4):272–282, 1989.

Johnson, RH, Lambie, DG, and Spalding, JMK: The autonomic nervous system. In Joynt, RJ (ed): Clinical Neurology, Vol 4. Philadelphia: JB Lippincott, 1994.

Jongkees, LBW: Cervical vertigo. Laryngoscope 79:1473–1484, 1969.

Kamei, T, and Kornhuber, H: Spontaneous and head-shaking nystagmus in normals and in patients with central lesions. Can J Otolaryngol 3:372–380, 1974.

Kamerer, DB, Furman, JM, and Whitney, SL: Vestibular System Evaluation and Rehabilitation. St. Louis: Mosby-Year Book, 1991.

Kandell, ER, and Schwartz, JH (eds): Principles of Neural Science, ed 2. Elsevier, New York, 1985.

Kasai, T, and Zee, DS: Eye-head coordination in labyrinthine-defective human beings. Brain Res 144:123–141, 1978.

Katz, J (ed): Handbook of Clinical Audiology. Baltimore: Williams & Wilkins, 1994.

Kayan, A, and Hood, JD: Neuro-otological manifestations of migraine. Brain 107:1123–1142, 1984.

Kemink, JL, et al: Transmatoid labyrinthectomy: Reliable surgical management of vertigo. Otolaryngol Head Neck Surg 101:5–10, 1989.

Kogeorgos, J, Scott, DF, and Swash, M: Epileptic dizziness. Br Med J 282:687–689, 1981.

Komaroff, AL: Clinical presentation of chronic fatigue syndrome. In Bock, GR, and Whelan, J (eds): Chronic Fatigue Syndrome. New York: Wiley, 1993, pp 43–61.

Komaroff, AL: Experience with sporadic and "epidemic" cases. In Dawson, DM, and Sabin, TD (eds): Chronic Fatigue Syndrome. Boston: Little, Brown, 1993.

Konrad, HR: Intractable vertigo—When not to operate. Otolaryngol Head Neck Surg 95:482–484, 1986.

Korzec, K, et al: Gadolinium-enhanced magnetic resonance imaging of the facial nerve in herpes zoster oticus and Bell's palsy: Clinical implication. Am J Otol 12(3):163–168, 1991.

Koziol-McLain, J, et al: Orthostatic vital signs in emergency department patients. Ann Emerg Med 20:806–810, 1991.

Krejcova, H, et al: Otoneurological symptomatology in Lyme disease. Adv Otorhinolaryngol 42:210–212, 1988.

Kubala, MJ, and Millikan, CH: Diagnosis, pathogenesis, and treatment of "Drop Attacks." Arch Neurol 11:107–113, 1964.

Lafarga, M, et al: Cytology and organization of reactive astroglia in human cerebellar cortex with severe loss of granule cells: A study of the ataxic form of Creutzfeldt-Jakob disease. Neuroscience 40(2):337–352, 1991.

Langman, AW, Kemink, JL, and Graham, MD: Titration streptomycin therapy for bilateral Meniere's disease. Ann Otol Rhinol Laryngol 99:923–926, 1990.

Lanzi, G, et al: Benign paroxysmal vertigo of childhood: A long follow-up. Cephalalgia 14:458–460, 1994.

Lawrence, M: Possible influence of cochlear otosclerosis on inner ear fluids. Ann Otol Rhinol Laryngol 75:553–558, 1966.

Leigh, RJ, and Zee, DS: The Neurology of Eye Movements, ed 2. Philadelphia: FA Davis, 1991.

LeLiever, WC: Comparative repositioning maneuvers for benign paroxysmal positional vertigo. Proceedings from the COSM Meeting, Palm Beach, Florida, May 7–13, 1994.

LeLiever, WC, and Barber, HO: Recurrent vestibulopathy. Laryngoscope 91:1–6, 1981.

Levenson, MJ, et al: The large vestibular aqueduct syndrome in children. Arch Otolaryngol Head Neck Surg 115:54–58, 1989.

Lin, J, et al: Direction-changing positional nystagmus: Incidence and meaning. Am J Otolaryngol 7:306–310, 1986.

Longridge, NS, and Mallinson, AI: A discussion of the dynamic illegible "E" test: A new method of screening for aminoglycoside vestibulotoxicity. Otolaryngol Head Neck Surg 92:671–677, 1984.

Longridge, NS, and Mallinson, AI: The dynamic illegible E-test. Acta Otolaryngol (Stockh) 103:273–279, 1987.

Luetje, CM: Theoretical and practical implications for plasmapheresis in autoimmune inner ear disease. Laryngoscope 99:1137–1146, 1989.

Lundborg, T: Diagnostic problems concerning acoustic tumors. Acta Otolaryngol (Stockh) (Suppl)99:1–111, 1950.

Mackenzie, M, and Wolfenden, N: Otosclerosis. J Laryngol Otol 69:437–456, 1955.

Manolidis, LS, and Balojannis, SJ: Ultrastructural alterations of the vestibular nuclei in Jacob-Creutzfeld disease. Acta Otolaryngol (Stockh) 95:508–521, 1983.

McCabe, BF: Autoimmune inner ear disease: Therapy. Am J Otolaryngol 10(3):196–197, 1989.

McCabe, BF: Otosclerosis and vertigo. Trans Pacific Coast Oto-Ophthalmol Soc Ann Meeting 47:37–42, 1966.

McClure, JA: Horizontal canal BPV. J Otolaryngol 14(1):30–35, 1985.

McClure, JA, Copp, JC, and Lycett, P: Recovery nystagmus in Meniere's disease. Laryngoscope 91:1727–1737, 1981.

McKenna, MJ, and Mills, BG: Immunohistochemical evidence of measles virus antigens in active otosclerosis. Otolaryngol Head Neck Surg 102(4):415–421, 1989.

Melvill Jones, G: Adaptive modulation of VOR parameters by vision. In Berthoz, A, and Melvill Jones, G (eds): Adaptive Mechanisms in Gaze Control: Reviews in Oculomotor Research. Amsterdam: Elsevier, 1985, pp 21–50.

Melvill Jones, G, and Berthoz, A: Mental control of the adaptive process. In Berthoz, A, and Melvill Jones, G (eds): Adaptive Mechanisms in Gaze Control. Amsterdam: Elsevier, 1985.

Meyerhoff, WL, et al: Progressive sensorineural hearing loss in children. Otolaryngol Head Neck Surg 110(6):569–579, 1994.

Meyerhoff, WL, Paparella, MM, and Shea, D: Meniere's disease in children. Laryngoscope 88:1504–1511, 1978.

Moller, AR: Auditory Neurophysiology. J Clin Neurophysiol 11(3):284–308, 1994.

Moller, AR, and Jannetta, PJ: Neural generators of the brainstem auditory evoked potentials. In Nodar, RH, and Barber, C (eds): Evoked Potentials II: The Second International Evoked Potentials Symposium. Boston: Butterworth Publishers, 1984.

Moller, MB, et al: Microvascular decompression of the eighth nerve in patients with disabling positional vertigo: Selection criteria and operative results in 207 patients. Acta Neurochir (Wien) 125:75–82, 1993.

Monday, LA, and Tetrault, L: Hyperventilation and vertigo. Laryngoscope 109:1003–1010, 1980.

Money, K, Johnson, W, and Corlett, R: Role of semicircular canals in positional alcohol nystagmus. Am J Physiol 208(6):1065–1070, 1965.

Monsell, EM, Brackmann, DE, and Linthicum, FH: Why do vestibular destructive procedures sometimes fail? Otolaryngol Head Neck Surg 99:472–479, 1988.

Monsell, EM, Cass, SP, and Rybak, LP: Chemical labyrinthectomy: Methods and results. In Brackmann, DE (ed): Otologic Surgery, Philadelphia: WB Saunders, 1994.

Monsell, EM, and Wiet, RJ: Endolymphatic sac surgery: Methods of study and results. Am J Otol 9(5):396–402, 1988.

Monsell, EM, et al: Surgical treatment of vertigo with retrolabyrinthine vestibular neurectomy. Laryngoscope 98:835–839, 1988.

Moore, BE, and Atkinson, M: Psychogenic vertigo. Arch Otolaryngol 67:347–353, 1958.

Morales-Garcia, C: Cochleo-vestibular involvement in otosclerosis. Acta Otolaryngol (Stockh) 73:484–492, 1972.

Moriarty, B, Rutka, J, and Hawke, M: the incidence and distribution of cupular deposits in the labryrinth. Laryngoscope 109:56–59, 1992.

Moscatello, AL, et al: Otolaryngologic aspects of Lyme disease. Laryngoscope 101:592–595, 1991.

Moscicki, RA, et al: Serum antibody to inner ear proteins in patients with progressive hearing loss. JAMA 272(8):611–616, 1994.

Murphy, TP: Mal de débarquement syndrome: A forgotten entity? Otolaryngol Head Neck Surg 109:10–13, 1993.

Nakada, T, and Kwee, I: Oculopalatal myoclonus. Brain 109:431–441, 1986.

National Institute on Deafness and Other Communication Disorders, NIH: A Report of the Task Force on the National Strategic Research Plan, April 1989, 1983, pp 74, 168.

Nedzelski, JM: Cerebellopontine angle tumors: Bilateral flocculus compression as cause of associated oculomotor abnormalities. Laryngoscope 93:1251–1260, 1983.

Nedzelski, JM, Barber, HO, and McIlmoyl, L: Diagnoses in a dizziness unit. J Otolaryngol 15(2):101–104, 1986.

Neuhuber, WL, and Zenker, W: Central distribution of cervical primary afferents in the rat, with emphasis on proprioceptive projects to vestibular, perihypoglossal, and upper thoracic spinal nuclei. J Comp Neurol 280:231–253, 1989.

NeuroCom International Inc. EquiTest System Operator's Manual (Version 4.0), Clackamas, Oregon.

Nielsen, JM: Tornado epilepsy simulating Meniere's syndrome. Neurology 9:794–796, 1959.

Niklasson, M, et al: Effects of toluene, styrene, trichloroethylene, and trichloromethane on the vestibulo- and opto-oculo motor system in rats. Neurotoxicol Teratol 15:327–334, 1993.

Oas, JG, and Baloh, RW: Vertigo and the anterior inferior cerebellar artery syndrome. Neurology 42:2274–2279, 1992.

Odkvist, LM, et al: Vestibular and oculomotor disturbances caused by industrial solvents. J Otolaryngol 9:53–59, 1980.

Odkvist, LM, et al: Vestibulo-oculomotor disturbances in humans exposed to styrene. Acta Otolaryngol (Stockh) 94:487–493, 1982.

Odkvist, LM, Moller, C, and Thuomas, K-A: Otoneurologic disturbances caused by solvent pollution. Otolaryngol Head Neck Surg 106:687, 1992.

Olsson, J: Neurotologic findings in basilar migraine. Laryngoscope 101:1–41, 1991.

Oosterveld, WJ, et al: Electronystagmographic findings following cervical whiplash injuries. Acta Otolaryngol (Stockh) 111:201–205, 1991.

Pagnini, P, Nuti, D, and Vannucchi, P: Benign paroxysmal vertigo of the horizontal canal. ORL J Otorhinolaryngol Relat Spec 51:161–170, 1989.

Paige, GD: Senescence of human visual-vestibular interactions. J Vest Res 2:133–151, 1992.

Paparella, MM: The cause (multifactorial inheritance) and pathogenesis (endolymphatic malabsorption) of Meniere's disease and its symptoms (mechanical and chemical). Acta Otolaryngol (Stockh) 99:445–451, 1985.

Paparella, MM, and Chasen, WD: Otosclerosis and vertigo. J Laryngol Otol 80:511–517, 1966.

Paparella, MM, Mancini, F, and Liston, SL: Otosclerosis and Meniere's syndrome: Diagnosis and treatment. Laryngoscope 94:1414–1417, 1984.

Parisier, SC, and Birken, EA: Recurrent meningitis secondary to idiopathic oval window CSF leak. Laryngoscope 86:1503–1515, 1976.

Parnes, LS, and McClure, JA: Posterior semicircular canal occlusion for intractable benign paroxysmal positional vertigo. Ann Otol Rhinol Laryngol 99:330–334, 1990.

Parnes, LS, and McClure, JA: Posterior semicircular canal occlusion in the normal hearing ear. Otolaryngol Head Neck Surg 104:52–57, 1991.

Parnes, LS, and McClure, JA: Free-floating endolymph particles: A new finding during posterior semicircular canal occlusion. Laryngoscope 102:988–992, 1992.

Parnes, LS, and Price-Jones, R: Particle repositioning maneuver for benign paroxysmal positional vertigo. Ann Otol Rhinol Laryngol 102:325–331, 1993.

Peitersen, E: Vestibulospinal reflexes. Arch Otolaryngol 79:481–486, 1976.

Peppard, SB: Effect of drug therapy on compensation from vestibular injury. Laryngoscope 96:878–898, 1986.

Peterka, R, and Black, F: Age-related changes in human posture control: Sensory organization tests. J Vest Res 1:73–85, 1990.

Peterka, R, Black, F, and Schoenhoff, M: Age-related changes in human vestibulo-ocular reflexes: Sinusoidal rotation and caloric tests. J Vest Res 1:49–59, 1990.

Pierrot-Deseilligny, C, et al: The "one-and-a-half" syndrome. Brain 104:665–699, 1981.

Platzer, W (ed): PERNKOPF, Atlas der topographischen und angewandten Anatomie des Menschen, ed 3. Munchen–Wien–Baltimore: Urban & Schwartzenberg, 1989.

Proctor, B, Guadjian, ES, and Webster, JE: The ear in head trauma. Laryngoscope 66:17–50, 1956.

Prusiner, SB: Prions and neurodegenerative diseases. N Engl J Med 317(25):1571–1581, 1987.

Pullen, FW: Perilymphatic fistula induced by barotrauma. Am J Otol 13(3):270–272, 1992.

Pyykko, I, et al: Intratympanic gentamicin in bilateral Meniere's disease. Otolaryngol Head Neck Surg 110:162–167, 1994.

Rauch, SD, Merchant, SN, and Thedinger, BA: Meniere's syndrome and endolymphatic hydrops: Double-blind temporal bone study. Ann Otol Rhinol Laryngol 98:873–882, 1989.

Reid, WH: The treatment of psychologic disorders (revised for the DSM-III-R). New York: Brunner/Mazel, 1945.

Rhoton, AL: Microsurgical anatomy of posterior fossa cranial nerves. In Barrow, DL (ed): Surgery of the Cranial Nerves of the Posterior Fossa. American Association of Neurological Surgeons, 1993.

Richter, E: Quantitative study of human Scarpa's ganglion and vestibular sensory epithelia. Acta Otolaryngol (Stockh) 90:199–208, 1980.

Richter, E, and Schuknecht, HF: Loss of vestibular neurons in clinical otosclerosis. Arch Otorhinolaryngol 234:1–9, 1982.

Rintelmann, WF (ed.): Hearing Assessment. Perspectives in Audiology Series. Austin: Pro-ed, 1991.

Rizvi, SS, and Boston, MA: Investigations into the cause of canal paresis in Meniere's disease. Laryngoscope 86:1258–1271, 1986.

Robinson, DA, et al: Alexander's law: Its behavior and origin in the human vestibulo-ocular reflex. Ann Neurol 16:714–722, 1984.

Robinson, D: A method of measuring eye movement using a scleral search coil in a magnetic field. IEEE Trans Bio-Med Electronics 10:137–145, 1963.

Rosenhall, U, and Rubin, W: Degenerative changes in the human vestibular sensory epithelia. Acta Otolaryngol (Stockh) 79:67–80, 1975.

Ross, MD, et al: Observations on normal and degenerating human otoconia. Ann Otol 85:310–326, 1976.

Rutka, JA, and Barber, HO: Recurrent vestibulopathy: Third review. J Otolaryngol 15(2):105–107, 1988.

Ryan, GMS, and Cope, S: Cervical vertigo. Lancet 2:1355–1358, 1955.

Rybak, LP, and Matz, GJ: Auditory and vestibular effects of toxins: Manifestations of systemic disease. In Cummings, CW, et al (eds): Otolaryngology—Head and Neck Surgery, Vol. 4. St. Louis: Mosby-Year Book, 1986, pp 3161–3172.

Sando, I, et al: Vestibular pathology in otosclerosis temporal bone histopathological report. Laryngoscope 84(4):593–605, 1974.

Schluederberg, A, et al: Chronic fatigue syndrome research. Ann Intern Med 117:325–331, 1992.

Schmid, R, and Jeannerod, M: Vestibular habituation: An adaptive process? In Berthoz, A, and Melvill Jones, G (eds): Adaptive Mechanisms in Gaze Control. Amsterdam: Elsevier, 1985.

Schuknecht, HF: A clinical study of auditory damage following blows to the head. Ann Otol Rhinol Laryngol 59:331–359, 1950.

Schuknecht, HF: Positional vertigo: Clinical and experimental observations. Trans Am Acad Ophthalmol Otolaryngol 66:319–332, 1962.

Schuknecht, HF: Cupulolithiasis. Arch Otolaryngol 90:113–126, 1969.

Schuknecht, HF: Pathology of the Ear. Cambridge, MA: Harvard University Press, 1974.

Schuknecht, HF: Mondi dysplasia: A clinical and pathological study. Ann Otol Rhinol Laryngol 89 (Suppl 65), 3–23, 1980.

Schuknecht, HF, and Kitamura, K: Vestibular neuritis. Ann Otol Rhinol Laryngol (Suppl)78(90):1–19, 1981.

Schuknecht, HF, Neff, WD, and Perlman, HD: An experimental study of auditory damage following blows to the head. Ann Otol Rhinol Laryngol 60:273–289, 1951.

Schwaber, MK, and Whetsell, WO: Cochleovestibular nerve compression syndrome. II. Vestibular nerve histopathology and theory of pathophysiology. Laryngoscope 102:1030–1036, 1992.

Selesnick, SH, and Jackler, RK: Atypical hearing loss in acoustic neuroma patients. Laryngoscope 103:437–446, 1993.

Semont, A, Greyss, G, and Vitte, E: Curing the BPPV with a liberatory maneuver. 42:290–293, 1988.

Sharpe, JA, and Fletcher, WA: Saccadic intrusions and oscillations. Can J Neurol Sci 11:426–433, 1984.

Sharpe, JA, et al: Paralytic pontine exotropia. Neurology 24:1076–1081, 1974.

Shea, JJ, Ge, X, and Orchik, DJ: Endolymphatic hydrops associated with otosclerosis. Am J Otol 15(3):348–357, 1994.

Sheehy, JL, and Hughes, RL: The ABC's of impedance audiometry. Laryngoscope 134(11):1935–1949, 1974.

Shone, G, Kemink, JL, and Telian, SA: Prognostic significance of hearing loss as a lateralizing indicator in the surgical treatment of vertigo. J Laryngol Otol 105:618–620, 1991.

Shumway-Cook, A, and Horak, FB: Assessing the influence of sensory interaction on balance. J Am Phys Ther Assoc 66(10):1548–1550, 1986.

Shumway-Cook, A, and Horak, FB: Rehabilitation strategies for patients with vestibular deficits. In Arenberg, IK (ed): Dizziness and Balance Disorders. New York: Kugler Publications, 1993, pp 677–691.

Silverstein, H: Streptomycin treatment for Meniere's disease. Ann Otol Rhinol Laryngol (Suppl)112(2):44–47, 1984.

Silverstein, H, and Norell, H: Retrolabyrinthine vestibular neurectomy. Otolaryngol Head Neck Surg 90:778–782, 1982.

Silverstein, H, Smouha, E, and Jones, R: Natural history vs. surgery for Meniere's disease. Otolaryngol Head Neck Surg 100:6–16, 1989.

Silverstein, H, Wolfson, RJ, and Rosenberg, S: Diagnosis and management of hearing loss. Clin Symposia 44(3):2–32, 1992.

Skedros, DG, et al: Sources of errors in use of beta 2 transferrin analysis for diagnosing perilymphatic and cerebral spinal fluid leaks. Otolaryngol Head Neck Surg 109:861–864, 1993.

Smith, BH: Vestibular disturbances in epilepsy. Neurology 10:465–469, 1960.

Smith, PF, and Curthoys, IS: Mechanisms of recovery following unilateral labyrinthectomy: A review. Brain Res 14:155–180, 1989.

Soliman, AM: Experimental autoimmune inner ear disease. Laryngoscope 99:188–194, 1989.

Steele, JC, Richardson, JC, and Olszewski, J: Progressive supranuclear palsy. Arch Neurol 10:333–359, 1964.

Stockwell, CW: Vestibular function testing: Four year update. In Cummings, CW, et al (eds): Otolaryngol Head Neck Surg. St. Louis: Mosby-Year Book, 1990, p 39.

Stolz, SE, Chatrian, G-E, and Spence, A: Epileptic Nystagmus. Epilepsia 32(6):910–918, 1991.

Supance, JS, and Bluestone, CD: Perilymph fistulas in infants and children. Otolaryngol Head Neck Surg 91:663–671, 1983.

Theunissen, EJM, Huygen, PLM, and Folgering, HTH: Vestibular hyperreactivity and hyperventilation. Clin Otolaryngol 11:161–169, 1986.

Tinetti, ME, Speechley, M, and Ginter, SF: Risk factors for falls among elderly persons living in the community. N Engl J Med 319(26):1701–1707, 1988.

Toglia, J, Thomas, K, and Kuritzky, A: Common migraine and vestibular function electronystagmographic study and pathogenesis. Ann Otol 90:267–271, 1981.

Traccis, S, et al: Successful treatment of acquired pendular elliptical nystagmus in multiple sclerosis with isoniazid and base-out prisms. Neurology 40:492–494, 1990.

Tusa, RJ, et al: Ipsiversive eye deviation and epileptic nystagmus. Neurology 40:662–665, 1990.

Tusa, RJ, Saada, AA, and Niparko, JK: Dizziness in childhood. J Child Neurol 9:261–274, 1994.

Uemura, T, et al: Neuro-Otological Examination. Baltimore: University Park Press, 1977.

Veldman, JE, et al: Autoimmunity and inner ear disorders: An immune-complex mediated sensorineural hearing loss. Laryngoscope 94:501, 1984.

Victor, M, Adams, RD, and Collins, GH: The Wernicke-Korsakoff Syndrome and Related Neurologic Disorders Due to Alcoholism and Malnutrition, ed 2. Philadelphia: FA Davis, 1989.

Vogel, H, Thumler, R, and Von Baumgarten, RJ: Ocular Counterrolling. Acta Otolaryngol (Stockh) 102:457–462, 1986.

Von Baumgarten, RJ: Plasticity in the nervous system at the unitary level. In Schmitt, FO (ed): The Neurosciences: Second Study Program. New York: Rockefeller University, 1970.

Voorhees, RL: Dynamic posturography findings in central nervous system disorders. Otolaryngol Head Neck Surg 103:96–101, 1990.

Wackym, PA, et al: Histopathologic findings in Meniere's disease. Otolaryngol Head Neck Surg 112(1)91, 1995.

Waespe, W, Cohen, B, and Raphan, T: Dynamic modification of the vestibulo-ocular reflex by the nodulus and uvula. Science 288:199–202, 1985.

Watson, CP, and Terbrugge, K: Positional nystagmus of the benign paroxysmal type with posterior fossa medullobastoma. Arch Neurol 39:601–602, 1982.

Watson, P, et al: Positional vertigo and nystagmus of central origin. Can J Neurol Sci 8(2):133–137, 1981.

Weber, PC, and Cass, SP: Clinical assessment of postural stability. Am J Otol 14(6):566–569, 1993.

Weber, PC, and Cass, SP: Neurotologic manifestation of Chiari 1 malformation. Otolaryngol Head Neck Surg 109:853–860, 1993.

Weller, TH: Varicella and herpes zoster: Changing concepts of the natural history, control, and importance of a not-so-benign virus. N Engl J Med 309:1434–1440, 1983.

Westheimer, G, and Blair, S: The ocular tilt reaction—A brainstem oculomotor routine. Invest Ophthalmol Vis Sci 14(11):833–839, 1975.

Wilson, DF, et al: The sensitivity of auditory brainstem response testing in small acoustic neuromas. Laryngoscope 102:961–964, 1992.

Wilson, FJ, and Melvill Jones, G: Mammalian Vestibular Physiology. New York: Plenum Press, 1979.

Wilson, WR, and Schuknecht, HF: Update on the use of streptomycin therapy for Meniere's disease. Am J Otol 2(2):108–111, 1980.

Wist, ER, Brandt, TH, and Krafczyk, S: Oscillopsia and retinal slip. Brain 106:153–168, 1983.

Yamanobe, S, and Harris, JP: Inner ear—Specific antibodies. Laryngoscope 103:319–326, 1993.

Yates, BJ: Vestibular influences on the sympathetic nervous system. Brain Res 17:51–59, 1992.

Yates, BJ, Jakus, J, and Miller, A: Vestibular effects on respiratory outflow in the decerebrate cat. Brain Res 629:209–217, 1993.

Yates, BJ, and Miller, AD (eds): Vestibular Autonomic Regulation. CRC Press (in press).

Yee, RD, Baloh, R, and Honrubia, V: Effect of Baclofen on congenital nystagmus. In Lennerstrand, G, Zee, D, and Keller, E (eds): Functional Basis of Ocular Motility Disorders. Oxford: Pergamon Press, 1982, pp 151–158.

Yee, RD, et al: Abnormal eye movements in Gerstmann-Straussler-Scheinker disease. Arch Ophthalmol 110:68–74, 1992.

Yoo, TJ: Etiopathogenesis of Meniere's disease: A hypothesis. Ann Otol Rhinol Laryngol (Suppl)113(93):6–12, 1984.

Yoo, TJ, et al: Type II collagen-induced autoimmune endolymphatic hydrops in guinea pig. Science 222:65–67, 1983.

Young, L, and Shenna, D: Eye movement measurement techniques. Am Psychol 30(3):315–330, 1975.

Zee, DS: Ophthalmoscopy in examination of patients with vestibular disorders. Ann Neurol 3:373–374, 1978.

Zee, DS, Friendlich, AL, and Robinson, DA: The mechanism of downbeat nystagmus. Arch Neurol 30:227–237, 1974.

Zee, DS, and Robinson, DA: A hypothetical explanation of saccadic oscillations. Ann Neurol 5:405–414, 1979.

Zee, DS, Yee, R, and Robinson, D: Optokinetic responses in labyrinthine-defective human beings. Brain Res 113(2):423–428, 1976.

Zilstorff-Pedersen, K, and Peitersen, E: Vestibulospinal reflexes. Arch Otolaryngol 77:237–245, 1963.

Appendix of Diagnoses

Diagnosis/Condition	Case No.
Anterior Inferior Cerebellar Artery Syndrome	U4
Anxiety Disorder	C2
Autoimmune Inner Ear Disease	C24
Benign Paroxysmal Vertigo of Childhood	C12
Benign Positional Vertigo	T1, C9, C15, U17
Bilateral Vestibular Loss	C6, C21
Brainstem Infarction	T4, U1, U4
Cerebellar Degeneration	C11
Cerebellopontine Angle Lesion	T6
Cervical Vertigo	C7
Chiari Malformation	C3, C18
Chronic Fatigue Syndrome	U13
Congenital Nystagmus	C22
Creutzfeldt-Jakob Disease	U15
Drop Attacks	U16
Disequilibrium of Aging	C17
Endolymphatic Hydrops (Meniere's Disease)	T3, T9, C10, C14, C16
Enlarged Vestibular Aqueduct Syndrome	U8
Herpes Zoster Oticus	U11
Horizontal Semicircular Canal Benign Positional Vertigo	U17
Idiopathic Orthostatic Hypotension	U10
Impaired Compensation	T8, C1, C16
Labyrinthine Concussion	T7, C8, C22
Mal de Débarquement Syndrome	U14
Malformation of the Inner Ear	U8
Meniere's Disease (Endolymphatic Hydrops)	T3, T9, C10, C14, C16
Migraine	C4, C12, U12, U16
Multiple Sclerosis	T2, C26
Multisensory Disequilibrium	C21
Nonspecific Vestibulopathy	C18
Ocular Flutter	U2
One and One-Half (1½) Syndrome	U6
Otitis Media and Cholesteatoma Formation	C19
Otosclerosis and Otosclerotic Inner Ear Syndrome	C20
Ototoxicity	C6
Perilymphatic Fistula	C19, C23
Posterior Inferior Cerebellar Artery Syndrome	T4
Progressive Supranuclear Palsy	U3
Ramsay Hunt Syndrome	U11
Recurrent Vestibulopathy	C25
Solvent Toxicity	C13

Index

Italics indicate figures or tables.

333

ISBN 0-8036-0166-2

EAN

9 780803 601666

90000